Biological Psychology:
An Illustrated Survival Guide

Biological Psychology
An Illustrated Survival Guide

Written by

Paul Aleixo

and

Illustrated by

Murray Baillon

(Lettering by Alex Oh!)

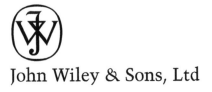

John Wiley & Sons, Ltd

© 2008   Paul Aleixo and Murray Baillon

Published in 2008   John Wiley & Sons Ltd, The Atrium, Southern Gate, Chichester
West Sussex, PO19 8SQ, England

Telephone   (+44) 1243 779777

With grateful thanks to Nat Gertler and Mark Lewis for their kind permission to reproduce Mister U.S. (Copyright and TM 1997 Nat Gertler and Mark Lewis).

Email (for orders and customer service enquiries): cs-books@wiley.co.uk
Visit our Home Page on www.wiley.com

Other Wiley Editorial Offices

John Wiley & Sons Inc., 111 River Street, Hoboken, NJ 07030, USA

Jossey-Bass, 989 Market Street, San Francisco, CA 94103-1741, USA

Wiley-VCH Verlag GmbH, Boschstr. 12, D-69469 Weinheim, Germany

John Wiley & Sons Australia Ltd, 42 McDougall Street, Milton, Queensland 4064, Australia

John Wiley & Sons (Asia) Pte Ltd, 2 Clementi Loop #02-01, Jin Xing Distripark, Singapore 129809

John Wiley & Sons Canada Ltd, 6045 Freemont Blvd, Mississauga, ONT, L5R 4J3, Canada

Wiley also publishes its books in a variety of electronic formats. Some content that appears in print may not be available in electronic books.

Library of Congress Cataloging-in-Publication Data

Aleixo, Paul.
  Biological psychology : an illustrated survival guide / written by Paul Aleixo and illustrated by Murray Baillon.
    p. cm.
  Includes bibliographical references and index.
  ISBN 978-0-470-87099-0 – ISBN 978-0-470-87100-3
  1. Psychobiology–Comic books, strips, etc. I. Baillon, Murray. II. Title.
  QP360.A44 2008
  612.8–dc22
                        2007050284

British Library Cataloguing in Publication Data

A catalogue record for this book is available from the British Library

ISBN 978-0-470-87099-0 (hbk) 978-0-470-87100-3 (pbk)

Typeset in 10/13pt Garamond by Thomson Digital

Special thanks with awe and admiration to
Scott McCloud for inspiration – PA

Contents

About the Authors

Paul Aleixo

Paul has worked as a lecturer in several British universities since completing his Doctoral degree in psychology in the early 1990s. Currently a Senior Lecturer in psychology, he has varied research interests including the application of psychological principles to educational practice. He has taught a number of psychology courses including Biological Psychology for many years. A lifelong interest in comics has led him to explore their use in education. This book is one of these explorations.

Murray Baillon

Murray first met Paul when they were both fresh-faced first year students at University. It was here that they took their first steps as creative partners, writing and performing sketches for student revues. They also both read a lot of comics, which created a shared frame of reference that proved invaluable for this book. After graduating with a B.Sc. in Psychology, Murray then moved into teaching, completing a PGCE at the University of Greenwich. It was while teaching in Singapore that Murray took on his first professional work as an illustrator. He continued to fit illustration work around teaching until recently, when he decided to fit teaching in around illustrating. His work includes fabric print design; logos; cartoons and comic strips for various publications; and children's book illustrations. He has really enjoyed the challenges that Paul set him in this book, as he has never tried to draw things like angry neurons before.

How to Use this Book

For each chapter there are notes that accompany the illustrated pages. They are connected to the pages by page number and panel number. Each cartoon 'box' is called a 'panel' and these are numbered from 1 starting at the top left of each page and increasing in number from left to right and from top to bottom of each page. For example:

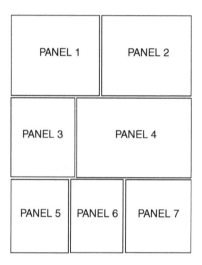

Please note that not all pages and/or panels will have accompanying notes.

Acknowledgements

There are a number of people that must be thanked for getting this book into print.

Firstly, to all at Wiley UK, who not only supported, but positively encouraged this book and for their patience in its production. Particular thanks must go to Gillian Leslie for supporting the idea from the beginning, and to Ruth Graham, Nicole Burnett and Sarah Tilley for production advice.

To all those at my day job who supported this project and offered advice along the way. Special thanks to Brown for his unending support.

To Alan Moore, Neil Gaiman, Nat Gertler *et al.* for inspiration.

To Nat Gertler and Mark Lewis for the use of Mister U.S.

To Comicraft for their excellent advice and fonts.

Finally, grateful thanks to my family.

P. Aleixo
June 2007

As well as to those mentioned above, I would like to express my thanks:

To great comic book artists and cartoonists, from Jack Kirby, John Byrne and Alan Davis to Charles Schultz and Bill Watterson, to whose lofty standards I will always aspire.

To Alison, my wife, for her endless encouragement and support, to my mother for her dedicated proof reading, and to my children for their enthusiasm and interest.

Murray Baillon
June 2007

Introduction

Psychology is a popular subject with students. There is just something about the study of the mind and behaviour that many find inherently interesting and fascinating. However, despite this popularity, there are also a number of areas within most psychology courses that are decidedly unpopular! The three that spring easily to mind are Research Methods, Cognitive Science and, yes, Biological Psychology. Many students of psychology simply find these areas too 'difficult'.

Unfortunately for most students, these areas are, in most cases, compulsory study elements of psychology courses. There is just no way to completely avoid them.

In many ways, the problem regarding biological psychology is easy to understand. The application of biology to studying behaviour involves biological principles that many students have never come across before and if they have only at a very superficial level. Furthermore, biology itself is based on the principles of chemistry and physics.

So to be able to understand biological psychology easily depends on understanding not only psychology but also biology, physics AND chemistry. Unfortunately, many students of psychology do not come to the study of psychology with a science background.

Furthermore, while there are some excellent textbooks on biological psychology available at the introductory level, these tend to make assumptions about the scientific knowledge of the reader.

The original idea for this book came from the experience of teaching undergraduate students on a course in biological psychology at the introductory level. Over several years, students would come and explain that they understood the class sessions but got lost when they hit the books back home.

This book is an attempt to help those who find themselves in a similar dilemma. It aims to bridge the gap between an introductory lecture course on biological psychology and the mainstream textbooks. The additional aim is to highlight that biological psychology is an interesting and fascinating subject in its own right.

Why Comics?

We chose to do this book in a comic book format because we felt that it was the best way to demystify what is perceived as a difficult subject. We are certainly not the first to deal with instructional material in this format. A pioneer of the comic medium, Will Eisner, was employed by the United States Army to produce technical instructional leaflets, in comics, during the Second World War. More recently, Scott McCloud has shown that serious analysis can be delivered in an entertaining and detailed manner through comics.

Furthermore, research in this area shows that comics are very useful for many teaching purposes.

We therefore thought that it was time to bring comics to psychology for teaching purposes.

Structure of this Book

This book covers the basic material needed to get a grasp of biological psychology. It is not meant to be an 'all-encompassing' text but instead is meant to support the excellent books that go into a great deal more depth. It is organised into ten chapters, each followed by notes that expand and detail some of the points made in the main chapters.

We've enjoyed producing this book and hope that you will enjoy reading it.

Paul Aleixo & Murray Baillon
June 2007

CHAPTER 1
THE BRAIN AND THE NERVOUS SYSTEM

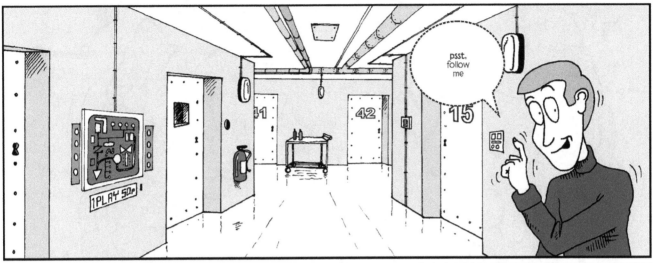

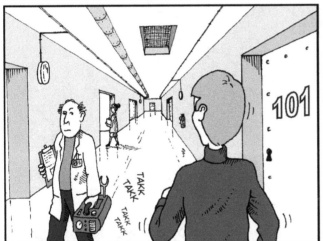

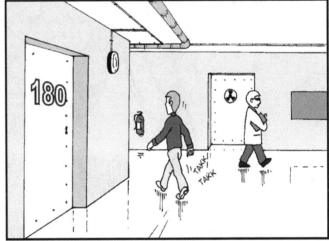

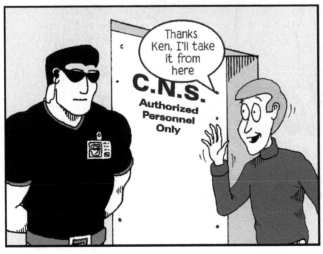

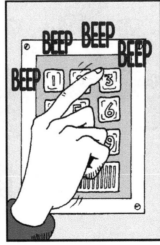

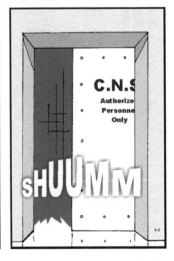

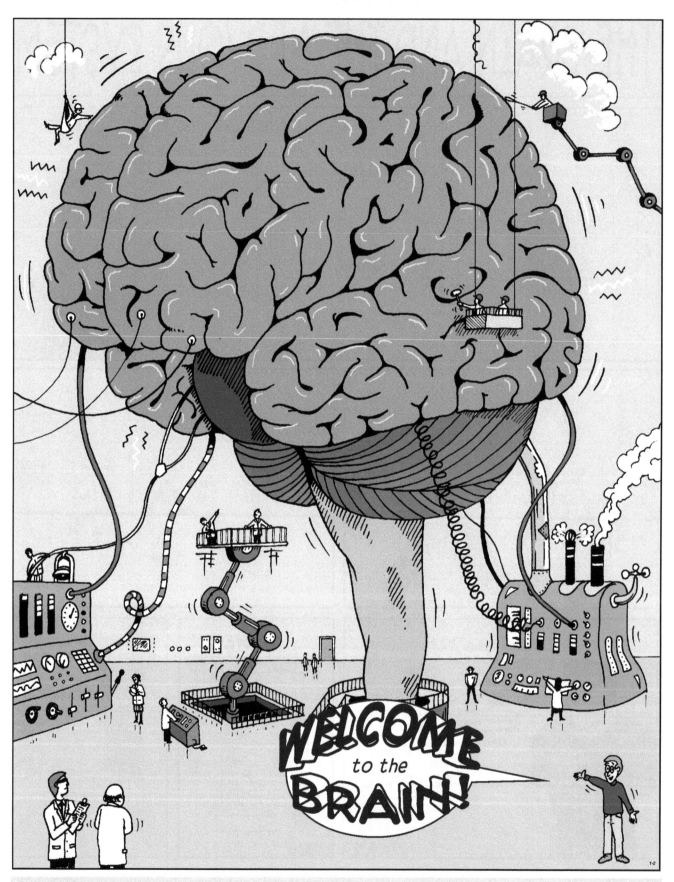

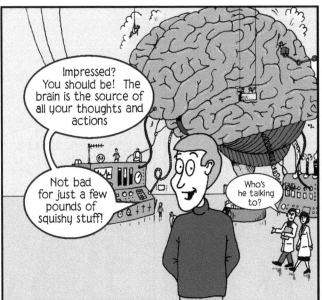

Impressed? You should be! The brain is the source of all your thoughts and actions

Not bad for just a few pounds of squishy stuff!

Who's he talking to?

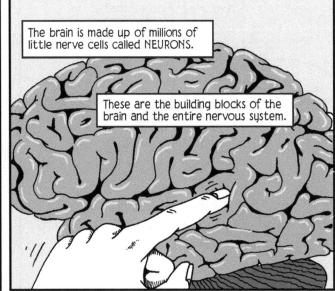

The brain is made up of millions of little nerve cells called NEURONS.

These are the building blocks of the brain and the entire nervous system.

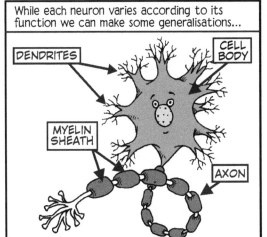

While each neuron varies according to its function we can make some generalisations...

DENDRITES

CELL BODY

MYELIN SHEATH

AXON

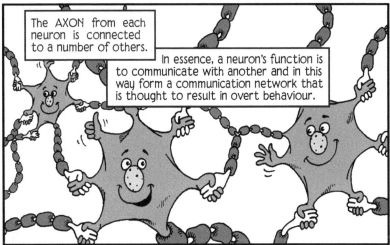

The AXON from each neuron is connected to a number of others.

In essence, a neuron's function is to communicate with another and in this way form a communication network that is thought to result in overt behaviour.

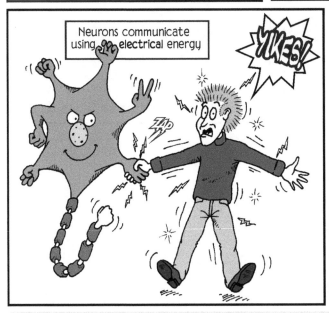

Neurons communicate using electrical energy

YIKES!

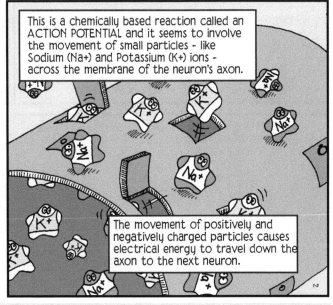

This is a chemically based reaction called an ACTION POTENTIAL and it seems to involve the movement of small particles - like Sodium (Na+) and Potassium (K+) ions - across the membrane of the neuron's axon.

The movement of positively and negatively charged particles causes electrical energy to travel down the axon to the next neuron.

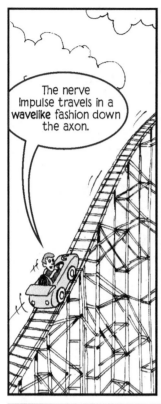

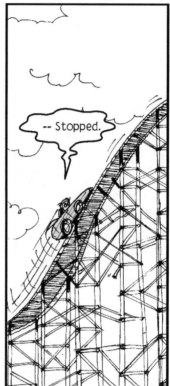

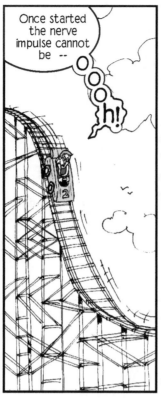

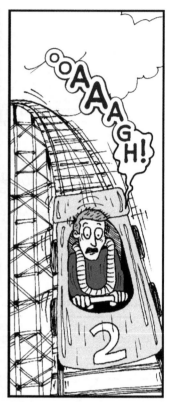

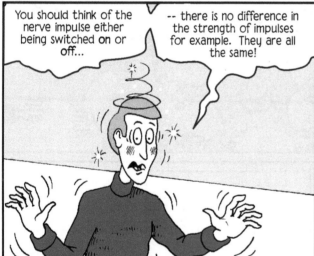

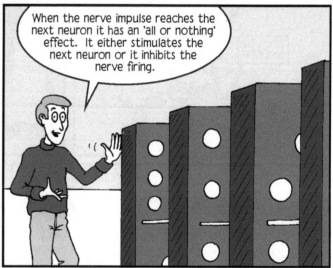

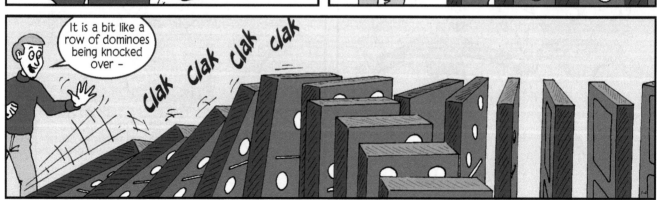

This network of neurons, all firing impulses, affect other neurons and an overall pattern of nerve impulses is formed that results in behaviour!

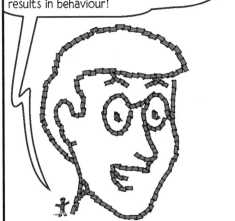

So, it's all very simple. Each axon is connected to the dendrites of another neuron that sends the signal on to another neuron it is connected to and so on....

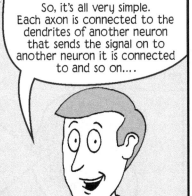

...or is it?

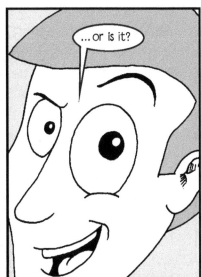

Actually, the majority of neurons do not touch any other neuron!

VERY TINY GAP

...so how is the nerve impulse carried across this gap?

When the nerve impulse reaches the end of the axon, this causes the release of chemicals known as neurotransmitters.

This gap is called a SYNAPSE

NEUROTRANSMITTER MOLECULES

SYNAPTIC GAP

RECEPTOR SITES

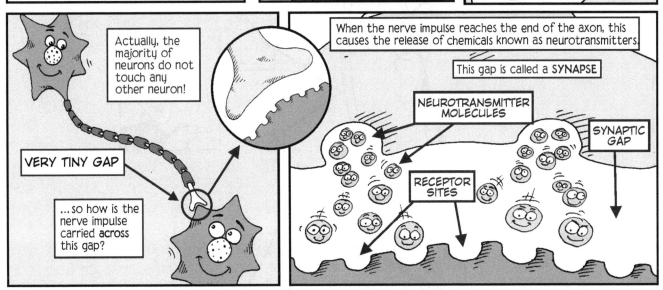

When the neurotransmitters reach receptor sites in the receiving neuron this causes a chemical reaction.

This sets up the action potential and sends the nerve impulse on, down that neuron's axon.

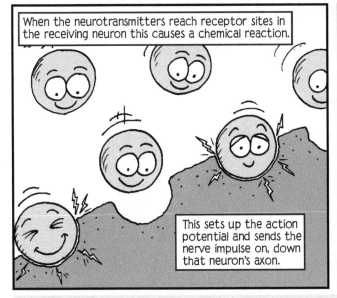

Since each neuron can be connected to many others and each impulse can either inhibit or stimulate a neuron next in line, this creates a very complex - and fast - system of neuronal circuitry.

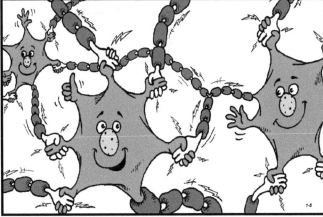

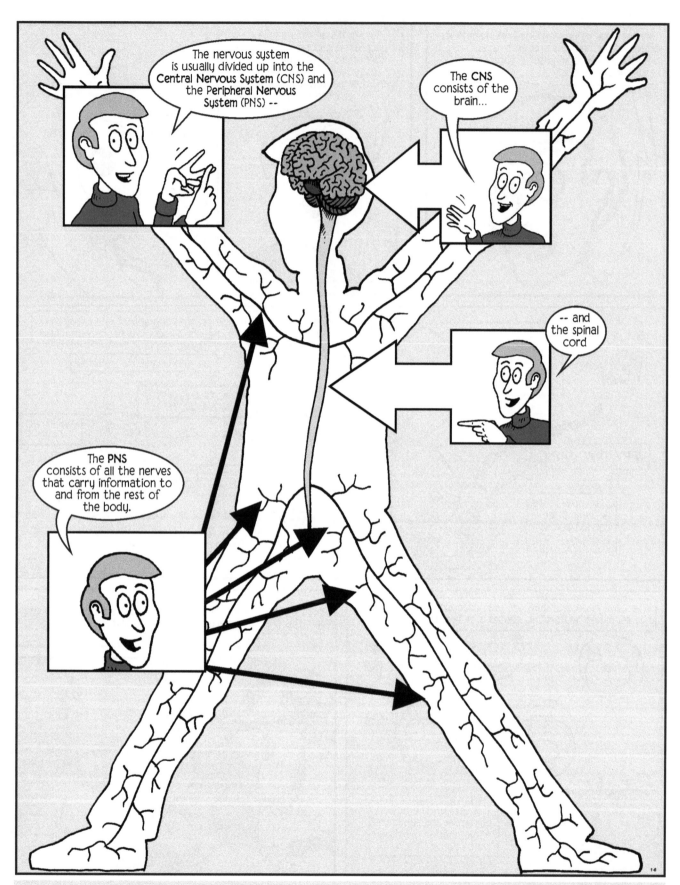

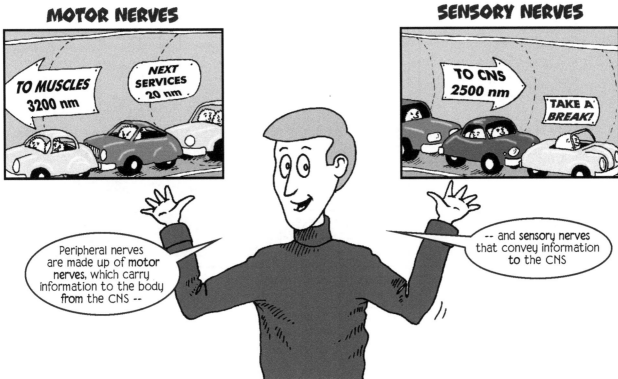

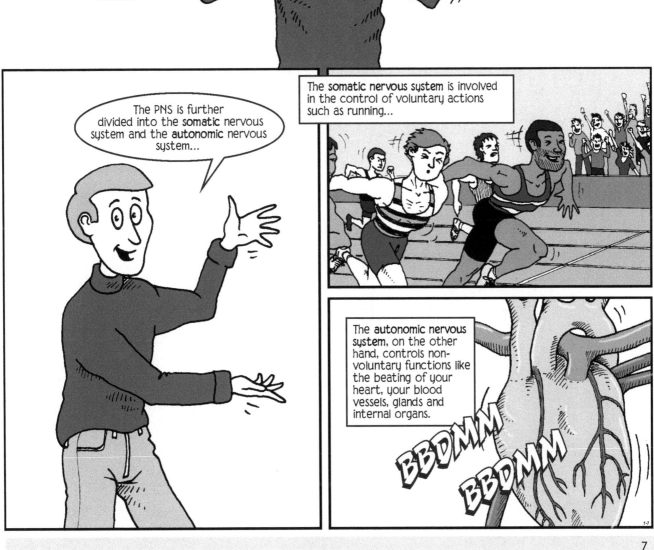

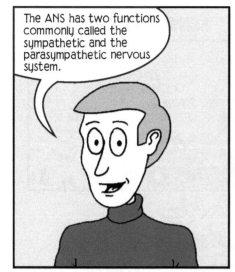

The ANS has two functions commonly called the sympathetic and the parasympathetic nervous system.

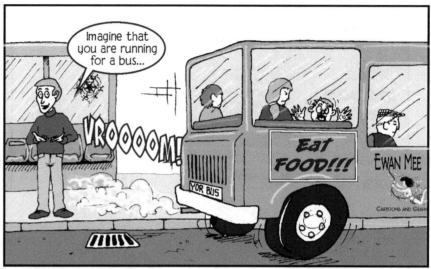

Imagine that you are running for a bus...

VROOOOM!

Eat FOOD!!!

EWAN MEE

YOR BUS

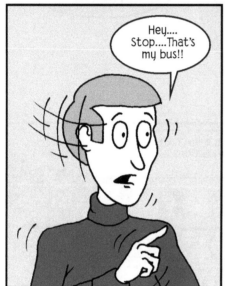

Hey.... Stop....That's my bus!!

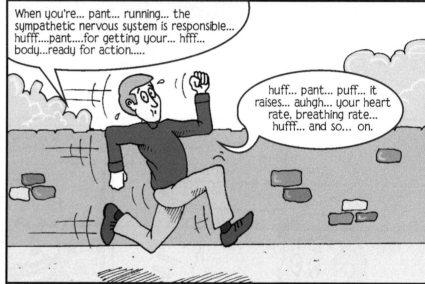

When you're... pant... running... the sympathetic nervous system is responsible... hufff....pant....for getting your... hfff... body...ready for action.....

huff... pant... puff... it raises... auhgh... your heart rate, breathing rate... hufff... and so... on.

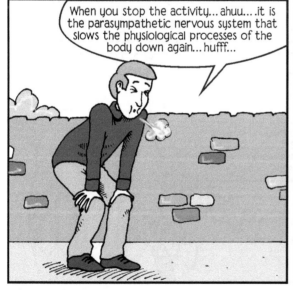

When you stop the activity...ahuu....it is the parasympathetic nervous system that slows the physiological processes of the body down again...hufff...

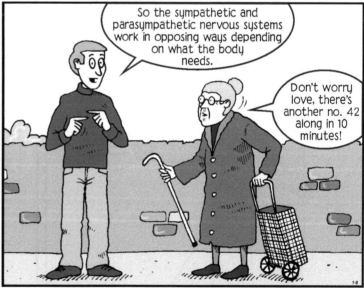

So the sympathetic and parasympathetic nervous systems work in opposing ways depending on what the body needs.

Don't worry love, there's another no. 42 along in 10 minutes!

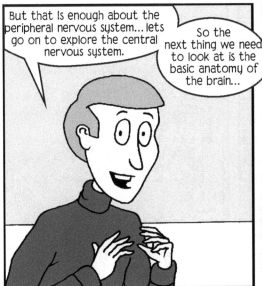

But that is enough about the peripheral nervous system... lets go on to explore the central nervous system.

So the next thing we need to look at is the basic anatomy of the brain...

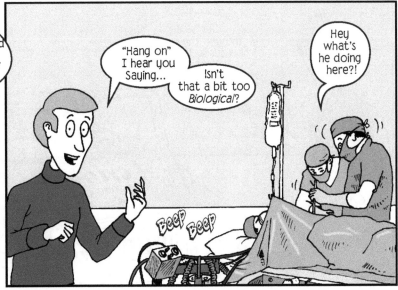

"Hang on" I hear you saying...

Isn't that a bit too *Biological*?

Hey what's he doing here?!

Beep Beep

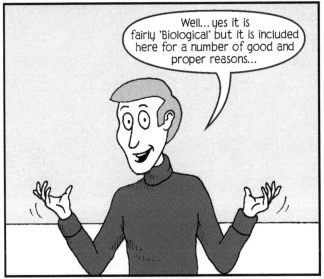

Well... yes it is fairly 'Biological' but it is included here for a number of good and proper reasons...

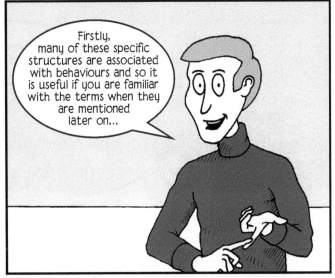

Firstly, many of these specific structures are associated with behaviours and so it is useful if you are familiar with the terms when they are mentioned later on...

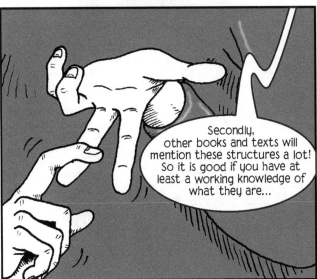

Secondly, other books and texts will mention these structures a lot! So it is good if you have at least a working knowledge of what they are...

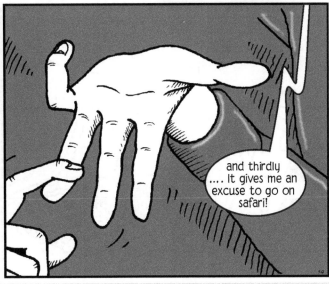

and thirdly .... It gives me an excuse to go on safari!

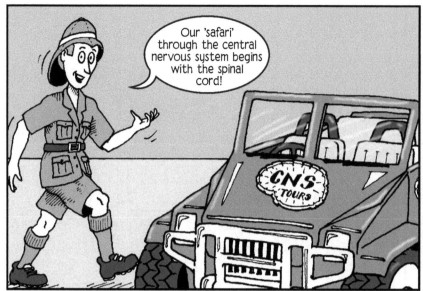

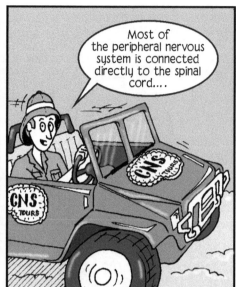

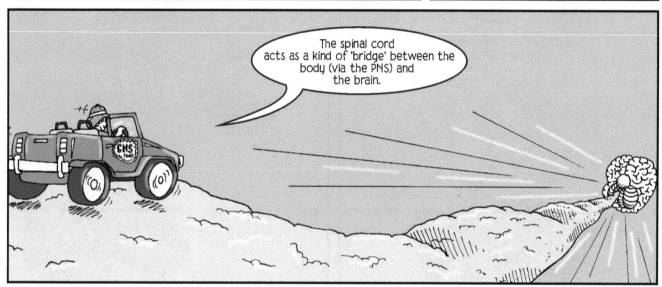

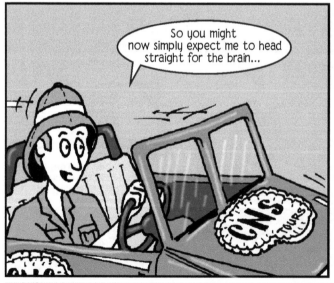

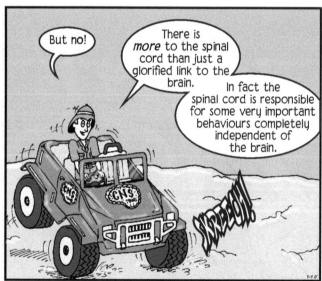

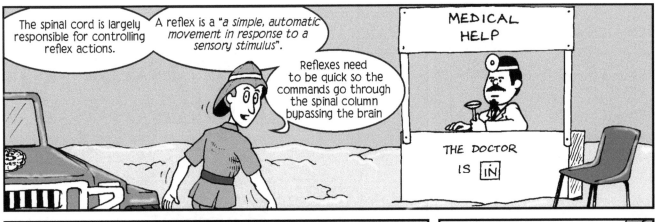

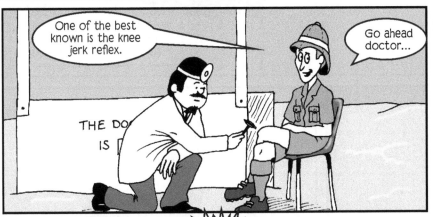

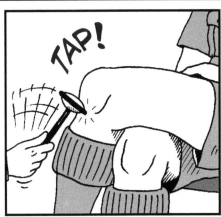

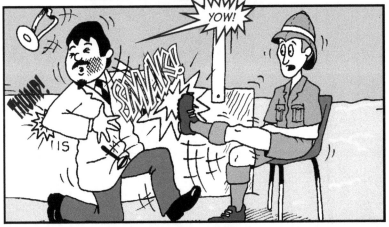

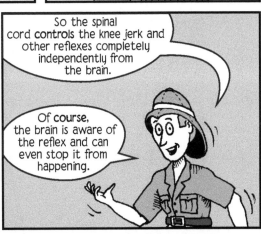

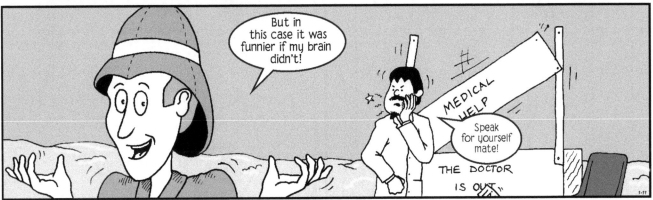

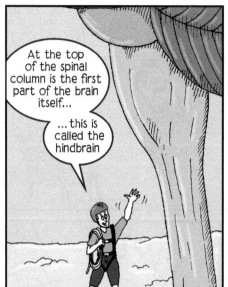

At the top of the spinal column is the first part of the brain itself...

...this is called the hindbrain

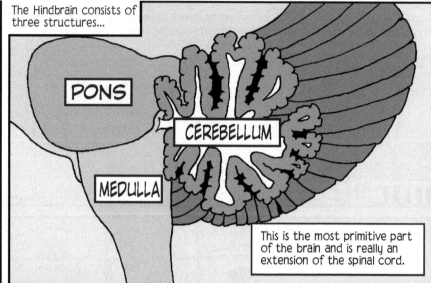

The Hindbrain consists of three structures...

PONS

CEREBELLUM

MEDULLA

This is the most primitive part of the brain and is really an extension of the spinal cord.

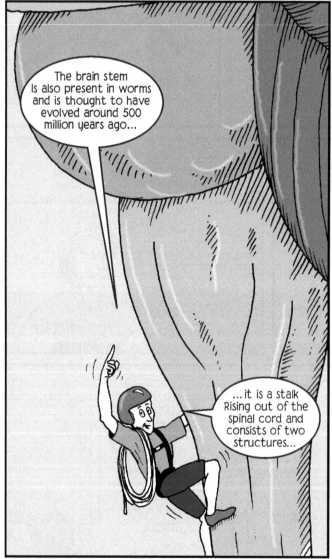

The brain stem is also present in worms and is thought to have evolved around 500 million years ago...

...it is a stalk Rising out of the spinal cord and consists of two structures...

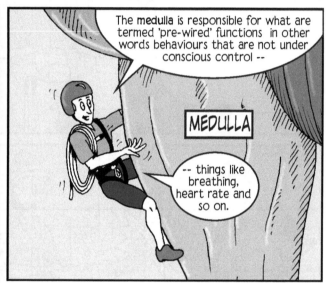

The medulla is responsible for what are termed 'pre-wired' functions in other words behaviours that are not under conscious control --

MEDULLA

-- things like breathing, heart rate and so on.

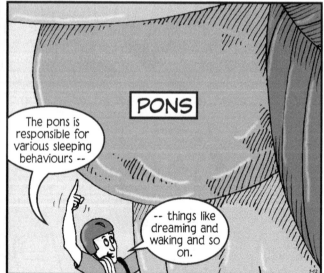

PONS

The pons is responsible for various sleeping behaviours --

-- things like dreaming and waking and so on.

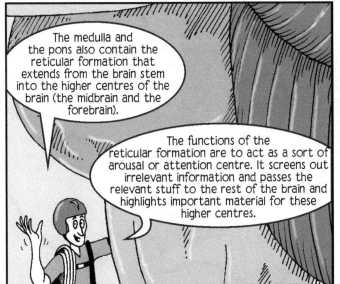

The medulla and the pons also contain the reticular formation that extends from the brain stem into the higher centres of the brain (the midbrain and the forebrain).

The functions of the reticular formation are to act as a sort of arousal or attention centre. It screens out irrelevant information and passes the relevant stuff to the rest of the brain and highlights important material for these higher centres.

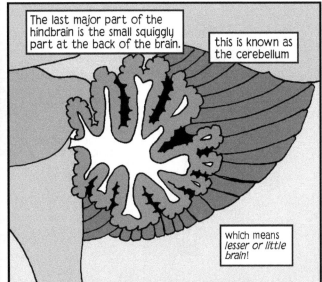

The last major part of the hindbrain is the small squiggly part at the back of the brain.

this is known as the cerebellum

which means *lesser or little brain*!

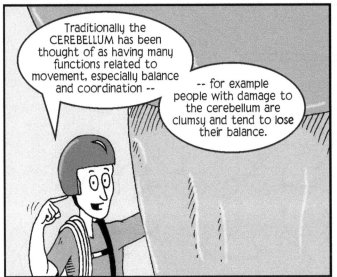

Traditionally the CEREBELLUM has been thought of as having many functions related to movement, especially balance and coordination --

-- for example people with damage to the cerebellum are clumsy and tend to lose their balance.

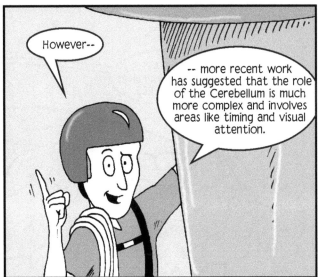

However--

-- more recent work has suggested that the role of the Cerebellum is much more complex and involves areas like timing and visual attention.

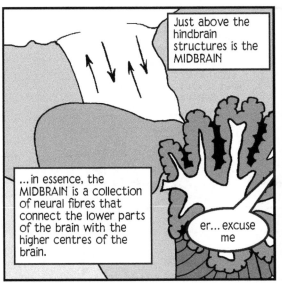

Just above the hindbrain structures is the MIDBRAIN

...in essence, the MIDBRAIN is a collection of neural fibres that connect the lower parts of the brain with the higher centres of the brain.

er... excuse me

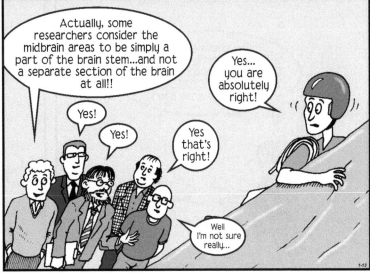

Actually, some researchers consider the midbrain areas to be simply a part of the brain stem...and not a separate section of the brain at all!!

Yes!

Yes!

Yes that's right!

Yes... you are absolutely right!

Well I'm not sure really...

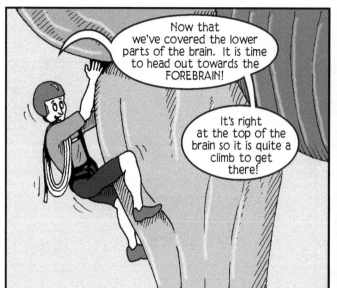

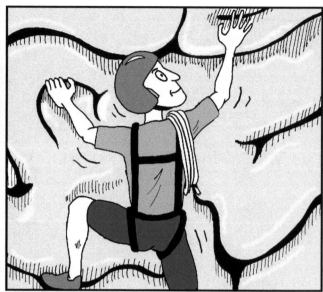

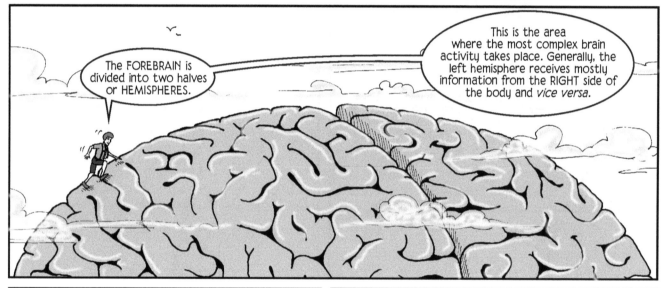

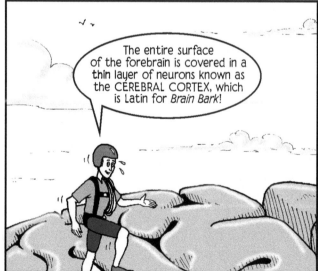

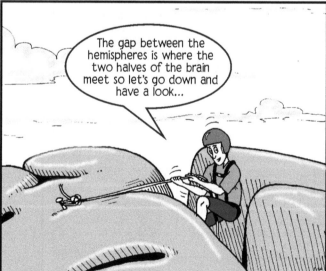

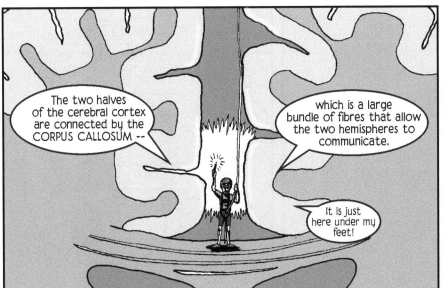

The two halves of the cerebral cortex are connected by the CORPUS CALLOSUM --

which is a large bundle of fibres that allow the two hemispheres to communicate.

It is just here under my feet!

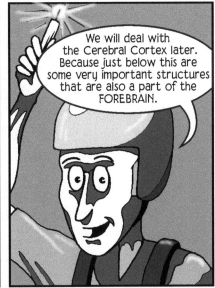

We will deal with the Cerebral Cortex later. Because just below this are some very important structures that are also a part of the FOREBRAIN.

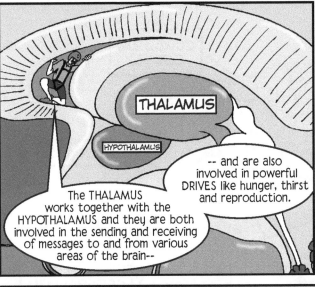

THALAMUS

HYPOTHALAMUS

-- and are also involved in powerful DRIVES like hunger, thirst and reproduction.

The THALAMUS works together with the HYPOTHALAMUS and they are both involved in the sending and receiving of messages to and from various areas of the brain--

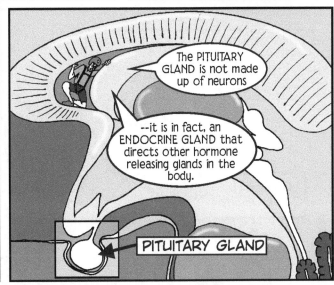

The PITUITARY GLAND is not made up of neurons

--it is in fact, an ENDOCRINE GLAND that directs other hormone releasing glands in the body.

PITUITARY GLAND

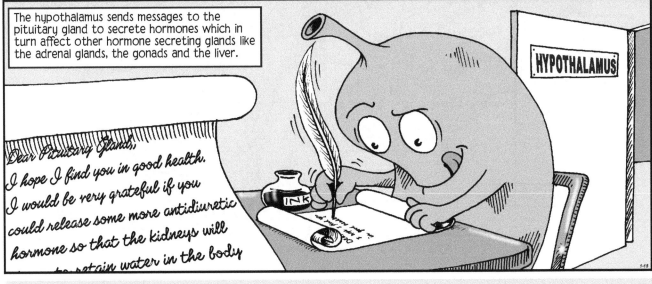

The hypothalamus sends messages to the pituitary gland to secrete hormones which in turn affect other hormone secreting glands like the adrenal glands, the gonads and the liver.

Dear Pituitary Glands,
I hope I find you in good health.
I would be very grateful if you
could release some more antidiuretic
hormone so that the kidneys will
to retain water in the body

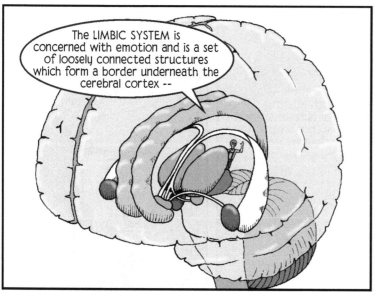

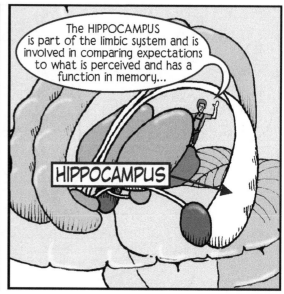

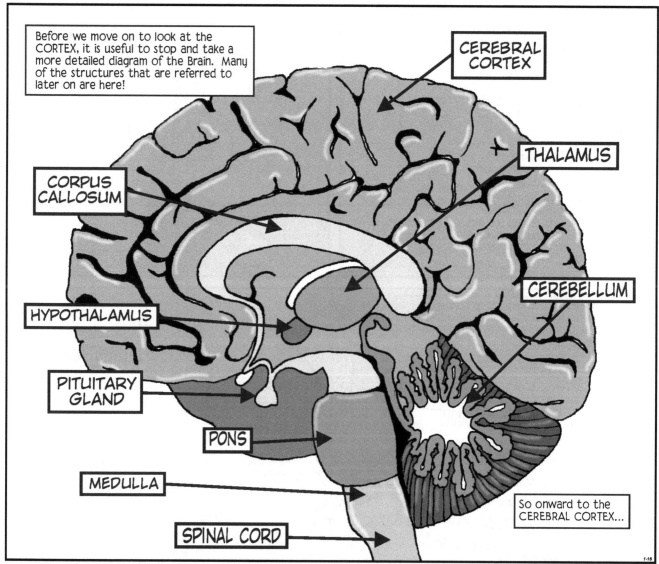

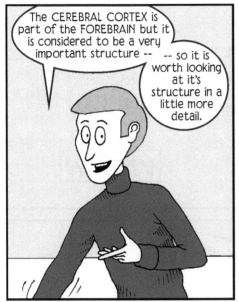

The CEREBRAL CORTEX is part of the FOREBRAIN but it is considered to be a very important structure -- -- so it is worth looking at it's structure in a little more detail.

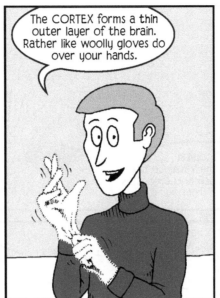

The CORTEX forms a thin outer layer of the brain. Rather like woolly gloves do over your hands.

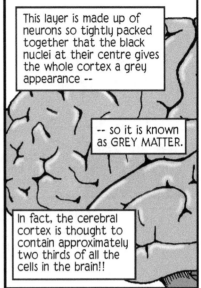

This layer is made up of neurons so tightly packed together that the black nuclei at their centre gives the whole cortex a grey appearance --

-- so it is known as GREY MATTER.

In fact, the cerebral cortex is thought to contain approximately two thirds of all the cells in the brain!!

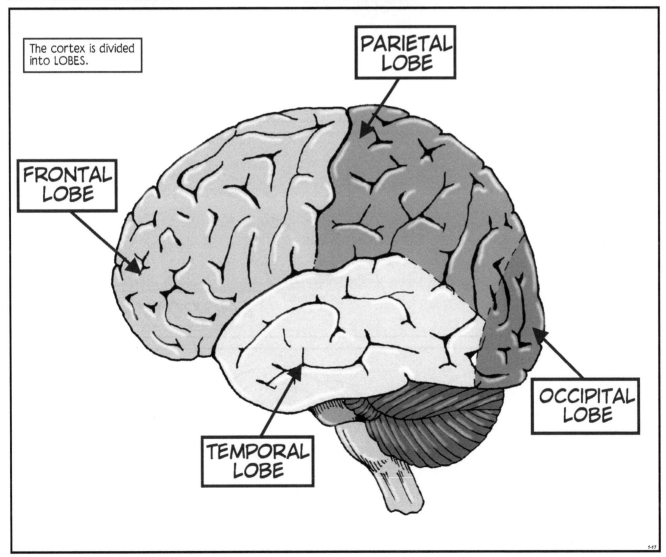

The cortex is divided into LOBES.

PARIETAL LOBE

FRONTAL LOBE

OCCIPITAL LOBE

TEMPORAL LOBE

1-17

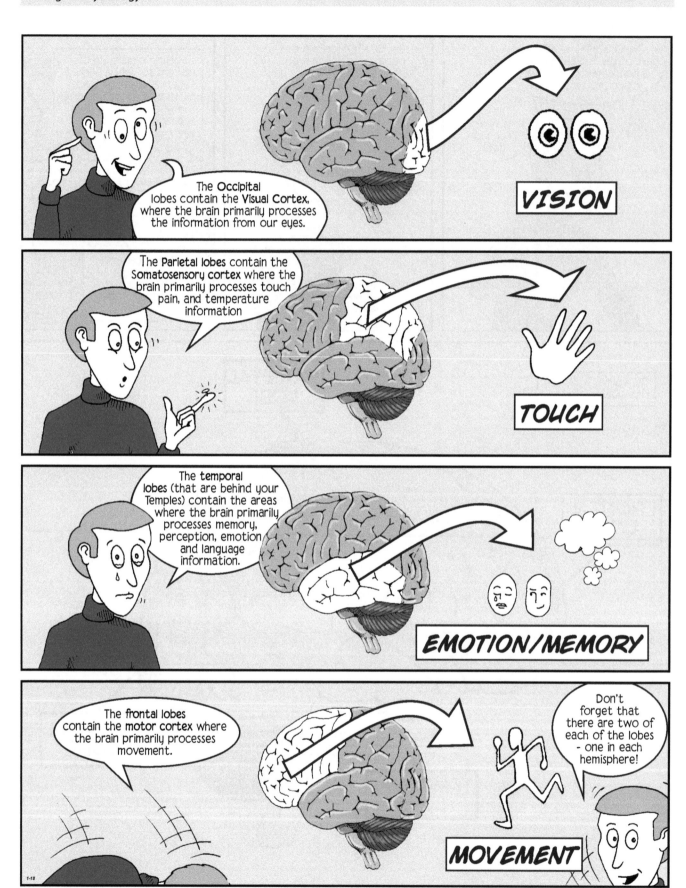

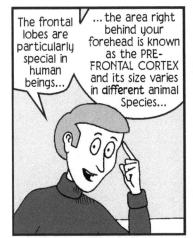

The frontal lobes are particularly special in human beings...

...the area right behind your forehead is known as the PRE-FRONTAL CORTEX and its size varies in **different** animal Species...

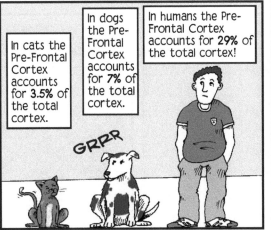

In cats the Pre-Frontal Cortex accounts for **3.5%** of the total cortex.

In dogs the Pre-Frontal Cortex accounts for **7%** of the total cortex.

In humans the Pre-Frontal Cortex accounts for **29%** of the total cortex!

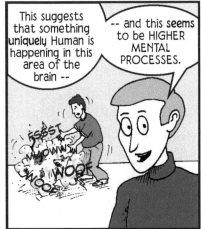

This suggests that something **uniquely** Human is happening in this area of the brain --

-- and this **seems** to be HIGHER MENTAL PROCESSES.

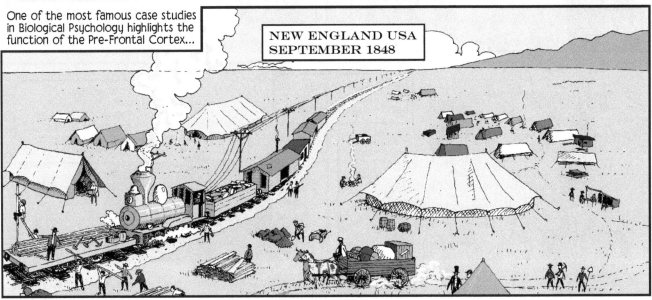

One of the most famous case studies in Biological Psychology highlights the function of the Pre-Frontal Cortex...

NEW ENGLAND USA
SEPTEMBER 1848

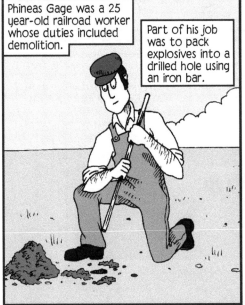

Phineas Gage was a 25 year-old railroad worker whose duties included demolition.

Part of his job was to pack explosives into a drilled hole using an iron bar.

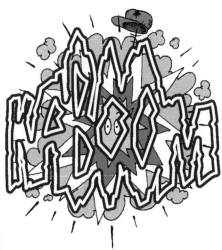

Unfortunately, on this occasion, the explosives went off prematurely.

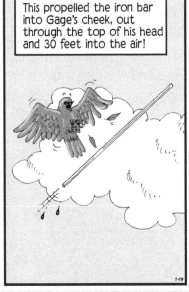

This propelled the iron bar into Gage's cheek, out through the top of his head and 30 feet into the air!

Remarkably, Gage survived and reportedly walked to the cart that took him to hospital.

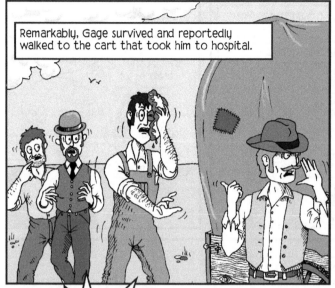

Even more remarkably, most of Gage's mental faculties remained unchanged and he attempted to return to work a while later.

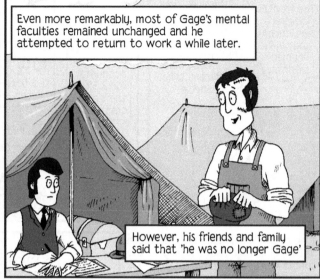

However, his friends and family said that 'he was no longer Gage'

He'd gone from being mild mannered and kind to being obnoxious and rude.

YOU CAN TAKE YOUR JOB AND SHOVE IT UP YOUR $%* !!!

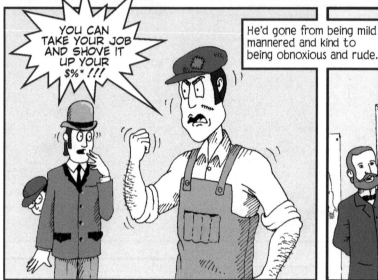

Although not widely accepted at the time, Dr. John Harlow suggested that Gage's personality change had been a result of damage to the frontal lobes of the brain.

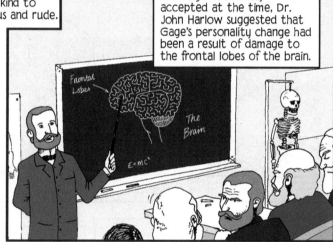

Phineas Gage died in May 1860 but his skull was kept at Harvard University.

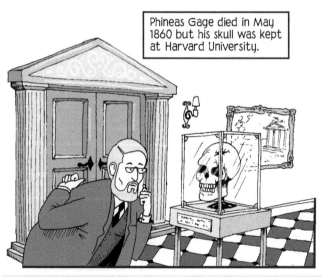

MODERN COMPUTER IMAGING WORK BY HANNA DAMASIO AND HER COLLEAGUES CONFIRMED THAT HARLOW WAS INDEED CORRECT: THE DAMAGE TO GAGE'S BRAIN WAS CONFINED TO THE PART OF BOTH FRONTAL LOBES THAT DEAL WITH EMOTIONS AND MAKING DECISIONS IN SOCIAL SETTINGS.

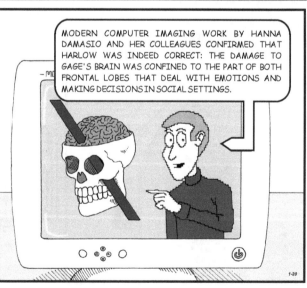

The case study of Phineas Gage was the first clue that suggested that the pre-frontal lobes of the brain are responsible for higher mental processes like personality, the ability to plan behaviours, set goals and intention behaviour.

The case of Phineas Gage also highlights the **early** thinking on what is known as the *Localisation of Function* in the brain.

In other words it shows that some behaviours can be *localised* to specific parts of the brain.

PAUL BROCA was an early pioneer of localisation of function. He discovered that damage to a small area on the left side of the brain had caused his patient to lose the ability to speak.

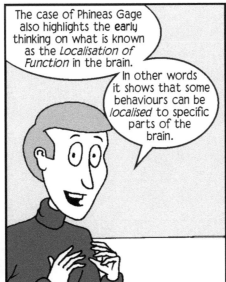
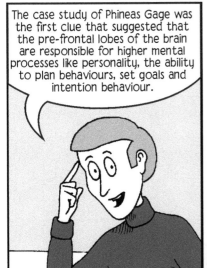
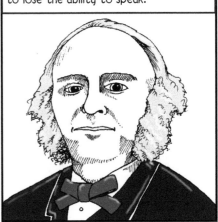

This area is now known as BROCA's AREA and is an area of the brain important for language production.

By the 1880s most researchers in the area were convinced of the concept of localisation of function in the brain...

...although, it was later discovered that the extent of the localisation is not as great as was once thought!

These and other case studies led early researchers to see the brain as *explainable*.

This meant that studying the brain **could** provide answers for what had, up to that point, been seen as the domain of a separate concept - 'the *mind*.'

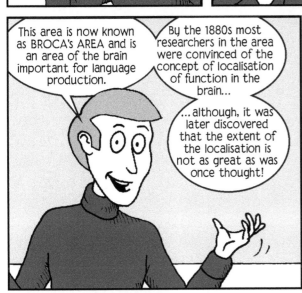
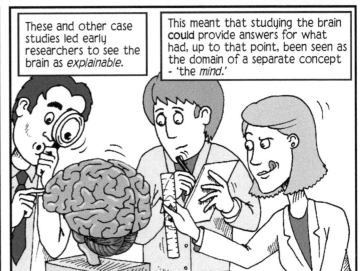

The rest of this book will discuss the various functions of the brain in more detail and at times we will refer to specific parts of the brain to understand how things 'work'.

THIS BOOK!

For now, I just want you to take a few moments to think about the brain in all its glory and the amazing things you are capable of simply because you have one of your very own!

Er...you do own one, don't you?

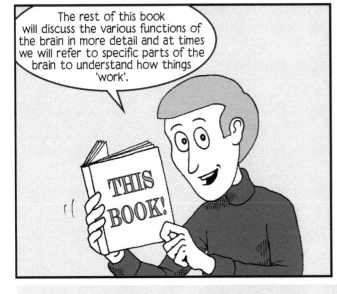
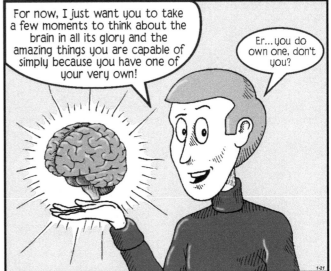

The brain and the nervous system

▶ **PAGE 1**

Biological Psychology is the application of biological principles to the study of behaviour. The term *behaviour* refers to a wide variety of phenomena including both internal events like thinking and emotion as well as overt behaviour that can be seen by others.

A great deal of biological psychology is concerned with the physiology of the nervous system and especially the brain. Other terms are used to describe the same area of research: Physiological Psychology, Psychophysiology, Biopsychology, Biological Bases of Behaviour and so on.

▶ **PAGE 2**

The average adult human brain is actually around the size of a grapefruit or a small melon and is pinkish-grey in colour. It has many folds and creases and looks a little like a large walnut.

▶ **PAGE 3**

Panel 1

These days we are quite accustomed to seeing the brain as the source of our thoughts and actions. However, this was not always the dominant idea. Ancient cultures, including the Egyptian, Indian and Chinese, considered the *heart* to be the seat of thoughts and emotions. The ancient Greek philosophers Hippocrates (460–370 BC) and Galen (AD 130–200) both suggested the brain as the source of these phenomena whilst Aristotle (384–322 BC) believed the brain was there to cool the passions of the heart!

French philosopher Renée Descartes (1596–1650) was one of the first people to see the human body as a machine and he suggested that a separate entity called the *mind* controlled the brain and nervous system and it worked as a sort of hydraulic pump.

The next major innovation was in the late 1700s by Italian philosopher Luigi Galvani who discovered that he could make a frog's leg twitch by stimulating a nerve with electricity. Later on, Fritsch and Hitzig (1870) succeeded in producing movement in dogs by stimulating their brains with electricity. German physicist Herman von Helmholtz (1821–94) later discovered that the nerves were not simply 'wires' since he calculated that the speed of nerve conduction of around 30 to 40 metres per second was far slower than the flow of electricity or around 3×10^8 metres per second (the speed of light).

All of these pioneering ideas led to the concept that the brain behaved like a biological machine and that this could be investigated using scientific principles.

The adult brain weighs around 1400 grams and has a gelatinous consistency. A living brain is so soft and squidgy that it can be cut with a blunt knife.

Panel 2

There are approximately 100 billion neurons in the human brain (Williams & Herrup, 1988). However, neurons only make up approximately 10 per cent of the cells in the brain. The rest are known as *glial* cells, and these provide a supporting role for the neurons themselves. Neurons are larger than glial cells however and make up about 50 per cent of the volume of the brain.

The idea that the neuron is the unit of brain was suggested by the Spanish Nobel prize winner Santiago Ramón y Cajal from work carried out between 1887 and 1903.

Panel 3

It should be noted that there are a number of different types of neuron. The type depicted here is based on a 'typical' motor neuron. Oh and just for clarity's sake, neurons do not have faces!

The cell body of a neuron contains (amongst other things) the cell nucleus that contains the genetic material and the other structures that keeps the neuron alive.

The dendrites are points on a neuron where information from other neurons are received.

The axon is the long part of a neuron that sends the nerve impulse. Axons can be quite long.

The myelin sheath that surrounds the axon is the insulating material (rather like the plastic around an electric cable). It is made up of a fatty material and has a white appearance.

Panel 5

Technically, it needs to be pointed out that the nerve impulse only happens down the neuron's axon so you could not get a shock in this way. However, it should also be pointed out that this scene is impossible since neurons are microscopic cells and they do not have 'hands'!

Panel 6

Note: The explanation of the nerve impulse involves a complex number of disciplines including concepts from chemistry, physics and biology and many find these difficult to understand. The following explanation is unashamedly simplified although we are aware that some of the terms may appear like a foreign language that need some interpretation.

The concepts described in this explanation baffle even the most qualified individuals and this is not as a result of their intellect, but rather an issue with their background. The following description has been 'run by' an experienced psychologist with a Ph.D. who finds this area taxing and is assured that it is basic enough! Obviously, some may find the material overly simplistic and to these readers we recommend further reading.

Please note that this explanation concerns **only** the electrical nerve impulse *within* a single neuron. It does **not** deal with the conduction of impulses across different neurons.

The Nerve Impulse

The fluid inside body cells has certain chemicals that are electrically charged (this means that these chemicals are moving between positive and negative charges in currents, similar to that in the electricity in your home). These are called ions and the important ones for nerve conduction are sodium and potassium (that both have one positive charge), calcium (that has two positive charges), certain proteins called organic anions (that have a negative charge) and chloride (that has one negative charge). The positive ions are attracted to the negative ions and *vice versa*. Hence these chemicals tend to move towards each other. The fluid inside the cell is separated from fluid outside the cell by a cell membrane that allows some chemicals through and not others (it is known as a *semi-permeable* membrane). Therefore, not all the ions can move freely to where they are attracted.

At rest, a nerve cell (neuron) has a negative charge inside the cell and a positive charge outside the cell. This is because the membrane allows positive potassium ions (K^+) easily through to the inside while negative chloride ions (Cl^-) and positive sodium ions (Na^+) have more difficulty. Additionally, there are the organic anions (A^-) inside the cells. Furthermore, there is a pump mechanism that moves sodium ions out of the cell relative to the number of potassium ions within the cell (for those who want to know, the cell 'allows' one sodium ion for each potassium ion, the pump moves sodium out of the cell until this ratio is achieved). When the correct ratio of sodium and potassium ions is achieved, and thus the inside of the cell has a correct negative charge, the neuron is in a sate of balance that is called a *Resting Potential*. If you were to anthropomorphosise the neuron at this point it would be a 'very happy bunny'!

During this state of balance, this resting potential, it is possible to measure the amount of electricity being generated using a gadget called a voltmeter. When this is carried out, it is found that the resting potential of an average neuron is around -70 millivolts (mv) which means that the inside of the cell is 70mv less than the outside. Bear in mind that this is a very small amount of electricity. A portable CD player usually requires two 1.5 volt batteries to operate (a total of three volts, approximately forty times that in a neuron in a state of resting potential!).

Keeping the neuron in this 'happy' state requires a lot of work. In fact, the resting potential uses up approximately 40 per cent of the neuron's energy. However, despite using up such a great deal of the neuron's energy, this is worthwhile because the resting potential is absolutely essential in powering the actual nerve impulse.

When a neuron at rest is stimulated (by another neuron for example), this causes its voltage to move towards 0 mv (in other words from -70mv to 0mv). Before it reaches this, however, at around -55mv, this causes the nerve cell to *fire* or *spike*. This is called an *Action Potential*. When the neuron fires (i.e. it has an action potential) it sends an electrical impulse down its axon (which results in behaviour, for example the movement of a muscle). This value of -55mv is called a firing *threshold*. If it is not achieved, the neuron will not send a message.

The Action Potential

The action potential occurs because of an exchange of ions across the neuron's semi-permeable membrane. When the firing threshold level is reached (i.e. -55mv), this causes the cell to open sodium channels ('holes' in the semi-permeable membrane) that allow sodium ions to rush into the cell. This causes the rapid change from a negative charge of -55mv to a positive one of around $+30$mv. As soon as this happens, the cell tries to recover its resting potential state by closing sodium channels and opening potassium channels. The now negative charge on the outside of the cell then causes the movement of potassium ions to the outside of the cell, bringing the resting potential back. The final stage is for the sodium-potassium pump to help in the removal of sodium ions back to the outside of the cell.

What does this achieve?

All of this happens on one tiny spot on the cell membrane. However, the nerve impulse (which remember is carrying the message) has to travel the whole length of the neuron's axon. The 'struggle' that causes the action potential and then a return to the resting potential on one part of the membrane creates an imbalance in the spot on the membrane next to it. So, this next spot on the membrane opens the sodium channels and begins the action potential at that point. This creates a chain reaction of action potentials down the length of the neuron's axon. In the chapter, dominoes were used to highlight this wave of electricity that moves down the neuron's axon, but you could also see it as a worm's movement along the ground. One segment of its body pushes another segment which pushes on another and so on.

▶ **PAGE 4**

Panel 6

The 'all or nothing' effect is concerned with the *threshold* of -55mv. If this is not reached then the action potential does not occur. It often takes many neurons stimulating a single neuron to achieve this threshold.

▶ **PAGE 5**

Panels 2 to 6

Note: The following explanation deals with the transmission of the nerve impulse from one neuron to another.

Chemical transmission at the synapse

It was Ramón y Cajal who showed that neurons were not physically touching each other. These physical gaps are the reason von Helmholtz (see page 3 panel 1 above) did not find the nervous system transmitting electrical messages at the speed of light. The synaptic gaps slow down the message considerably.

Up until the 1920s, it was thought that the synapse was bridged by an electrical impulse. It took German physiologist Otto Loewi (1953) to show that synapses are bridged by sending chemicals across the gap. Chemical transmission is how most synapses are bridged.

We now know that there are a few neurons that **do** bridge the gap electrically by sending ions across the synapse. In other words, the action potential is physically carried from one neuron to the next. These are called *Electric Synapses* and are present in situations where very fast nerve transmission is very important. Electric synapses are rare and tend to occur in invertebrate animals. The crayfish, for example, has electric synapses that control the movement of its tail allowing it to escape from predators very quickly.

How is the chemical transmission achieved?

The end of a neuron's axon ends in what is described as the synaptic knob or the *pre-synaptic terminal* (it is called **pre**-synaptic because it is found *before* the synaptic gap). The pre-synaptic terminal is a sort of swelling at the end of the axon. Inside this swelling, there are small pockets that contain certain chemicals. These are called synaptic *vesicles* ('vesicle' means 'little bladder' – which is a very good description of what they are actually like!). The chemicals inside these 'little bladders' are called *neurotransmitters* and these are the chemicals that cross the synaptic gap and pass on the message from one neuron to another.

When the action potential arrives at the pre-synaptic terminal this causes calcium channels to open in the terminal's membrane (remember, these are 'holes' in the semi-permeable membrane that temporarily open to allow certain ions – in this case calcium – into the inside of the neuron). The calcium causes the vesicles near the terminal's membrane to fuse with it and thus open into the synapse. This allows the neurotransmitters inside them to spill out of the neuron into the synaptic gap.

What happens next?

The neurotransmitter chemicals flow or *diffuse* across the gap and reach the receiving part of the next neuron. This is called the **post**-synaptic neuron since it is *after* the synaptic gap. The neurotransmitter molecules fit into small 'holes' called *receptor sites* on the surface of the receiving neuron. This is rather like a key fitting into a lock so that the neurotransmitter molecules are the 'keys' shaped in such a way that they fit into the corresponding 'locks' of the receptor sites. This chemical 'jump' across a synapse takes only about 2 milliseconds (a millisecond is a millionth of a second!).

The locking of a neurotransmitter at a receptor site can have one of three effects:

1) *Ionotropic* effects
    Some neurotransmitters cause the postsynaptic neuron to open ion channels to allow a particular ion into the neuron.
    The neurotransmitter *glutamate*, for example, causes the sodium channels to open and therefore initiate an action potential. This is called an *excitatory* effect. The neurotransmitter *Gama-amniobutyric acid* (GABA) opens chloride gates that make the inside of the neuron more negative and hence stops an action potential taking place. This is called an *inhibitory* effect. However, both glutamate and GABA have ionotropic effects. Ionotropic effects are fast and are used when a quick response is needed such as in moving muscles.

2) *Metabotropic* effects
    Metabotropic effects are much slower and longer lasting than ionotropic effects. Metabotropic effects take place by creating a sequence of chemical (metabolic) reactions. When a neurotransmitter locks onto a metabotropic receptor this causes chemical changes inside the neuron that can have a variety of effects from opening an ion channel to switching on the effect of a chromosome. *Dopamine* is an example of a neurotransmitter that can have metabotropic effects.

3) *Modulatory* effects
    Some neurotransmitters act as what are known as *Neuromodulators*. Neuromodulators diffuse to more than one neuron. They then lock to all the correct receptor sites of the neurons close by. This is rather like a radio signal reaching all the radios that are tuned in to it.
    The effects of neuromodulators on neurons are quite small. They alter (modulate) the effect of the neurotransmitters (Millhorn *et al.*, 1989). Some neuromodulators, for example, can prolong or limit the effect of a neurotransmitter whilst others can limit the release of neurotransmitters. Endorphins (see Chapter 3) are examples of neuromodulators that have the effect of reducing pain responses.

Stopping the effect of neurotransmitters

Once the neurotransmitter has locked onto the receptor site and the desired message has been transmitted, it makes sense for the synapse to return back to its normal state in readiness for the next message. In order for this to be achieved, the neurotransmitter must be removed from the receptor sites and any that may be left in the synaptic gap. There are four ways in which the effect of the neurotransmitter is removed. Firstly, some of the neurotransmitter left in the gap simply flows away from the synaptic gap and is unable to bind to the receptors. Secondly, there are other chemicals called *enzymes* that are released into the gap that break up the neurotransmitters. Thirdly, there are chemicals that bind to the neurotransmitter molecules and absorb them back into the presynaptic neuron to be used again later (this is called the *reuptake* mechanism). And fourthly, there are supporting cells (glial cells) that absorb the neurotransmitter into themselves for re-use by the neuron.

Why have chemical transmission at synapses?

The chemical transmission at a synapse significantly slows down the nerve impulse. This must therefore have an important purpose. Given that neurons are either activated or not (in other words there is only a 'yes' or a 'no' response from each neuron) the chemicals at the synapse provide a great deal of complexity to the communication system. By using many different types of neurotransmitter molecules and different types of receptor sites on many different synapses, the nervous system can create a complicated code rather like having many letters in an alphabet to create a language.

▶ **PAGE 10**

Panel 3

The spinal cord is a segmented structure. Each segment has on each side a sensory nerve that receives information from the body and a motor nerve that sends information to the body. A cross-section through the spinal cord shows a darker 'H' in the centre that represents the tightly packed neurons. The white matter around this 'H' is made up mainly of axons with white myelin sheaths around them. The core of the spinal cord is a fluid-filled channel called the *central canal*.

Each segment of the spinal cord receives information from the brain and sends information to the brain. If the spinal cord is cut at a specific segment, then the brain loses all sensation from that segment and any segments below that one. Similarly, all motor control is also lost to the part of the body connected to this segment and the ones beneath it.

Protection for the central nervous system

The spinal cord and the brain are protected by fluid filled membranes called the *meninges*. The space between the meninges and the brain and spinal cord is filled with a liquid called *cerebrospinal fluid*. The brain and spinal cord therefore float in a bag of fluid. This protects the delicate structures from damage by impact. Sometimes the meninges become infected and this results in the condition known as *meningitis*.

In addition, the brain is protected from harmful chemicals by the *blood-brain barrier*. This is a set of tightly packed tiny blood vessels that prevent chemicals with large molecules from entering the brain. Anything that dissolves in fat can pass freely into the brain but there are many chemicals that only dissolve in water that need to be actively transported across the blood-brain barrier in order to reach the brain.

▶ **PAGE 11**

Panel 1

This definition of a reflex is from Garrett (2003, p.74).

▶ **PAGE 12**

Panel 1

The hindbrain is also sometimes referred to as the *rhombencephalon.*

▶ **PAGE 13**

Panel 5

The midbrain is also known as the *mesencephalon* and consists of two structures the *tectum* and the *tegmentum.* The important structures in the tectum are the *superior colliculi* that are involved in vision and the *inferior colliculi* that are concerned with audition. One important structure in the tegmentum is the *substantia nigra* that contains neurons that produce dopamine. It is the death of neurons in this area that is believed to be largely responsible for the movement disorder called Parkinson's disease (see Chapter 5).

The midbrain is relatively small in humans. In birds, reptiles, amphibians and fish the midbrain structures are much more noticeable.

▶ **PAGE 14**

Panel 1

The forebrain is sometimes referred to as the *prosencephalon.*

▶ **PAGE 15**

Panel 1

The *Corpus Callosum* is the largest of the *cerebral commisures.* These are dense fibres that carry information between the two cerebral hemispheres. The two hemispheres carry out slightly different tasks and therefore need to communicate with each other. Additionally, information from the senses is often directed to one specific hemisphere. For example, visual information on the left is sent to the right hemisphere while visual information on the right is sent to the left hemisphere. This information needs to be shared with the other hemisphere through the corpus callosum and the other comissures. Sometimes, surgeons cut the corpus callosum so that those suffering from epilepsy can confine their fits to just one cerebral hemisphere (this is only done in the most serious of cases). These individuals therefore have no internal communication between the cerebral hemispheres and have been studied to determine the different functions of the two hemispheres. These studies have shown that, for example, the left hemisphere is generally more involved in language than the right hemisphere and that the right hemisphere is more involved in spatial tasks and face recognition (e.g. Gazzaniga, 1967; McKeever, Seitz, Krutsch, & Van Eys, 1995; Nebes, 1974).

▶ **PAGE 16**

Panel 3

What this diagram omits are the brain *ventricles.* The ventricles are hollow spaces inside the brain filled with cerebrospinal fluid. There are four ventricles in the brain connected to the central canal of the spinal cord (see notes for page 10 panel 3 above) and to the meninges.

▶ **PAGE 19 (Panels 4 to 7) and PAGE 20 (Panels 1 to 5)**

The case of Phineas Gage

At the time of his accident, Phineas Gage was 25 and working as a railroad construction foreman near the town of Cavendish in Vermont, USA. One of his duties was to drill holes in rock in order to place explosive charges in them so that the rocks could be removed. The drilled hole had to be filled with the explosive powder and then sand placed on top. This mixture was then packed together using a three and a half foot (approximately 1.07 m) long iron rod. On the fatal day (13 September 1848 at about 4.30pm) Phineas Gage either forgot to add the sand or was packing the explosives before adding the sand when he was distracted and this caused a spark that ignited the explosive powder. The force of the explosion caused the iron rod to fly up through Gage's skull and into the air. The 3 cm diameter metal rod passed through his skull and caused damage to his brain (Damasio, 1994; Macmillan, 1986).

After his recovery from the accident, Gage failed to be re-employed by the railroad company and in 1850 he spent about a year as a side-show attraction at P.T. Barnum's New York museum displaying his injury (and the tamping iron!) to paying customers. He later spent some time in Chile as a coach driver before returning to his home in San Francisco in 1859 to become a farm worker before his death in 1860.

The type of deficit suffered by Phineas Gage is actually open to some debate. It is often stated that Gage suffered personality changes. This is usually referenced back to John Harlow (1868), the doctor who attended to Gage's injuries. He stated that:

> 'His contractors, who regarded him as the most efficient and capable foreman in their employ previous to his injury, considered the change in his mind so marked that they could not give him his place again. He is fitful, irreverent, indulging at times in the grossest profanity (which was not previously his custom), manifesting but little deference for his fellows, impatient of restraint or advice when it conflicts with his desires, at times pertinaciously obstinate, yet capricious and vacillating, devising many plans of future operation, which are no sooner arranged than they are abandoned in turn for others appearing more feasible. In this regard his mind was radically changed, so decidedly that his friends and acquaintances said he was 'no longer Gage' ". (Harlow, 1868 in Neylan, 1999, p. 280).

However, MacMillan (2000) has cast some doubt over the scientific accuracy of the personality changes ostensibly suffered by Gage. He points to the fact that at the time of the injury Harlow (writing in 1848, see Neylan, 1999) did not mention much regarding psychological changes. Similarly, Bigelow (1850), who was professor of medicine at Harvard University and examined Gage after his recovery, stated that he had recovered both in body and in mind and made no note of psychological changes. It was Harlow's quote above in 1868 (eight years after Gage's death) that seems to have been embellished by later writers and coupled with Gage's sensationalistic appearances at Barnum's museum. We therefore cannot be certain about the details of the case of Phineas Gage since, as MacMillan has pointed out; very few of the deficits attributed to Gage have been based on original sources written at the time. Many deficits have been suggested based on modern ideas of frontal lobe damage instead.

Panel 6

Damasio *et al.* (1994) conducted neural imaging studies on the surviving skull of Phineas Gage and reconstructed the path of the iron bar through his skull. They suggested that the accident damaged the part of both frontal lobes involved in making decisions in personal and social matters. More recent work by Ratiu *et al.* (2004) using computed tomography scanning (CAT scan) has cast some doubt over Damasio *et al.*'s conclusion, however. Ratui *et al.*'s work suggests that the damage to Gage's brain was much less extensive than was hitherto believed as they suggest that only Gage's left frontal lobe was actually damaged.

Despite these controversies, the case of Phineas Gage really does represent a milestone in terms of 'tipping the balance' in favour of the idea of localisation of function in the brain.

Phineas Gage – another perspective

Most introductory psychology textbooks mention the case of Phineas Gage (approximately 60 per cent according to MacMillan, 2000). However, in reading some of these, the case is generally described in a sanitised way. In these sources' excitement to place the case of Phineas Gage in its deserved important historical context, Phineas Gage the human being is lost. Little mention is made of Gage's horrific injuries except to say that the hot iron rod 'cauterised' the wound on its way through Gage's skull. Much is made of Gage walking to the cart that took him to the town, implying that despite the injury, Gage came away relatively unscathed, at least physically.

However, the reality seems very different if you read the original account from Harlow (1848; see Neylan, 1999). Phineas Gage suffered a great deal. Harlow attended to Gage about one and a half hours after the accident at approximately 6pm. This is his description of how he found his patient:

> 'He seemed perfectly conscious, but was getting exhausted from the haemorrhage, which was very profuse both externally and internally, the blood finding its way into the stomach, which rejected it as often as every 15 or 20 minutes. Pulse 60, and regular. His person, and the bed on which he was laid, were literally one gore of blood' (Harlow, 1848 in Neylan, 1999, p. 281).

He also mentions that Gage's hands and forearms were deeply burned up to the elbow; something which is rarely mentioned in other sources.

Harlow also describes the subsequent recovery of his patient from the 13 September until the 18 November 1848. During this time he mentions further haemorrhaging, vomiting, severe swelling of the face, 'foetid' discharge from the scalp intermingled with particles of brain, the formation of an abscess on one of the facial muscles and fungal growth from within the wound. Ever the clinician, Harlow does not attempt to describe the level of pain that Gage must have suffered.

This level of 'gory detail' is included here to remind us that despite the controversies over Gage's deficits there is a man at the heart of this case. Whether you believe that Gage suffered personality changes or if the phrase 'he was no longer Gage' was indeed spoken by his friends or not, should not detract from the horrendous physical suffering that Phineas Gage endured as a result of what happened on 13 September 1848.

▶ **PAGE 21**

Panel 3

Broca's Area

Pierre Paul Broca (1824–80) was a French surgeon who in 1861 treated a patient for gangrene. This patient had earlier lost his ability to say anything except the word 'tan' and to utter an oath. Five days later the patient died and Broca was able to examine his brain. He found damage to a specific part of the left frontal lobe. On the basis of this and other cases, Broca concluded that this part of the brain must be intact for speech production despite intact vocal apparatus and normal language comprehension.

Broca is often cited as one of the first to show localisation of function in the brain although others also wrote about this area at around the same time (Finger & Roe, 1996). The area of the frontal lobe is now known as *Broca's Area* and is generally seen as a language production area of the brain. Any serious impairment of language production is known as *Broca's Aphasia* regardless of whether the damage is to Broca's Area or not. Aphasia is the term used for any language impairment.

We now know that speaking involves a large part of the cortex, especially in the left hemisphere and is certainly not confined to Broca's Area (Wallesch, Henriksen, Korhuber & Paulson, 1985).

Wernicke's Area

In 1874 Carl Wernicke discovered that damage to an area in the left temporal lobe of the cortex produced an aphasia that was very different to that discovered by Broca. This is known as *Wernicke's Aphasia* or *Fluent Aphasia*. In this case the language impairment is characterised by an inability to remember names of objects and general impairment of language comprehension. The person is often seen as speaking very fluently despite difficulties in finding certain words (known as *Anomia*). Additionally, these individuals find it very difficult to understand both spoken and written speech. Like with Broca's Aphasia, these types of deficit are called Wernicke's Aphasia regardless of whether the damage is in the same part of the brain.

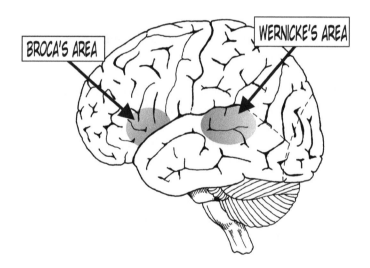

CHAPTER 2
VISION AND AUDITION

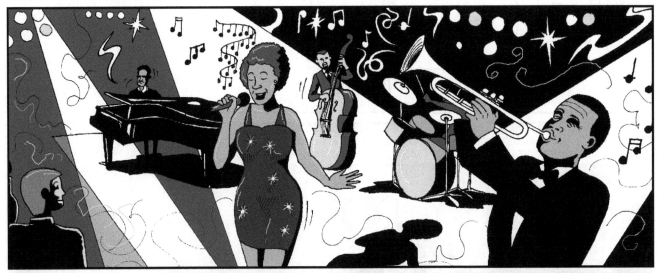

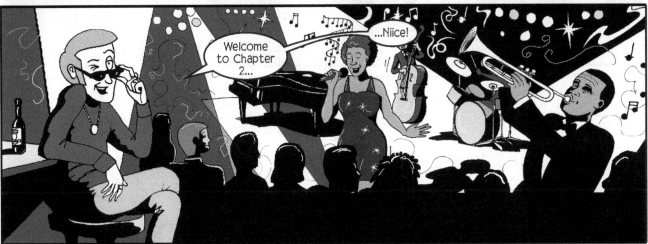

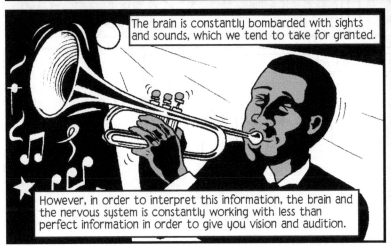

The brain is constantly bombarded with sights and sounds, which we tend to take for granted.

However, in order to interpret this information, the brain and the nervous system is constantly working with less than perfect information in order to give you vision and audition.

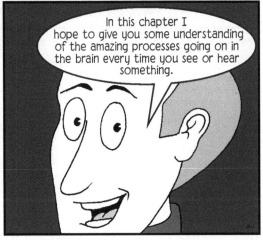

In this chapter I hope to give you some understanding of the amazing processes going on in the brain every time you see or hear something.

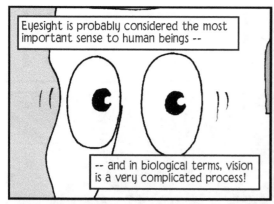

Eyesight is probably considered the most important sense to human beings --

-- and in biological terms, vision is a very complicated process!

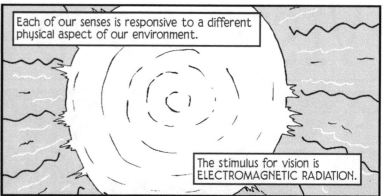

Each of our senses is responsive to a different physical aspect of our environment.

The stimulus for vision is ELECTROMAGNETIC RADIATION.

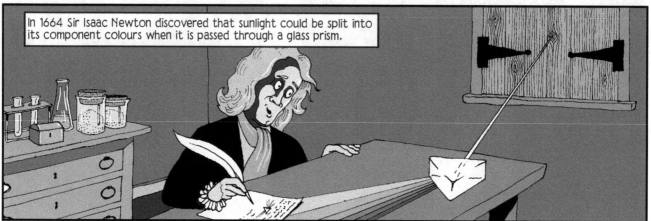

In 1664 Sir Isaac Newton discovered that sunlight could be split into its component colours when it is passed through a glass prism.

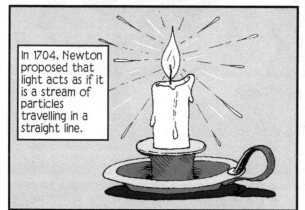

In 1704, Newton proposed that light acts as if it is a stream of particles travelling in a straight line.

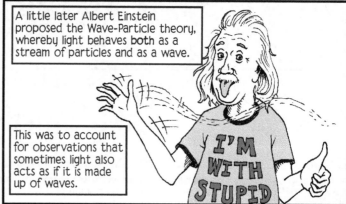

A little later Albert Einstein proposed the Wave-Particle theory, whereby light behaves **both** as a stream of particles and as a wave.

This was to account for observations that sometimes light also acts as if it is made up of waves.

I'M WITH STUPID

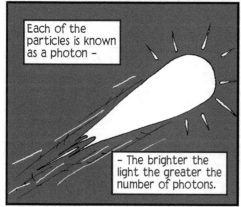

Each of the particles is known as a photon –

– The brighter the light the greater the number of photons.

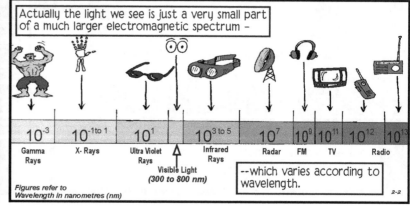

Actually the light we see is just a very small part of a much larger electromagnetic spectrum –

10^{-3}	10^{-1} to 1	10^1		10^3 to 5	10^7	10^9	10^{11}	10^{12}	10^{13}
Gamma Rays	X- Rays	Ultra Violet Rays	Visible Light (300 to 800 nm)	Infrared Rays	Radar	FM	TV	Radio	

Figures refer to Wavelength in nanometres (nm)

--which varies according to wavelength.

2-2

The wavelength is the distance between the peaks of the waves –

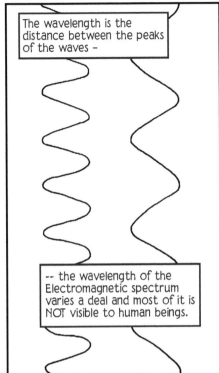

-- the wavelength of the Electromagnetic spectrum varies a deal and most of it is NOT visible to human beings.

Vision begins with light reflecting off things and entering the eyes –

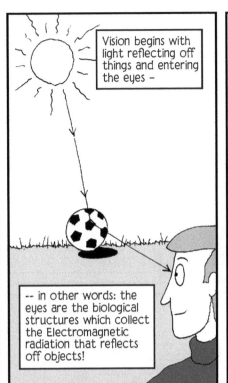

-- in other words: the eyes are the biological structures which collect the Electromagnetic radiation that reflects off objects!

It took first century philosopher Ibn Al-Haytham, to show that light rays bounce off any object in all directions but we only see those rays that hit our eyes at right angles --

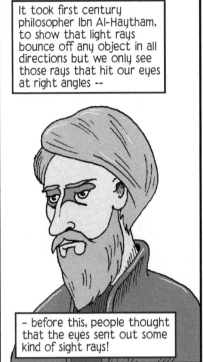

- before this, people thought that the eyes sent out some kind of sight rays!

Each eye contains a number of structures to collect and convert visible light into nerve impulses.

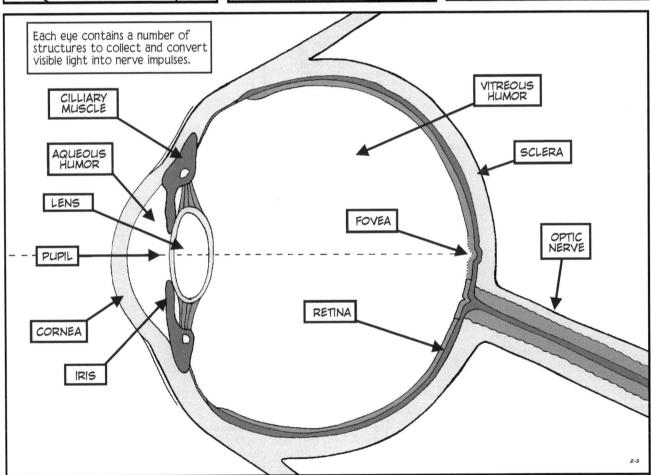

CILLIARY MUSCLE

AQUEOUS HUMOR

LENS

PUPIL

CORNEA

IRIS

VITREOUS HUMOR

SCLERA

FOVEA

OPTIC NERVE

RETINA

2-3

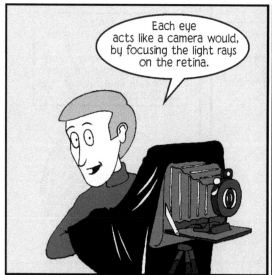

Each eye acts like a camera would, by focusing the light rays on the retina.

The lens focuses the light on the retina by changing its shape.

This is similar to the moving of a lens back and forth by a camera.

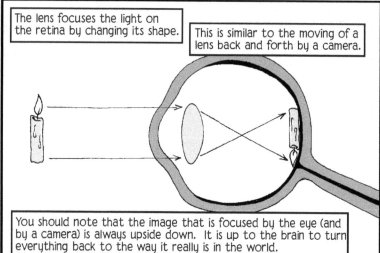

You should note that the image that is focused by the eye (and by a camera) is always upside down. It is up to the brain to turn everything back to the way it really is in the world.

The goal of the eye focusing the light is to create a clear image on the retina.

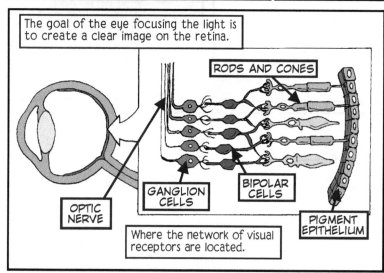

RODS AND CONES

OPTIC NERVE

GANGLION CELLS

BIPOLAR CELLS

PIGMENT EPITHELIUM

Where the network of visual receptors are located.

The most important parts of the retina are the visual receptors - the rods and the cones.

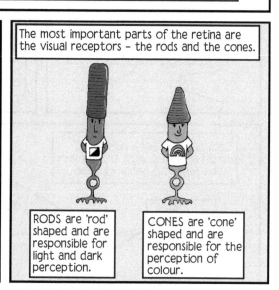

RODS are 'rod' shaped and are responsible for light and dark perception.

CONES are 'cone' shaped and are responsible for the perception of colour.

Like all sensory receptors, the function of the rods and cones is to convert or transduce the stimulus - in this case light - into nerve impulses.

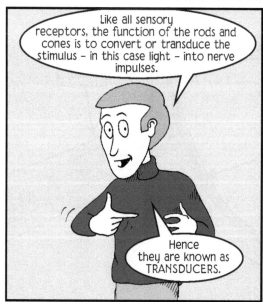

Hence they are known as TRANSDUCERS.

While not fully understood, the mechanism of transduction involves PHOTOPIGMENTS - chemicals which change when exposed to light.

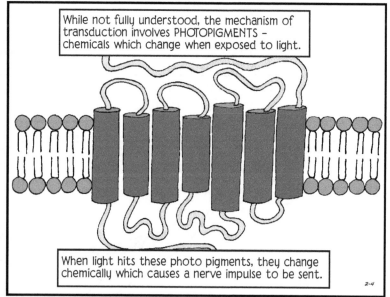

When light hits these photo pigments, they change chemically which causes a nerve impulse to be sent.

2-4

There are a number of differences between rods and cones.

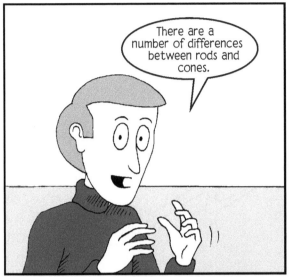

Firstly rods and cones are distributed differently in the retina.

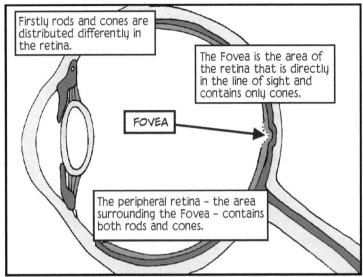

The Fovea is the area of the retina that is directly in the line of sight and contains only cones.

FOVEA

The peripheral retina - the area surrounding the Fovea - contains both rods and cones.

Rods outnumber cones in the retina by 20 to 1.

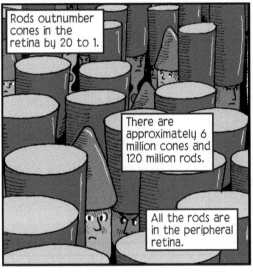

There are approximately 6 million cones and 120 million rods.

All the rods are in the peripheral retina.

The retina is made up of rods and cones and a network of other nerve cells.

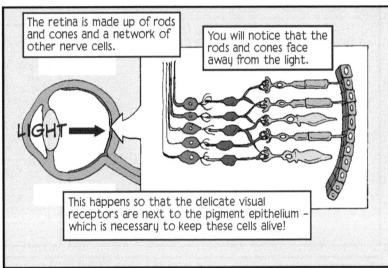

You will notice that the rods and cones face away from the light.

LIGHT

This happens so that the delicate visual receptors are next to the pigment epithelium - which is necessary to keep these cells alive!

This doesn't really cause any problems as most of the support cells are transparent.

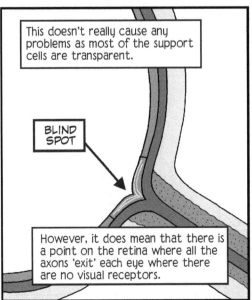

BLIND SPOT

However, it does mean that there is a point on the retina where all the axons 'exit' each eye where there are no visual receptors.

This results in each of our eyes having a 'blind spot' where we can't see anything!

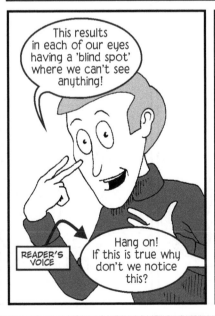

READER'S VOICE

Hang on! If this is true why don't we notice this?

Normally, we aren't aware of our blind spots because the brain fills them in or the overlap of the eyes means that one eye can usually see what the other cannot.

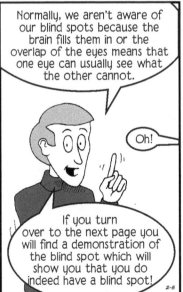

Oh!

If you turn over to the next page you will find a demonstration of the blind spot which will show you that you do indeed have a blind spot!

2-5

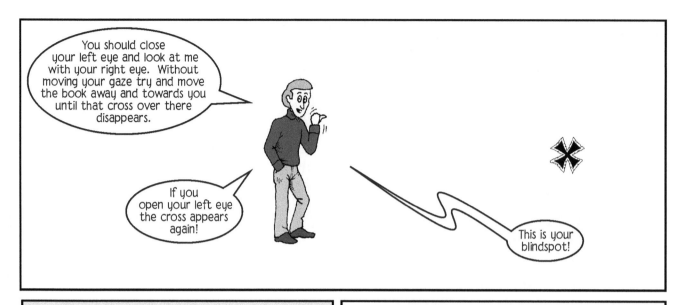

This is the route that the nerve fibres take from the eyes to the visual cortex in the brain.

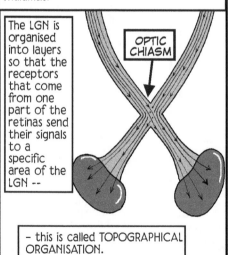

The first thing to note is that the visual fields 'cross over'. In other words everything you see on the left of your gaze is sent to the right brain hemisphere and everything on the right of your gaze is sent to the left hemisphere.

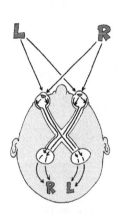

The cross-over occurs at the Optic Chiasm which sends most of the connections to each Lateral Geniculate Nucleus of the Thalamus.

The LGN is organised into layers so that the receptors that come from one part of the retinas send their signals to a specific area of the LGN --

OPTIC CHIASM

- this is called TOPOGRAPHICAL ORGANISATION.

One and a half million axons go from each LGN towards the occipital lobe of the cortex.

The area of the cortex responsible for vision is known as the VISUAL CORTEX. It is also known as the STRIATE CORTEX because (like the LGN) it is organised into layers and looks striped –

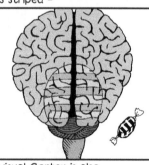

The visual Cortex is also topographically organised so that neurons in the LGN send their signals to a specific area of the visual cortex.

2-6

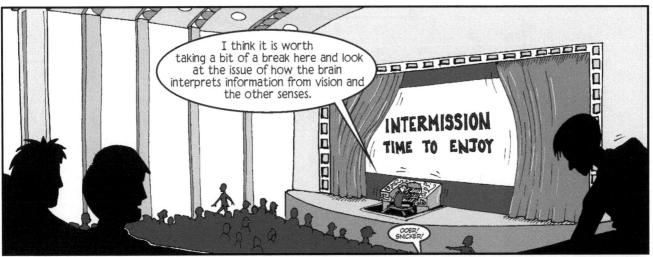

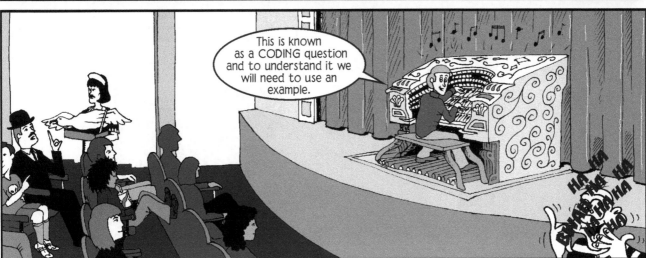

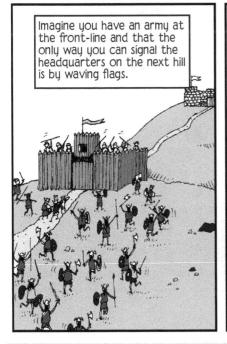

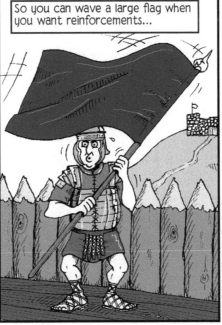

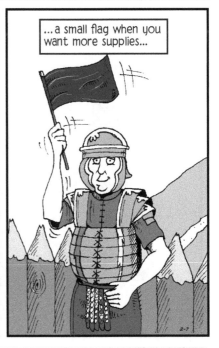

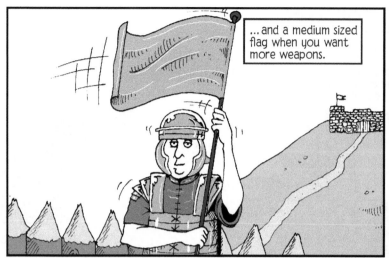

...and a medium sized flag when you want more weapons.

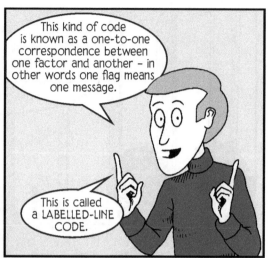

This kind of code is known as a one-to-one correspondence between one factor and another – in other words one flag means one message.

This is called a LABELLED-LINE CODE.

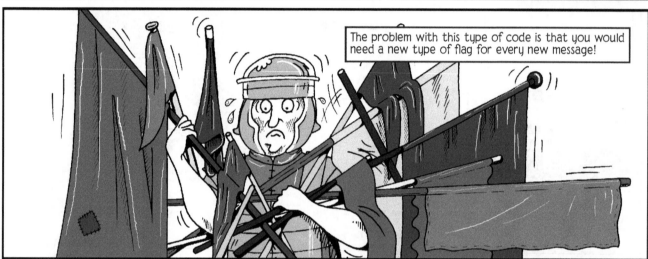

The problem with this type of code is that you would need a new type of flag for every new message!

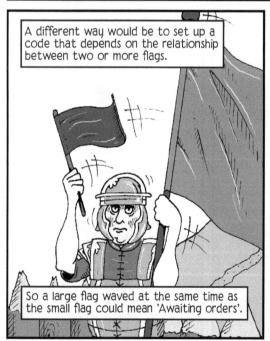

A different way would be to set up a code that depends on the relationship between two or more flags.

So a large flag waved at the same time as the small flag could mean 'Awaiting orders'.

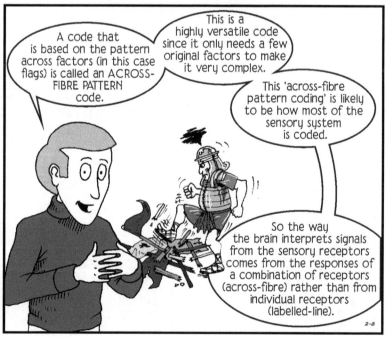

A code that is based on the pattern across factors (in this case flags) is called an ACROSS-FIBRE PATTERN code.

This is a highly versatile code since it only needs a few original factors to make it very complex.

This 'across-fibre pattern coding' is likely to be how most of the sensory system is coded.

So the way the brain interprets signals from the sensory receptors comes from the responses of a combination of receptors (across-fibre) rather than from individual receptors (labelled-line).

2-8

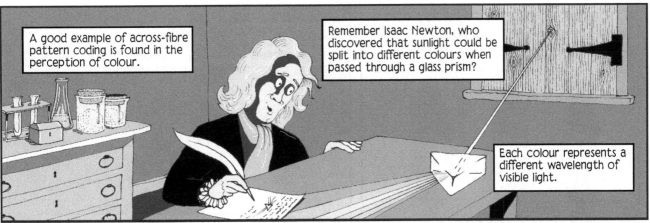

A good example of across-fibre pattern coding is found in the perception of colour.

Remember Isaac Newton, who discovered that sunlight could be split into different colours when passed through a glass prism?

Each colour represents a different wavelength of visible light.

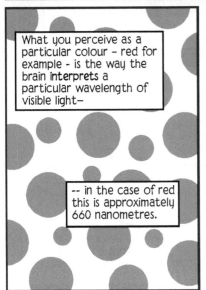

What you perceive as a particular colour - red for example - is the way the brain interprets a particular wavelength of visible light—

-- in the case of red this is approximately 660 nanometres.

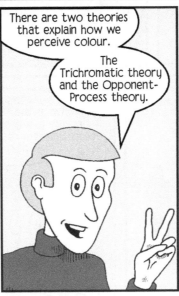

There are two theories that explain how we perceive colour.

The Trichromatic theory and the Opponent-Process theory.

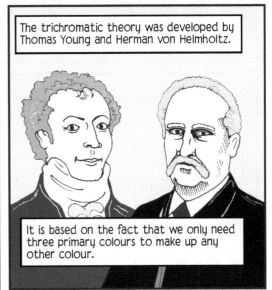

The trichromatic theory was developed by Thomas Young and Herman von Helmholtz.

It is based on the fact that we only need three primary colours to make up any other colour.

Through various experiments, Young and Helmholtz found that there appeared to be three primary colours - Red, Blue and Green - which when mixed in different proportions would produce all colours.

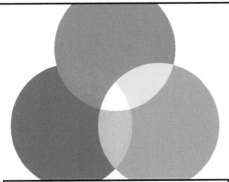

So if you mix red and green light together you get yellow light and if you mix blue and green light you get cyan coloured light and so on.

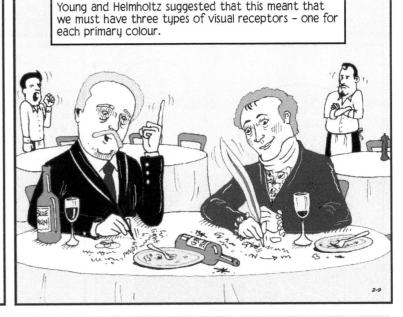

Young and Helmholtz suggested that this meant that we must have three types of visual receptors - one for each primary colour.

Dartnall and colleagues found three types of human cone pigments each having maximum absorption of light in the short (blue), middle (green) and long (red) wavelengths of visible light.

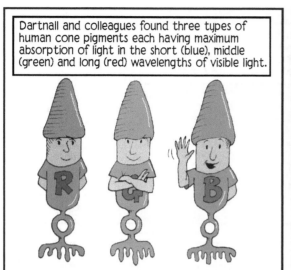

These three types of cone are arranged on the retina in groups so that they can detect the different wavelengths of all coloured light.

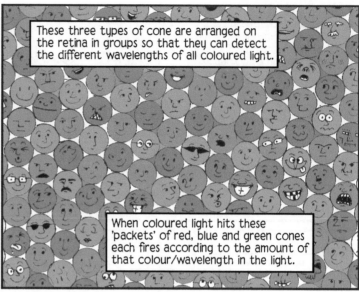

When coloured light hits these 'packets' of red, blue and green cones each fires according to the amount of that colour/wavelength in the light.

YELLOW LIGHT

So if yellow light stimulates the cones, this only causes the firing of the Red and Green cones NOT the blue cones. Thus the brain interprets these wavelengths as yellow light.

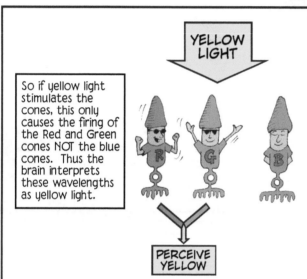

PERCEIVE YELLOW

This theory is known as the TRICHROMATIC theory because It suggests that our colour perception requires three different types of receptor.

The word 'trichromatic' means 'three colours'.

Because the perception of colour depends on the pattern of activity from the three types of cone cell – this is a great example of across-fibre pattern coding in the senses.

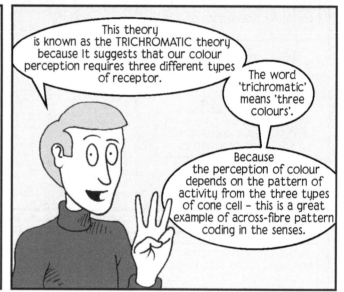

Hang on – what about this Opponent process theory you mentioned where does that fit in?

I'm glad you asked...

READER'S VOICE

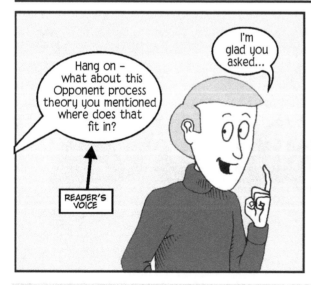

Ewald Hering's Opponent Process theory relied on two issues that could not be resolved by the trichromatic theory...

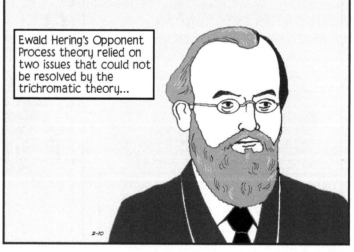

2-10

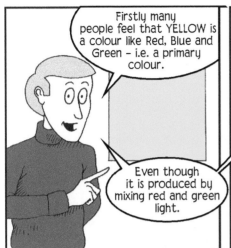

Firstly many people feel that YELLOW is a colour like Red, Blue and Green – i.e. a primary colour.

and secondly the concept of colour afterimages.

Even though it is produced by mixing red and green light.

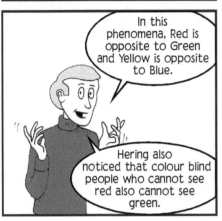

In this phenomena, Red is opposite to Green and Yellow is opposite to Blue.

Hering also noticed that colour blind people who cannot see red also cannot see green.

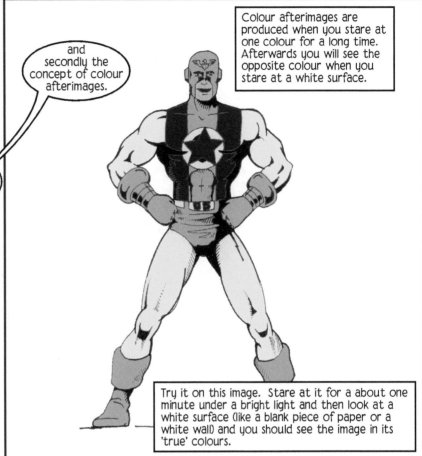

Colour afterimages are produced when you stare at one colour for a long time. Afterwards you will see the opposite colour when you stare at a white surface.

Try it on this image. Stare at it for a about one minute under a bright light and then look at a white surface (like a blank piece of paper or a white wall) and you should see the image in its 'true' colours.

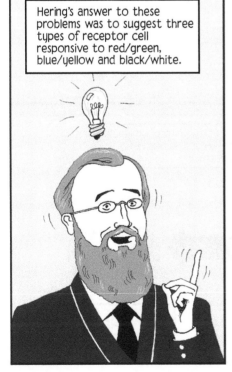

Hering's answer to these problems was to suggest three types of receptor cell responsive to red/green, blue/yellow and black/white.

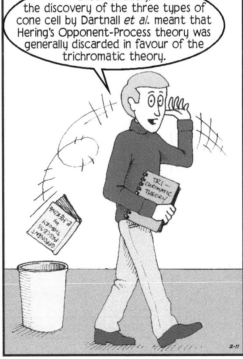

Unfortunately, the discovery of the three types of cone cell by Dartnall *et al.* meant that Hering's Opponent-Process theory was generally discarded in favour of the trichromatic theory.

2-11

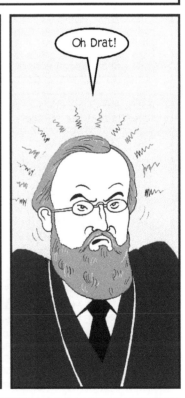

Oh Drat!

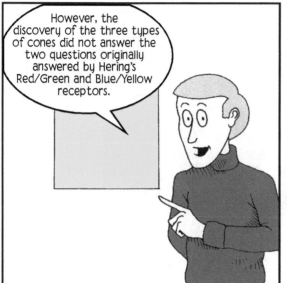

However, the discovery of the three types of cones did not answer the two questions originally answered by Hering's Red/Green and Blue/Yellow receptors.

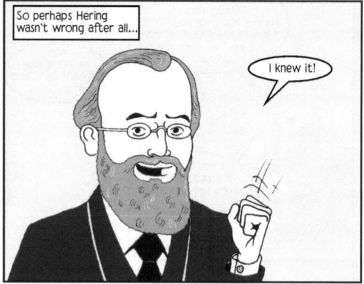

So perhaps Hering wasn't wrong after all...

I knew it!

More recent physiological evidence has found evidence for neurons that respond in opposite ways to different wavelengths of light.

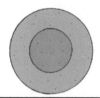

This cell for example responds mostly when red light hits its centre and green in its periphery. If red light hits the periphery and green the centre the cell hardly responds at all.

These types of 'opponent-process' cells have been found in the retina, the LGN as well as in the visual cortex.

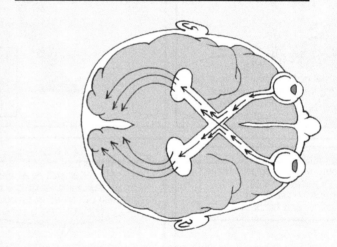

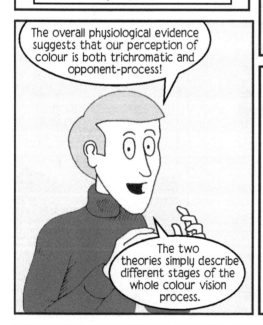

The overall physiological evidence suggests that our perception of colour is both trichromatic and opponent-process!

The two theories simply describe different stages of the whole colour vision process.

Trichromatic mechanisms occur at the receptor level – i.e. the retina – whilst opponent processes tend to occur further on in the visual pathway.

RODS AND CONES

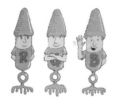

TRICHROMATIC THEORY

GANGLION CELLS

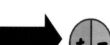

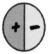

OPPONENT PROCESS THEORY

2-12

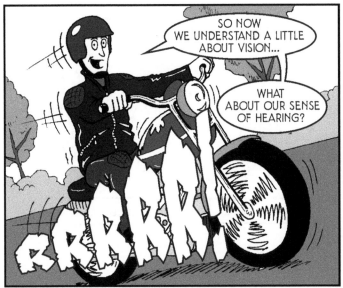

SO NOW WE UNDERSTAND A LITTLE ABOUT VISION...

WHAT ABOUT OUR SENSE OF HEARING?

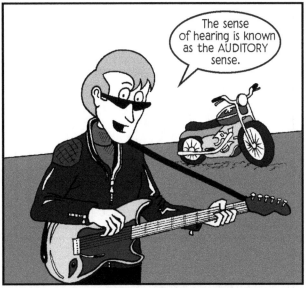

The sense of hearing is known as the AUDITORY sense.

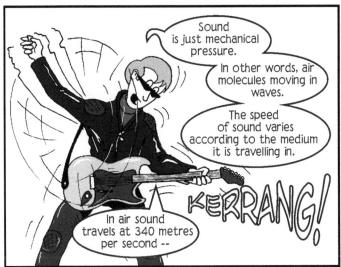

Sound is just mechanical pressure.

In other words, air molecules moving in waves.

The speed of sound varies according to the medium it is travelling in.

In air sound travels at 340 metres per second --

KERRANG!

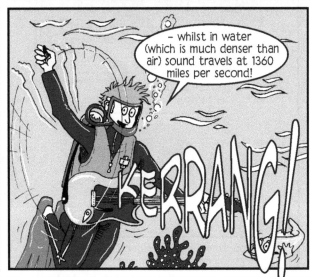

- whilst in water (which is much denser than air) sound travels at 1360 miles per second!

KERRANG!

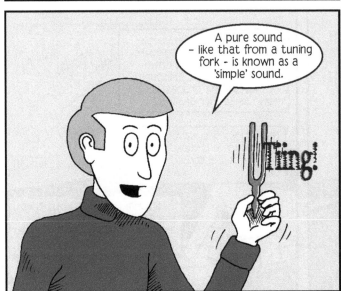

A pure sound - like that from a tuning fork - is known as a 'simple' sound.

Ting!

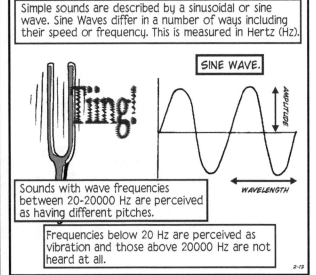

Simple sounds are described by a sinusoidal or sine wave. Sine Waves differ in a number of ways including their speed or frequency. This is measured in Hertz (Hz).

SINE WAVE.

AMPLITUDE

WAVELENGTH

Sounds with wave frequencies between 20-20000 Hz are perceived as having different pitches.

Frequencies below 20 Hz are perceived as vibration and those above 20000 Hz are not heard at all.

2-13

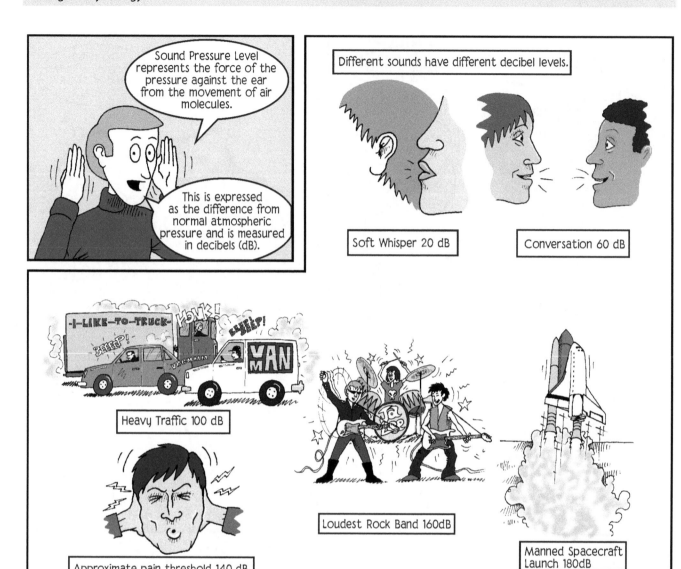

Sound Pressure Level represents the force of the pressure against the ear from the movement of air molecules.

This is expressed as the difference from normal atmospheric pressure and is measured in decibels (dB).

Different sounds have different decibel levels.

Soft Whisper 20 dB

Conversation 60 dB

Heavy Traffic 100 dB

Approximate pain threshold 140 dB

Loudest Rock Band 160dB

Manned Spacecraft Launch 180dB

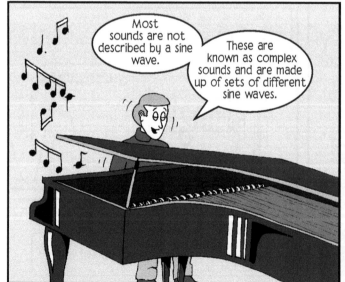

Most sounds are not described by a sine wave.

These are known as complex sounds and are made up of sets of different sine waves.

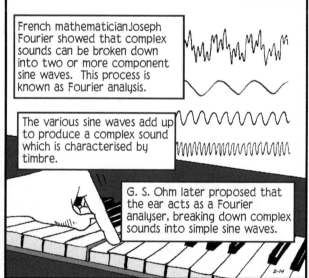

French mathematician Joseph Fourier showed that complex sounds can be broken down into two or more component sine waves. This process is known as Fourier analysis.

The various sine waves add up to produce a complex sound which is characterised by timbre.

G. S. Ohm later proposed that the ear acts as a Fourier analyser, breaking down complex sounds into simple sine waves.

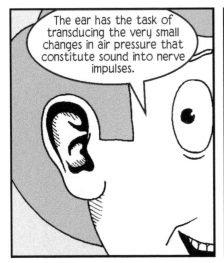

The ear has the task of transducing the very small changes in air pressure that constitute sound into nerve impulses.

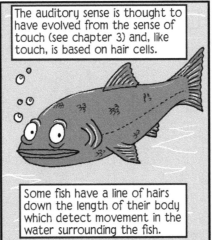

The auditory sense is thought to have evolved from the sense of touch (see chapter 3) and, like touch, is based on hair cells.

Some fish have a line of hairs down the length of their body which detect movement in the water surrounding the fish.

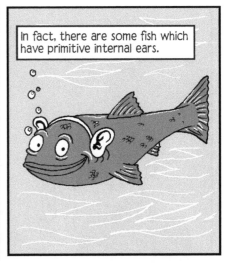

In fact, there are some fish which have primitive internal ears.

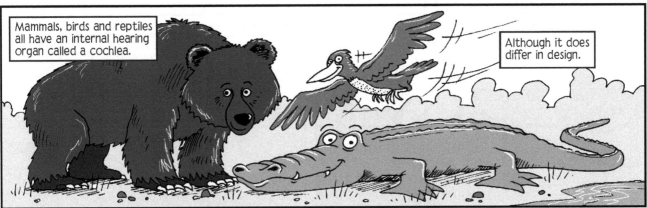

Mammals, birds and reptiles all have an internal hearing organ called a cochlea.

Although it does differ in design.

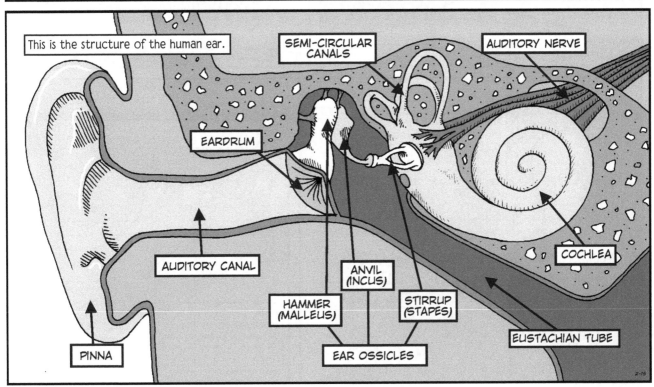

This is the structure of the human ear.

SEMI-CIRCULAR CANALS

AUDITORY NERVE

EARDRUM

AUDITORY CANAL

ANVIL (INCUS)

HAMMER (MALLEUS)

STIRRUP (STAPES)

EAR OSSICLES

COCHLEA

EUSTACHIAN TUBE

PINNA

2-15

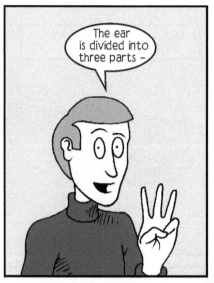

The ear is divided into three parts –

The Outer Ear:

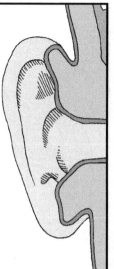

Which consists of the PINNA – the fleshy part on the outside of the body that is only found in mammals - channels sound into the auditory canal and helps to localise sounds.

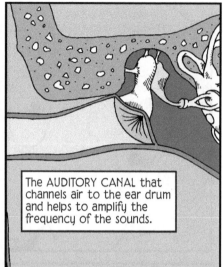

The AUDITORY CANAL that channels air to the ear drum and helps to amplify the frequency of the sounds.

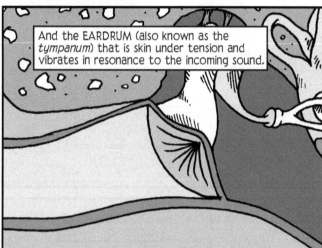

And the EARDRUM (also known as the *tympanum*) that is skin under tension and vibrates in resonance to the incoming sound.

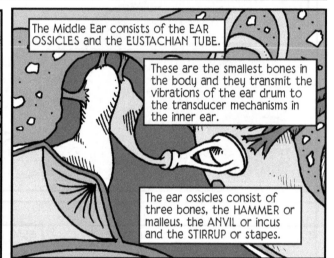

The Middle Ear consists of the EAR OSSICLES and the EUSTACHIAN TUBE.

These are the smallest bones in the body and they transmit the vibrations of the ear drum to the transducer mechanisms in the inner ear.

The ear ossicles consist of three bones, the HAMMER or malleus, the ANVIL or incus and the STIRRUP or stapes.

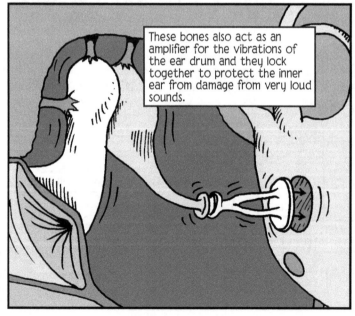

These bones also act as an amplifier for the vibrations of the ear drum and they lock together to protect the inner ear from damage from very loud sounds.

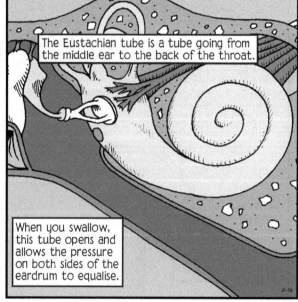

The Eustachian tube is a tube going from the middle ear to the back of the throat.

When you swallow, this tube opens and allows the pressure on both sides of the eardrum to equalise.

The Inner Ear consists of the OVAL WINDOW and the COCHLEA.

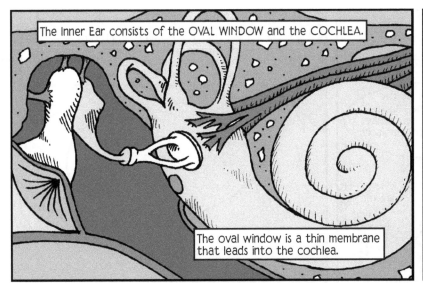

The oval window is a thin membrane that leads into the cochlea.

The foot of the stirrup rests on the oval window and thus transmits the vibrations of the eardrum to the internal structures of the cochlea.

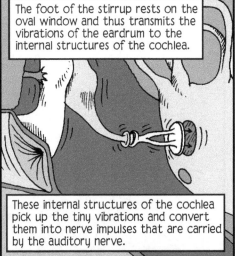

These internal structures of the cochlea pick up the tiny vibrations and convert them into nerve impulses that are carried by the auditory nerve.

If you looked at a cross-section of the inside of the cochlea you would see that it is made up of three chambers.

VESTIBULAR CANAL

COCHLEA CANAL

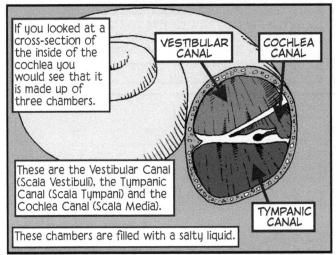

TYMPANIC CANAL

These are the Vestibular Canal (Scala Vestibuli), the Tympanic Canal (Scala Tympani) and the Cochlea Canal (Scala Media).

These chambers are filled with a salty liquid.

The most important chamber is the Cochlea Canal –

ORGAN OF CORTI

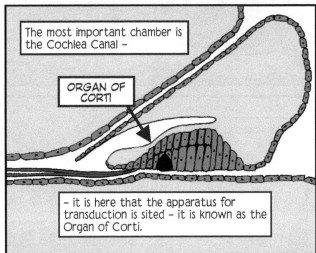

– it is here that the apparatus for transduction is sited – it is known as the Organ of Corti.

The Organ of Corti sits on the basilar membrane – the membrane that separates the tympanic canal from the cochlea canal

Poking out from the basilar membrane are tiny hair cells covered by a flap of tissue called the Tectorial membrane.

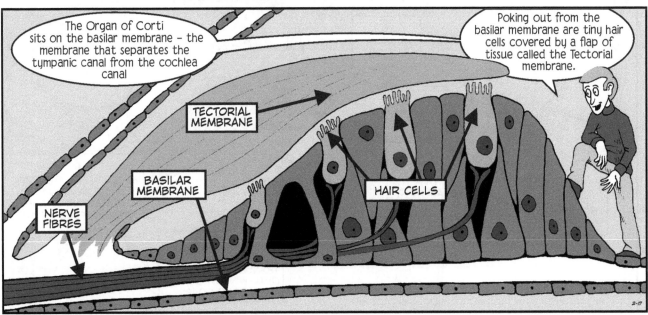

TECTORIAL MEMBRANE

BASILAR MEMBRANE

HAIR CELLS

NERVE FIBRES

2-17

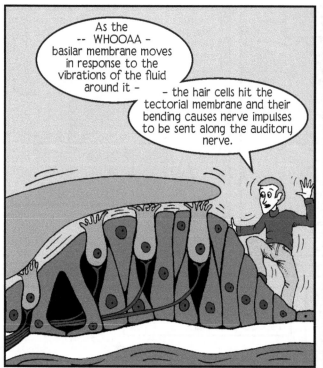

As the -- WHOOAA - basilar membrane moves in response to the vibrations of the fluid around it -

- the hair cells hit the tectorial membrane and their bending causes nerve impulses to be sent along the auditory nerve.

Bear in mind that the organ of corti runs along the whole length of the basilar membrane of the coiled cochlea. The Human cochlea has about 15500 hair cells all arranged in rows along its length.

It is also important to note that the tympanic and vestibular canals are joined at the end of the cochlea at a point called the helicotrema.

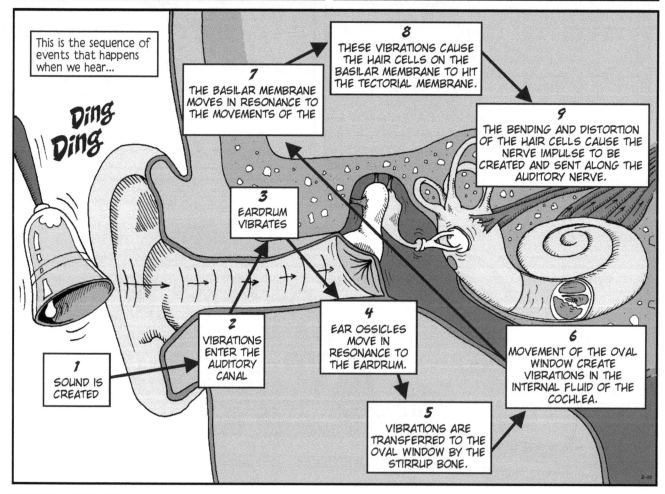

This is the sequence of events that happens when we hear...

Ding Ding

1 SOUND IS CREATED

2 VIBRATIONS ENTER THE AUDITORY CANAL

3 EARDRUM VIBRATES

4 EAR OSSICLES MOVE IN RESONANCE TO THE EARDRUM.

5 VIBRATIONS ARE TRANSFERRED TO THE OVAL WINDOW BY THE STIRRUP BONE.

6 MOVEMENT OF THE OVAL WINDOW CREATE VIBRATIONS IN THE INTERNAL FLUID OF THE COCHLEA.

7 THE BASILAR MEMBRANE MOVES IN RESONANCE TO THE MOVEMENTS OF THE

8 THESE VIBRATIONS CAUSE THE HAIR CELLS ON THE BASILAR MEMBRANE TO HIT THE TECTORIAL MEMBRANE.

9 THE BENDING AND DISTORTION OF THE HAIR CELLS CAUSE THE NERVE IMPULSE TO BE CREATED AND SENT ALONG THE AUDITORY NERVE.

The two auditory nerves (one from each cochlea) enter the brain on either side of the brain stem and pass through a series of structures before reaching the Primary Auditory Cortex in each temporal lobe.

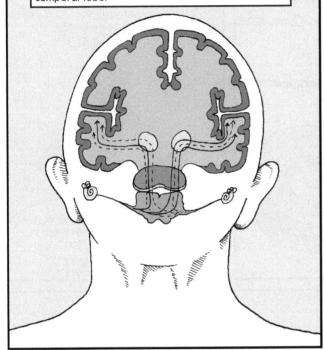

The majority of the auditory cortex is hidden under a fold on the temporal lobe.

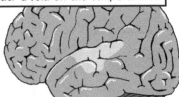

Like the visual cortex, the auditory cortex is topographically organised so that signals from specific hair cells in the cochlea end up in the same spot in the cortex.

The majority (but not all) of the nerves from each ear go to the opposite side of the brain hemispheres.

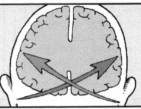

So most of the sounds from the left ear are processed in the right auditory cortex and the sounds in the right ear are processed in the left auditory cortex.

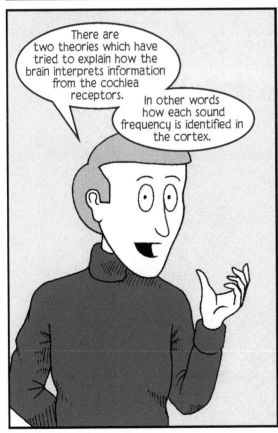

There are two theories which have tried to explain how the brain interprets information from the cochlea receptors.

In other words how each sound frequency is identified in the cortex.

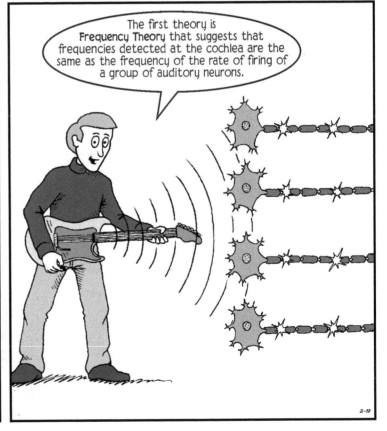

The first theory is **Frequency Theory** that suggests that frequencies detected at the cochlea are the same as the frequency of the rate of firing of a group of auditory neurons.

2-19

The second theory is **Place theory.**

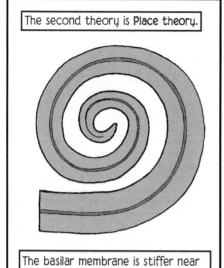

The basilar membrane is stiffer near to the oval window than it is at the other end. This means that different frequencies of sound can be detected at different points along the basilar membrane.

Most researchers now believe in a combination of both these theories to explain how the brain interprets sounds.

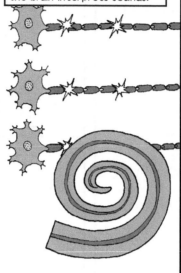

There is a lot more to the processing of sound information that is important to understand - like how the brain identifies where a sound is coming from and the specialised centres of the brain that are involved in language perception.

However, despite all this work, the auditory sense is still not fully understood!

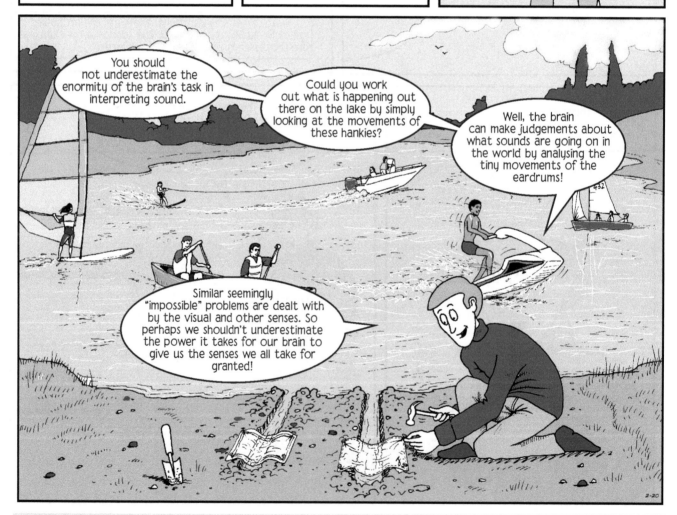

You should not underestimate the enormity of the brain's task in interpreting sound.

Could you work out what is happening out there on the lake by simply looking at the movements of these hankies?

Well, the brain can make judgements about what sounds are going on in the world by analysing the tiny movements of the eardrums!

Similar seemingly "impossible" problems are dealt with by the visual and other senses. So perhaps we shouldn't underestimate the power it takes for our brain to give us the senses we all take for granted!

Vision and audition

▶ **PAGE 33**

Panel 4

Our senses are the way that the nervous system gives us a picture of our environment. The way this is achieved is for each of our senses to be attuned to a different form of *energy* in the environment. While each sense is highly specialised for sensing specific types of stimuli, there are common elements to all of the biological mechanisms underlying them.

Firstly, all of the senses translate a particular physical stimulus into a nerve impulse. This is called *transduction*. Secondly, all the senses have *thresholds* below which you cannot sense anything. Thirdly, there is a decision to be made regarding whether the information is worth doing something about or not. This is usually referred to as *sensation* and involves both the intensity of the physical stimulation and the meaning that this has for a person.

Fourthly, the senses give us the ability to detect a change in the stimulus so that we know, for example, that a light has become brighter. This is known as a *difference threshold*. Lastly, the senses filter out material that continues without changing and is called *sensory adaptation*.

▶ **PAGE 34**

Panel 2

Each of our senses is responsive to a different aspect of our environment. In the case of sight it is a part of the electromagnetic spectrum and hearing is about detecting sound pressure waves. In later chapters, it will be seen that each of the senses detects other important stimuli. It is all our senses that give us a full impression of the most important aspects of what is happening 'out there' in the world.

Panel 3

Sir Isaac Newton lived from 1642 to 1727 and is often hailed as the greatest scientist of all time. He studied physics, mathematics, astronomy, philosophy and alchemy. Perhaps his greatest contribution was to describe universal laws of gravity and the three laws of motion that led to modern mechanics. His ideas on the nature of light were written by 1692 but were not published until 1704 in the book *Opticks*. This delay was made to ensure publication did not occur until most of Newton's critics on his ideas had died.

Panel 4

Newton called his light particles 'corpuscles'. At the time, there was disagreement about the nature of light. Christiaan Huygens, had suggested that light travels as a waveform – rather like ripples on a pond. However,

Newton argued that light must be made of particles since this explained the phenomenon of reflection. Because of Newton's status, his theory became the generally accepted one until the early 1800s.

In the early 1800s, diffraction of light was discovered that could be easily explained if light was seen as a wave. Further work by Frenel, Maxwell and Young at this time also provided evidence for light as a wave and Huygens' ideas were revived.

By the early twentieth century, there was an ongoing scientific debate about whether light was made up of particles or was a wave.

Panel 5

Albert Einstein is widely considered the greatest physicist of all time. He is mostly known for his theory of relativity and more specifically the theory that connects mass and energy which is exemplified by the formula $E=MC^2$. In 1905 he provided an explanation for the phenomena known as the *photoelectric effect*. He explained this by suggesting that light acts both as a stream of particles and waves. Einstein called the particles *photons*. Under some circumstances light acts as a stream of particles **and** under others as a wave. It really depends on what you are observing. This combined theory of the nature of light is called the *wave-particle theory*. Einstein received the Nobel Prize for Physics in 1921 for his explanation of the photoelectric effect.

In 1924 de Broglie suggested that *all* matter, not just light, also has wave-like properties. This is known as the de Broglie hypothesis. The only reason we cannot observe wave-like properties in all matter is due to size. The larger the matter, the less the wave form can be observed. The de Broglie hypothesis is the origin of what is referred to as *Quantum Mechanics* which is a cornerstone of modern physics.

Panel 6

Photons are packets of electromagnetic energy. Photons have no mass and no electric charge.

Panel 7

Human beings can only detect a very small aspect of the total electromagnetic spectrum. The narrow band of radiation that we can see is called the *visible spectrum* (for obvious reasons!). Other animals have a wider range of sensitivity. Some snakes, for example, can detect the infra-red radiation that is emitted from heat sources. This allows them to detect warm blooded animals (that are their prey) in low light situations. Some insects are also sensitive to ultra-violet light. Certain flowers attract insects by displaying ultra-violet patterns.

▶ PAGE 35

Panel 3

Ibn Al-Haytham was born in the year 965 in Basra, then part of the Persian empire and died (probably in Cairo) in 1040. He is also known by his Latinised name Alhacen. He was an Islamic mathematician, astronomer and physicist and is considered the father of modern optics for his work on lenses, mirrors, refraction and reflection. He is also considered one of the first scholars to devise hypotheses and use experiments to test them. As such he is often seen as the originator of the modern scientific method.

Prior to Al-Haytham, ancient Greek philosophers were divided on how the eyes functioned. Ptolemy and Euclid thought that the eyes sent out sight rays. Aristotle believed in the alternative theory that light entered the eyes. Al-Haytham looked at the evidence around him and observed that eyes could be dazzled or even injured with very bright light. He also argued logically that it seemed unlikely that sight rays could reach distant objects, like the stars, quickly enough. He therefore suggested that Aristotle was correct and he elaborated a theory that explained how light reflected off objects and bounced into the eyes.

His book on optics written from 1015 to 1021 was translated into Latin in the twelfth or beginning of the thirteenth century. This and other works were very influential on western writers from the Middle Ages onwards.

▶ **PAGE 36**

Panel 6

This panel shows a diagrammatic representation of a photo pigment molecule.

Photo pigments are chemicals that are sensitive to light. They are embedded in the thin membrane layers (called *lamellae*) of rod and cone cells. Photo pigment molecules contain two parts. The first is *opsin* (a protein) and the second is *retinal* (a molecule of fat). There are different types of opsin. Human rods contain *rhodopsin* and human cones contain *iopsin*. Retinal is made from vitamin A. Carrots are rich in vitamin A and is the reason carrots are said to be good for your eyesight!

When a photo pigment is exposed to light it breaks down into its constituent parts: opsin and retinal. At the same time the colour of the opsin is *bleached* by the light. In other words it becomes paler. In rhodopsin it changes from a reddish colour to a pale yellow colour. This bleaching causes a chain reaction of events that results in an action potential being produced not in the photoreceptors themselves but in the bipolar cells to which they are connected.

The photo pigments recombine in darkness or dim light. Rhodopsin, the rod opsin, is very sensitive to light compared to *Iopsin*, the cone opsin. In bright light conditions, rhodopsin, stays broken down so that rods do not contribute much to vision. In contrast, iopsin needs a great deal of light to work so cones are not very functional in dim light. So rods work in dim light when cones do not.

There are three varieties of Iopsin that are maximally responsive to different wavelengths of light. These three types account for the *trichromatic* theory of colour vision.

▶ **PAGE 38**

Panel 4

The majority (approximately 90 per cent) of the nerve fibres from the ganglion cells of the retina go to the Lateral Geniculate Nucleus (LGN) of the thalamus and then on to the visual cortex. Most of the remaining 10 per cent go to the *superior colliculus*. This is a clump of neurons in the midbrain. In less complex animals this structure is the main visual centre. In humans, the superior colliculus controls eye movements. In addition Stein and Meredith (1990) found that the superior colliculus is also involved in combining basic auditory and visual information so that our gaze can turn towards a sound.

The idea of topographical organisation is important since it means that the LGN preserve the map of our visual space in the retina.

Panel 6

The visual (or striate) cortex in the occipital lobes of the cortex is where most of the visual information is processed. The majority of the neurons in the visual cortex are devoted to processing the information from the fovea (Drasdo, 1977). The function of the neurons in the visual cortex was investigated by Hubel and Wiesel (1959, 1979). They discovered that there are neurons in the visual cortex that send a nerve impulse only when an image in a specific part of the visual field matches a certain pattern or orientation. These neurons are called *feature detectors*. Hubel and Wiesel identified three types of feature detectors and received the 1981 Nobel Prize for 'Physiology or Medicine' for their work on the visual system (in fact they shared it with Roger Sperry for his work on specialisation in the cerebral hemispheres).

The three main types of feature detectors are:

Simple Cells are neurons in the visual cortex that respond mostly to lines of a particular orientation. Each simple cell has a specific type of orientated line that it 'likes' the most. For example, one simple cell may fire the most when their visual field is presented with a line like this:

Another simple cell may be most responsive to a line in a different orientation:

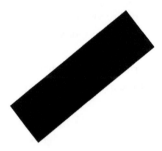

Complex Cells are neurons that are maximally responsive to a larger visual field compared to the simple cells. These complex cells will fire when a stimulus of the particular orientation falls anywhere inside its particular visual field. In addition, some complex cells respond to movement of the stimulus in a specific direction.

Hyper complex Cells will fire when lines are of a specific orientation but also have inhibitory regions at the end of the lines so they are mostly responsive to the location of ends of lines. This means that hyper complex cells tend to respond to lines of a more specific length than the other cells of the visual cortex.

▶ **PAGES 39 and 40**

Coding in the brain

The issue of coding is a complicated but important one. As the chapter explains, the issue is to answer the following question:

'If neurons have an 'all or nothing' response how can this create the complexity that exists in the senses?'

The answer is to refer to the two possible theories of *labelled-line* coding and *across-fibre pattern* coding. The first refers to a one-to-one correspondence between a sensory neuron and the brain cortex. In this case when the neuron sends a signal this means one thing. This would be quite a wasteful use of neurons and the nervous system would theoretically need one neuron for every possible sensory experience. This seems highly unlikely. Across-fibre pattern coding, however, means that several neurons interact together to produce different messages, rather like the different sized flags in the example.

In the human (and indeed mammalian) sensory code it is thought that there are no pure labelled-line codes. These sensory systems are just too complex. In addition, it is known that the response of each neuron varies a little and the brain gets a better idea of what is going on from a combination of neuronal responses (Pouget, Dayan & Zemel, 2000).

▶ **PAGE 41**

Panel 2

It is important to note that coloured light is simply the sensory experience of a particular wavelength of light. There is nothing inherently 'red' about red light or any other coloured light.

Panel 5

This diagram shows what happens when coloured lights are mixed. The three *primary* colours are Red, Green and Blue. They are called primary because they cannot be created by mixing any other coloured light. The full range of our colour experience is due to mixing all the primary colours and creating secondary colours: cyan, created by mixing green and blue; yellow, created by mixing green and red; and magenta, created by mixing red and blue. When all three primary colours are mixed we get white light.

You may be wondering why this combination of mixing light seems different to what happens when you mix coloured paints. The difference between light and paint is that light mixing is *additive* mixing whilst paint mixing is *subtractive*. When we add light together we *add* wavelengths of light and when we mix paint, more wavelengths of light are absorbed by the paint pigments. So in paints, when red, blue and green are mixed together the result is a paint that absorbs all light: in other words black paint.

Panel 6

In fact, this scene could never have happened as Young and Helmholtz never actually met. Thomas Young died in 1829 and Helmholtz was not born until 1821. It was Helmholtz who revived one of Young's ideas from fifty years earlier.

Thomas Young was born in 1773 and is often referred to as a 'polymath' as he contributed to many different scholarly areas in addition to his suggestions about colour vision. He is said to have been a child prodigy, learning Greek and Latin at the age of 14, established himself as a doctor at the age of 26 and was made a professor of the Royal Institution at the age of 28. His many contributions to science included providing evidence for the wave theory of light; devising a mathematical theory that continues to help modern engineering calculate the level of stress on a structure; contributed to the understanding of blood flow in the body; and devised a rule of thumb for determining the correct drug dosage for children. In addition, he also found time to compare the grammar and vocabulary of 400 different languages; made important contributions to the early deciphering of Ancient Egyptian hieroglyphs and developed a method for tuning musical instruments.

▶ **PAGE 42**

Panel 1

Please bear in mind that each colour cone is *maximally* responsive to wavelengths in the blue, green and red range. The actual response does vary a little.

Panel 2

A similar effect is found in colour television sets or computer monitors. They have small 'dots' made up of red, blue and green that when seen from a distance give the correct colour impression.

▶ **PAGE 43**

Panel 2

Mister U.S. is Copyright and TM 1997 Nat Gertler and Mark Lewis and is used here by their kind permission.

▶ **PAGE 44**

Panel 6

For a long time the Trichromatic and the Opponent-Process theories were in opposition since each explained things the other did not. Hurvich and Jameson (1957) resolved the issue by combining the two theories. They suggested that we do have three types of cone: each one responsive to red, blue and green light. They further suggested that these cones were connected in an opponent-process fashion at the ganglion cells. This scheme explains why yellow light is perceived as a 'pure' colour because both the red and green cones are excited AND both the opponent ganglion cells are also excited. Additionally, this theory explains complimentary colours since there are Red-Green and Blue-Yellow ganglion cells (as well as White-Black cells).

▶ **PAGE 45**

Panel 3

Sound is just the pushing of air or any another medium like water. When something falls over and hits the ground, the vibrations are transferred to the air and we can hear a noise. If there was no air, like on the moon, no vibrations could be transferred and we would therefore not hear a noise.

Panel 6

Sound waves vary in terms of amplitude (the 'height' of the wave) and frequency (the 'speed' of the wave). Amplitude has an influence on the loudness of a sound but is not an exact correspondence. Many factors influence loudness beyond the amplitude of the sound wave. The frequency of the wave is mostly related to the pitch of a sound. Generally speaking, the higher the frequency, the higher the pitch. However, as with other senses, the physical stimulus and the perception of that stimulus are not directly related since your brain adjusts things slightly to allow for better perception. This applies both to the amplitude of the sound wave and its frequency.

▶ **PAGE 46**

Panel 1

Atmospheric pressure is the physical pressure exerted upon our bodies from the amount of air above us. This gets lower the higher up you go – in a plane for example. We don't normally notice this as our bodies are accustomed to this pressure.

▶ **PAGE 47**

Panel 5

Please note the *semi-circular canals*. These are not involved in hearing. They are part of the system of balance that is covered in Chapter 3.

▶ **PAGE 48**

Panel 2

Human *pinnas* are quite basic compared to other mammals. Cats and dogs for example, have pinnas that can move to help sound detection.

Panel 7

Infections in the Eustachian tube and middle ear can be quite serious and common, especially in children. This is called *otitis media* whereby fluid builds up in the middle ear and can cause the eardrum to burst. When we have a cold sometimes the Eustachian tube blocks and causes earache.

▶ **PAGE 50**

Panels 1 and 2

There are some people who have damage to the cochlea who have cochlea implants. These are devices that analyse the frequency of the sounds. The responses from the device are then sent along electrodes that are implanted into different points along the basilar membrane. Cochlea implants can provide some good results for people with certain hearing problems.

▶ **PAGE 51**

Panels 1 to 3

The pathways from the ear mechanisms to the brain are some of the most complex of the sensory systems. Approximately 70 per cent of the pathways are *contralateral*, in other words the connections from the left ear go to the right brain hemisphere and those from the right ear go to the left hemisphere. The remaining 30 per cent of the connection are *ipsilateral*. In other words those connections from the right ear go to the right hemisphere and those from the left ear go to the left hemisphere.

▶ **PAGE 52**

Panel 1

Place theory is the reason we can hear through bone conduction. The vibrations from sound can enter the cochlea from the bone around it rather than through the oval window. Garrett (2003) describes how Thomas Edison, who was nearly deaf, invented the phonograph. He used to grasp the handle of the phonograph in his teeth in order to detect the sounds being played through bone conduction.

Panel 2

Most researchers subscribe to what is referred to as the *frequency-place* theory. This is a combination of the frequency and place theories whereby the frequency of the sound accounts for the processing of sounds up to approximately 200 hertz and all remaining sound frequencies are dependent on where on the basilar membrane there is the greatest movement.

Chapter 3
THE MECHANICAL SENSES

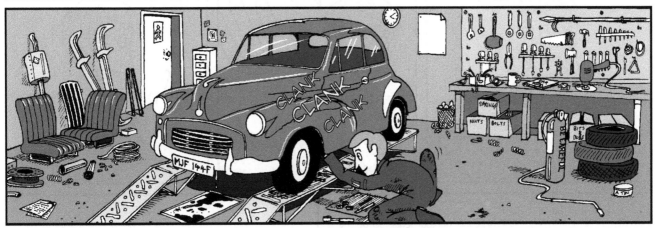

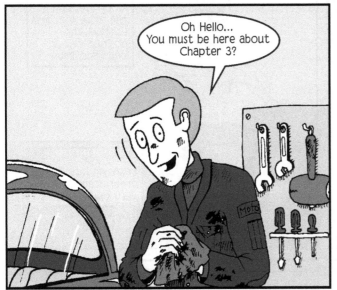

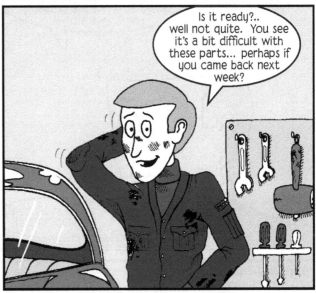

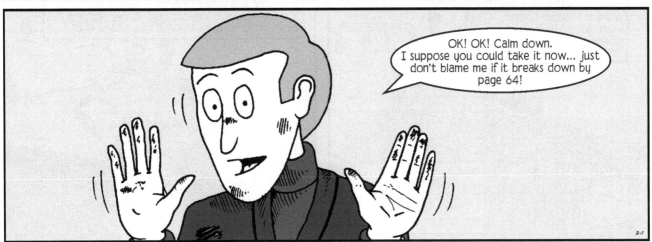

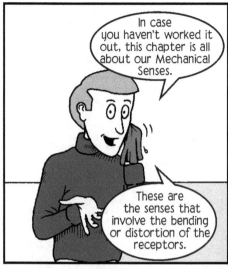

In case you haven't worked it out, this chapter is all about our Mechanical Senses.

These are the senses that involve the bending or distortion of the receptors.

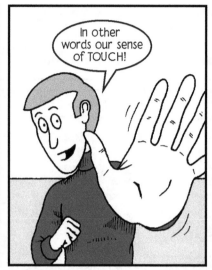

In other words our sense of TOUCH!

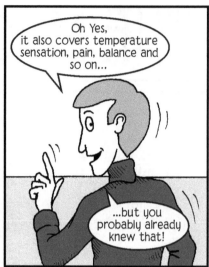

Oh Yes, it also covers temperature sensation, pain, balance and so on...

...but you probably already knew that!

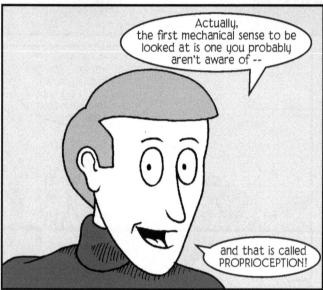

Actually, the first mechanical sense to be looked at is one you probably aren't aware of --

and that is called PROPRIOCEPTION!

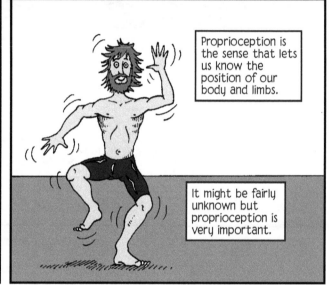

Proprioception is the sense that lets us know the position of our body and limbs.

It might be fairly unknown but proprioception is very important.

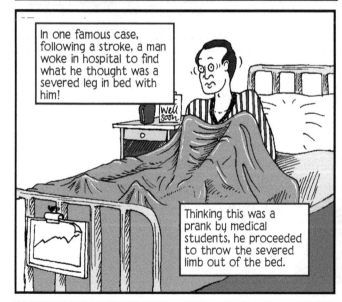

In one famous case, following a stroke, a man woke in hospital to find what he thought was a severed leg in bed with him!

Thinking this was a prank by medical students, he proceeded to throw the severed limb out of the bed.

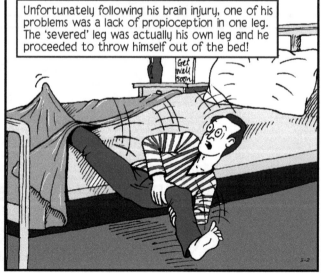

Unfortunately following his brain injury, one of his problems was a lack of propioception in one leg. The 'severed' leg was actually his own leg and he proceeded to throw himself out of the bed!

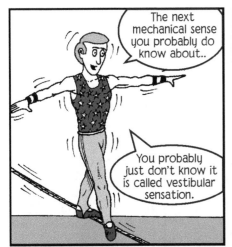

The next mechanical sense you probably do know about..

You probably just don't know it is called vestibular sensation.

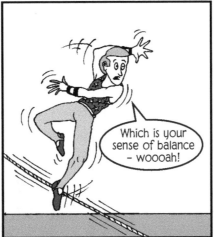

Which is your sense of balance - woooah!

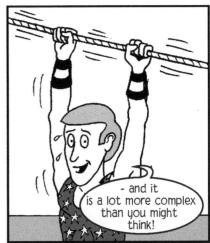

- and it is a lot more complex than you might think!

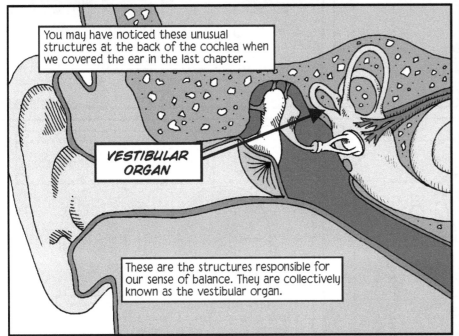

You may have noticed these unusual structures at the back of the cochlea when we covered the ear in the last chapter.

VESTIBULAR ORGAN

These are the structures responsible for our sense of balance. They are collectively known as the vestibular organ.

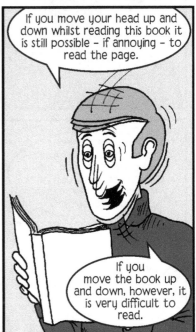

If you move your head up and down whilst reading this book it is still possible - if annoying - to read the page.

If you move the book up and down, however, it is very difficult to read.

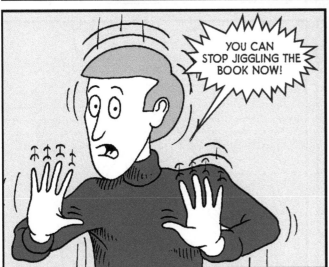

YOU CAN STOP JIGGLING THE BOOK NOW!

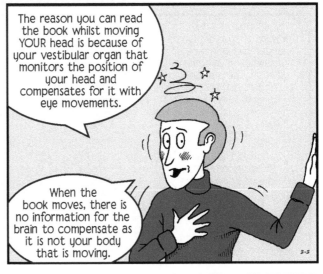

The reason you can read the book whilst moving YOUR head is because of your vestibular organ that monitors the position of your head and compensates for it with eye movements.

When the book moves, there is no information for the brain to compensate as it is not your body that is moving.

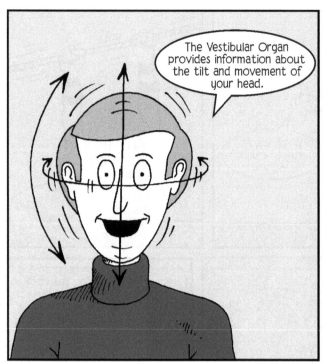

The Vestibular Organ provides information about the tilt and movement of your head.

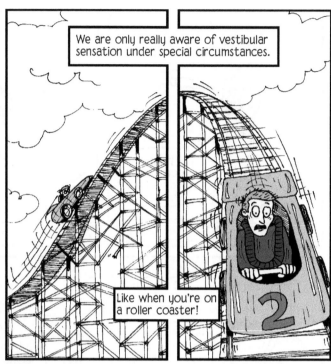

We are only really aware of vestibular sensation under special circumstances.

Like when you're on a roller coaster!

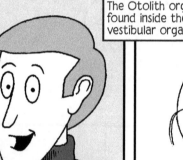

The Vestibular organ consists of the semi-circular canals and the **Otolith** organ (or vestibule) which both contain modified touch receptors.

These structures provide the brain with information about three aspects of our balance and position:

Position, Speed and Acceleration!

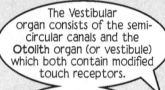

The Otolith organ is found inside the vestibular organ.

There are two parts to the otolith organ, oriented at right angles to each other. One is called the saccule and the other the utricle.

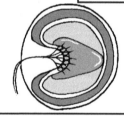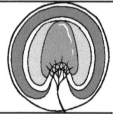

Each one is filled with a fluid called endolymph. Small lumps of chalk sit on top of a jelly like material in which are embedded hair cells.

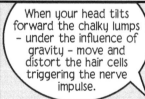

When your head tilts forward the chalky lumps – under the influence of gravity – move and distort the hair cells triggering the nerve impulse.

This gives the brain information about the position of the head.

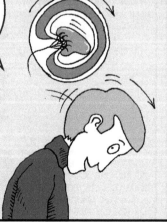

Because there are two sets of otolith organs they provide the brain with a wealth of information about the position of your head!

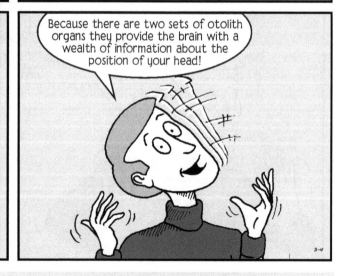

The Semi-Circular canals are oriented on three planes.

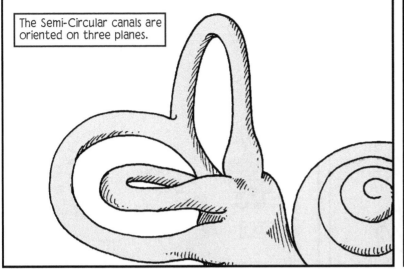

Each semi-circular canal is filled with a fluid called endolymph and has a small bump known as the crista ampularis that contains the hair cells.

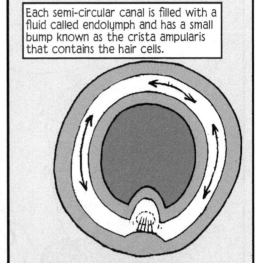

When your head moves, the liquid within the semi-circular canals also moves which in turn causes the crista ampularis gel fluid to move and trigger the hair cells.

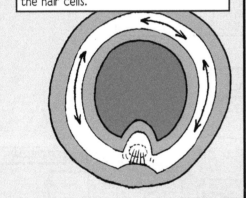

Because the semi-circular canals are on three different orientations the comparative stimulation of the different hair cells gives the brain information about the movement of your head.

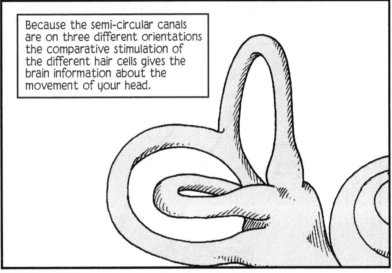

When you spin around, this causes some problems –

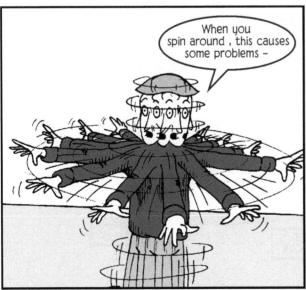

When you stop, the endolymph carries on moving inside the semi-circular canals and this confuses the vestibular system.

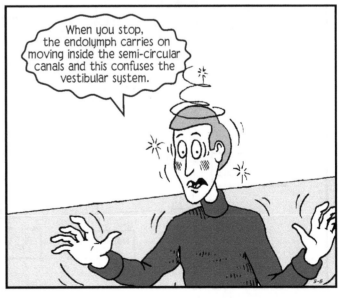

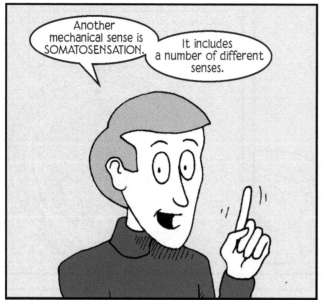

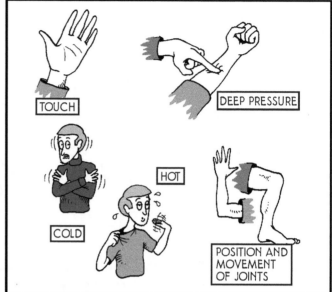

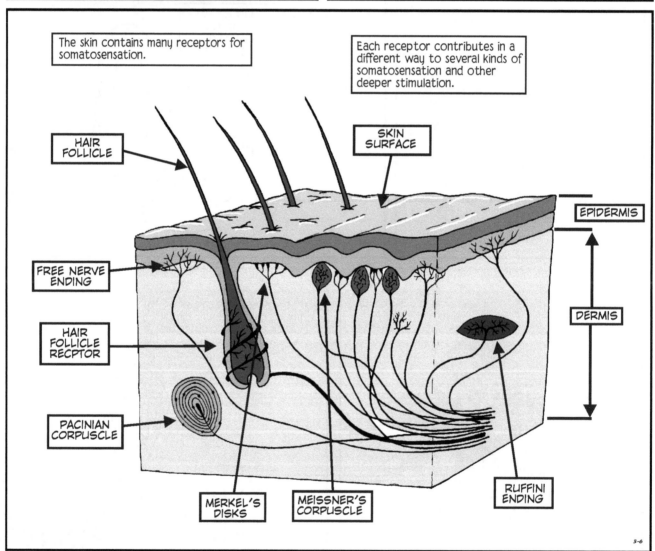

The skin contains many receptors for somatosensation.

Each receptor contributes in a different way to several kinds of somatosensation and other deeper stimulation.

HAIR FOLLICLE

SKIN SURFACE

EPIDERMIS

FREE NERVE ENDING

DERMIS

HAIR FOLLICLE RECPTOR

PACINIAN CORPUSCLE

MERKEL'S DISKS

MEISSNER'S CORPUSCLE

RUFFINI ENDING

3-6

The information from somatosensory receptors in the head enters the CNS through cranial nerves whilst that from receptors below the neck enter through the spinal cord.

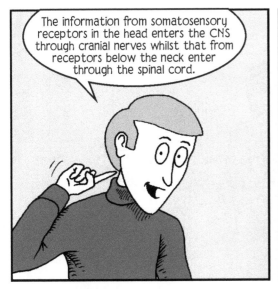

All the information from the touch receptors are sent to the primary somatosensory cortex in the parietal lobes.

Other areas of the cortex are also involved in the processing of touch information.

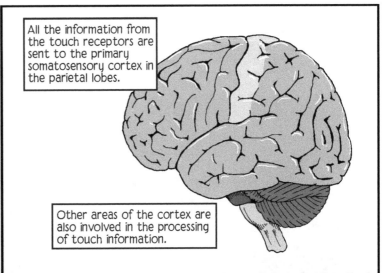

The somatosensory cortex receives input primarily from the contralateral side of the body.

In other words, touch information from the left side of the body goes mostly to the right hemisphere and that on the right goes mostly to the left hemisphere.

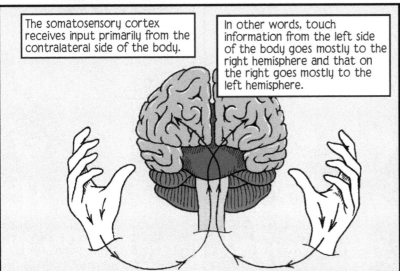

Tickling – ha ha ha – is an interesting case of touch information – – it appears – HEEE HEEE HEEE – to be an automatic response.

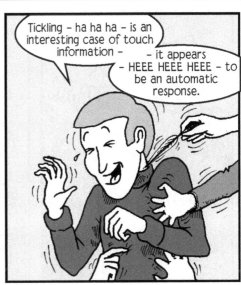

Most people can't tickle themselves.

This is because the brain knows that it is you tickling you and there is a mechanism that stops you surprising yourself every time one part of your body touches another.

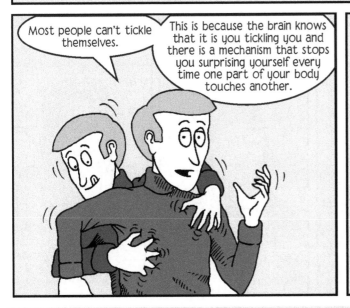

You can teach yourself to tickle yourself at least a little.

As long as you tickle the opposite side of your body!

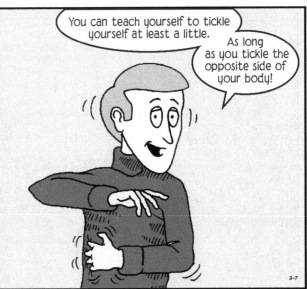

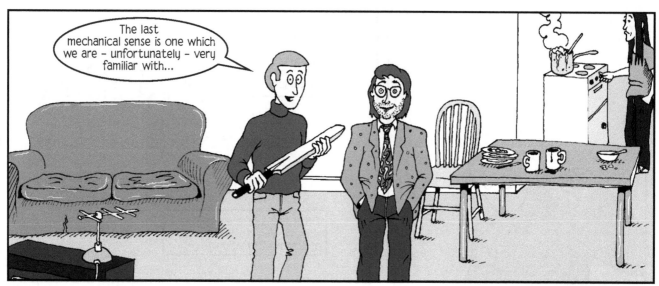

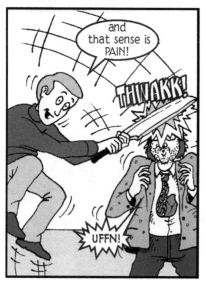

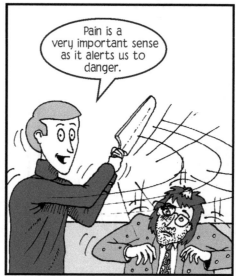

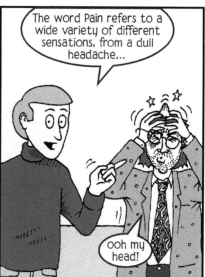

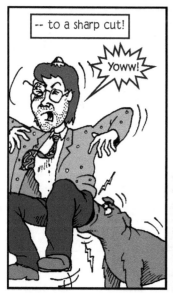

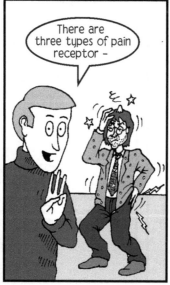

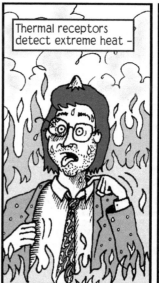

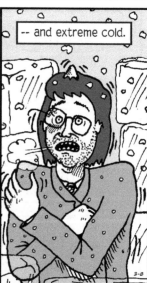

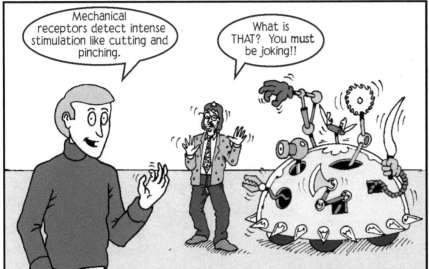

Mechanical receptors detect intense stimulation like cutting and pinching.

What is THAT? You must be joking!!

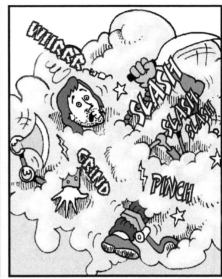

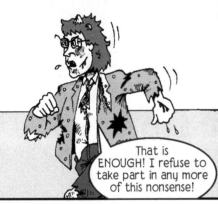

Polymodal receptors detect both thermal AND mechanical pressure as well as detecting chemicals that are released when body tissue is injured.

That is ENOUGH! I refuse to take part in any more of this nonsense!

Signals from pain receptors are sent partly along unmylenated and mylenated axons to the spinal cord.

The unmylenated axons are faster and carry sharp pain information so you feel sharp pain before other pain.

In the spinal cord neurons release SUBSTANCE P that helps to enhance the effects of neurotransmitters.

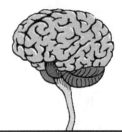

From the spinal cord, pain information goes firstly to the thalamus in the brain which then relays information to areas of the cortex and areas of the brain associated with emotional responses.

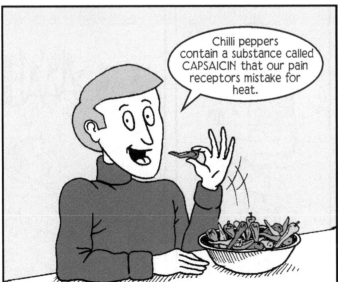

Chilli peppers contain a substance called CAPSAICIN that our pain receptors mistake for heat.

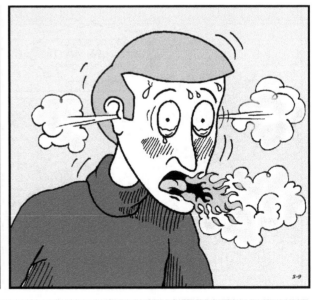

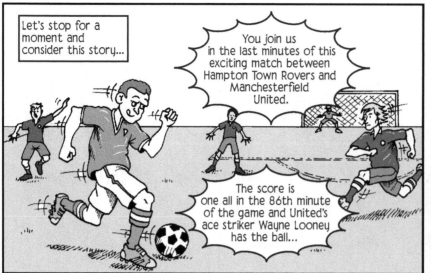

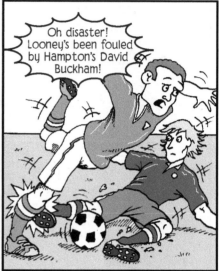

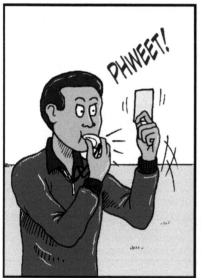

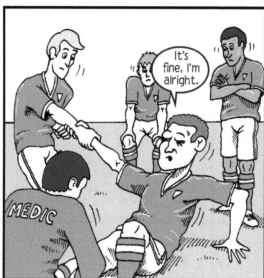

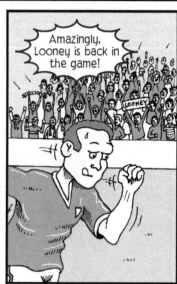

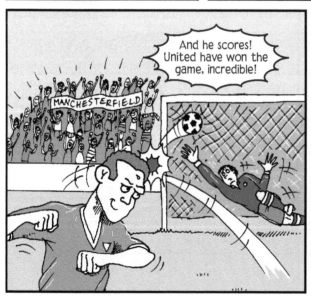

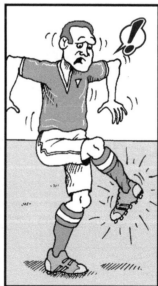

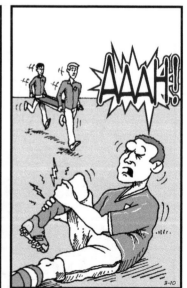

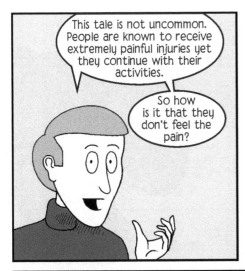

This tale is not uncommon. People are known to receive extremely painful injuries yet they continue with their activities.

So how is it that they don't feel the pain?

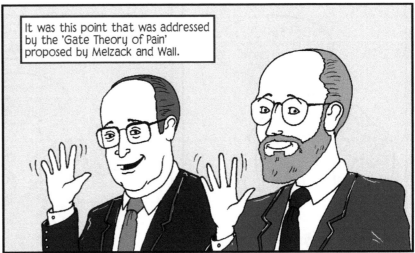

It was this point that was addressed by the 'Gate Theory of Pain' proposed by Melzack and Wall.

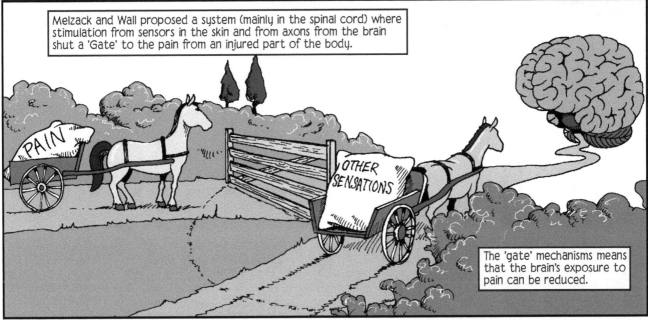

Melzack and Wall proposed a system (mainly in the spinal cord) where stimulation from sensors in the skin and from axons from the brain shut a 'Gate' to the pain from an injured part of the body.

PAIN

OTHER SENSATIONS

The 'gate' mechanisms means that the brain's exposure to pain can be reduced.

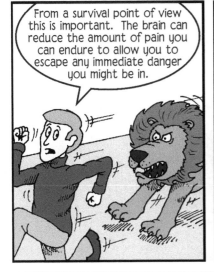

From a survival point of view this is important. The brain can reduce the amount of pain you can endure to allow you to escape any immediate danger you might be in.

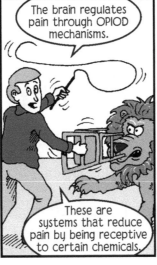

The brain regulates pain through OPIOD mechanisms.

These are systems that reduce pain by being receptive to certain chemicals.

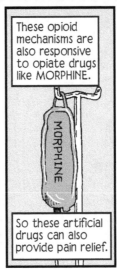

These opioid mechanisms are also responsive to opiate drugs like MORPHINE.

MORPHINE

So these artificial drugs can also provide pain relief.

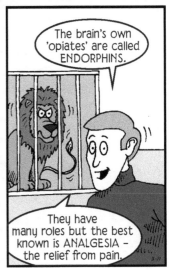

The brain's own 'opiates' are called ENDORPHINS.

They have many roles but the best known is ANALGESIA - the relief from pain.

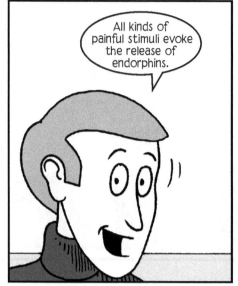

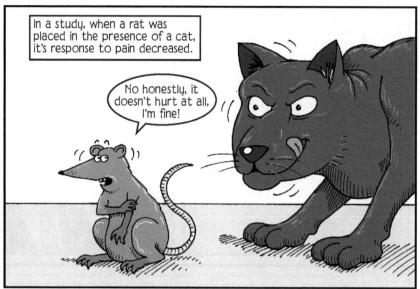

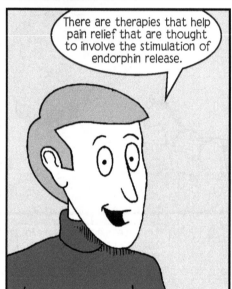

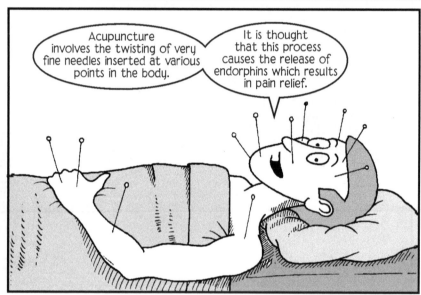

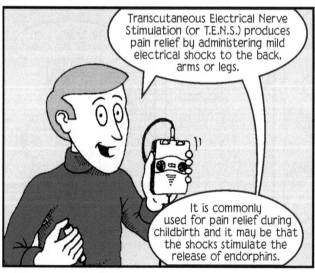

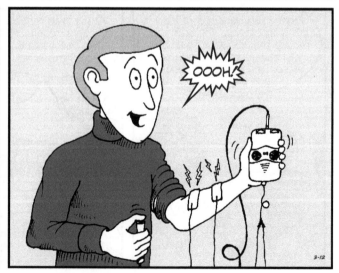

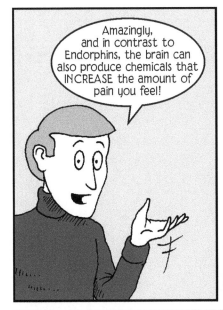

Amazingly, and in contrast to Endorphins, the brain can also produce chemicals that INCREASE the amount of pain you feel!

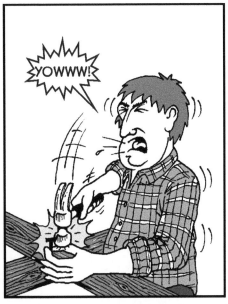

YOWWW!

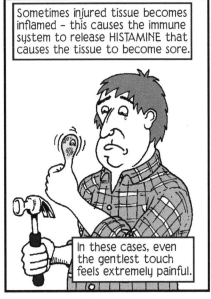

Sometimes injured tissue becomes inflamed - this causes the immune system to release HISTAMINE that causes the tissue to become sore.

In these cases, even the gentlest touch feels extremely painful.

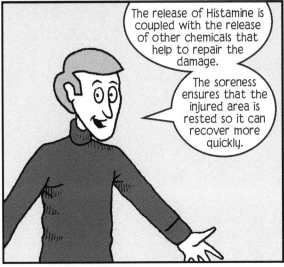

The release of Histamine is coupled with the release of other chemicals that help to repair the damage.

The soreness ensures that the injured area is rested so it can recover more quickly.

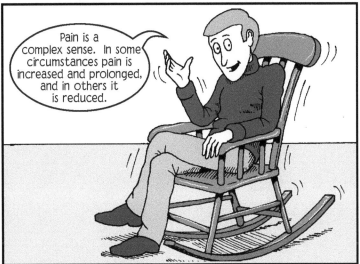

Pain is a complex sense. In some circumstances pain is increased and prolonged, and in others it is reduced.

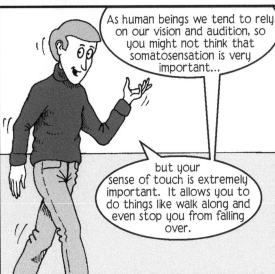

As human beings we tend to rely on our vision and audition, so you might not think that somatosensation is very important...

but your sense of touch is extremely important. It allows you to do things like walk along and even stop you from falling over.

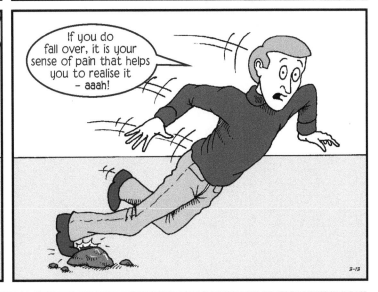

If you do fall over, it is your sense of pain that helps you to realise it - aaah!

The mechanical senses

▶ **PAGE 62**

Panel 2

The mechanical senses are primarily responsible for the detection of vibrations. These vibrations are different to those detected by the auditory sense. However, it is likely that the mechanical senses are the basis for the evolution of the detection of sound. Both audition and the mechanical senses involve the bending of hair-like receptors.

Panel 4

Proprioception is the sense that tells us about the position and movement of our arms and legs and the rest of our body. There are a number of different *proprioceptors* in the body. Normally these are connected to our muscles and tendons. One propioceptor is called a *muscle spindle*. This is parallel to a muscle and detects when the muscle stretches. When this happens, the muscle spindle sends a signal to a neuron in the spinal cord which then sends a signal to the muscles next to the spindle to cause it to contract resulting in a movement. This is what happens when there is a *stretch reflex* such as what happens in the knee jerk reflex (see Chapter 1). There are other types of propioceptor, each responsible for a different aspect of the detection of movement and location of the body.

Panels 6 to 7

This case was described by Oliver Sacks (1985) in his book *The Man who mistook his wife for a Hat*. This incident is in Chapter 4 called 'The man who fell out of bed' (an earlier account was also published in his book *A Leg to Stand On*, published in 1984). Sacks describes an incident when he met a patient as a medical student. The young man in question had fallen out of bed and become quite agitated and upset. When Oliver Sacks attended he was asked to explain what was happening. The story is as described in the chapter. The man had awoken and felt a severed leg in bed with him. He thought this was a prank by medical students so he tried to throw the leg out of his bed. To his great surprise he found himself following the leg and ended up on the floor. He had completely lost sensation in his leg – one of the things he had lost was 'proprioception' for the leg.

The rest of Sack's book provides a number of different descriptions of neurological cases that are also relevant to biological psychology. This and other books by Oliver Sacks are highly recommended.

▶ **PAGE 66**

Panel 3

This diagram shows a typical cross-section of the major somatosensory receptors found in the skin of mammals. Some receptors respond to more than one kind of stimulus and so each one probably contributes to a variety of different 'touch' like sensations.

▶ **PAGE 67**

Panel 4

Tickling is a very poorly understood aspect of touch sensation. It is very difficult to explain the purpose of tickling. Chimpanzees tend to pant rhythmically when they are tickled. This leads to the idea that they indeed 'laughing'. However, the link between humour and the response to tickling is not very clear. Most people do not enjoy being tickled for very long. Also, if you laugh at one joke you are more likely to laugh at the next one. But if you are tickled and laugh, this does not affect whether you laugh at a joke or not (Harris, 1999).

▶ **PAGE 68**

Panel 6

In fact, it is likely that we do not have specific 'pain' receptors at all (Green, 1994). They are simply somatosensory receptors that also respond to painful stimuli. The sensation of pain is connected to a number of different aspects of our behaviour, most notably emotions and motivation. The fear caused by pain, for example, can be very effective at teaching animals and people a number of responses. There is also the issue that normal somatosensory stimuli can be detected as painful if they are extreme. Stretching of the skin, for example, can range from mild to extremely painful but involves the same receptors.

▶ **PAGE 69**

Panel 6

Contrary to popular opinion, the hot part of a chilli is neither the skin, flesh nor the seeds. The capsaicin compounds that give chillies their heat are found only in the pith to which the seeds are attached. The redder the pith the hotter the chilli!

After the initial heat of a chilli, the area exposed becomes desensitised from the pain for a while. This has allowed the development of pain-killing creams that contain capsaicin. When an area of the body experiencing chronic pain (such as the joints in arthritis) is rubbed with capsaicin cream this is followed by a period of pain-free sensation in that area. It must be noted that the area must first be anaesthetised otherwise the heat and pain from the capsaicin would be unbearable.

▶ **PAGE 71**

Panel 2

The 'Gate Theory of Pain' is very complex but the basic idea is that pain signals in the periphery of the body do not always reach the higher centres of the brain. In the spinal cord there is a 'gate' mechanism that needs to be open for a pain signal to be sent on. There are a number of influences on whether the gate mechanism opens or not. These include both information from the skin that has to reach a certain threshold for pain to be detected and descending fibres from the brain. It is the signals from the brain that allow psychological motivation to decrease the experience of pain by closing the gate in the spinal cord.

▶ **PAGE 72**

Panel 1

The discovery of *endorphins* provided a physiological basis for the 'Gate Theory of Pain' suggested many years earlier.

Both pleasant and unpleasant stimuli can cause the release of endorphins. Sutton *et al.* (1997) found that inescapable pain is especially efficient at releasing very strong endorphins to block any more pain. Endorphins are also released during sex, during an athlete's 'high' and even when some people listen to particular types of music! (Goldstein, 1980). Additionally, placebo pain relief that is produced when people mistakenly believe they have taken pain relief medication, is known to be endorphin based in origin (Basbaum & Fields, 1984).

Panel 2

The study referred to here was conducted by Lester and Fanselow (1985).

▶ **PAGE 73**

Panel 3

Non-steroidal anti-inflammatory drugs, like ibuprofen, appear to work by reducing the amount of histamine released by the damaged tissue (Hunt & Mantyh, 2001).

CHAPTER 4
THE CHEMICAL SENSES

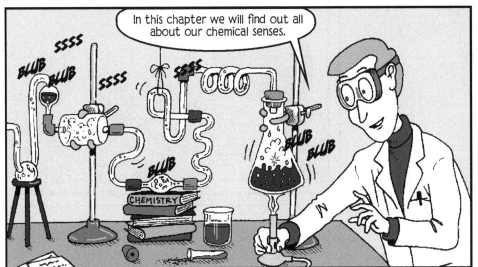

In this chapter we will find out all about our chemical senses.

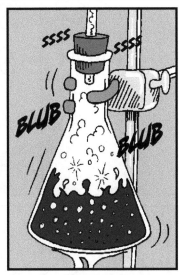

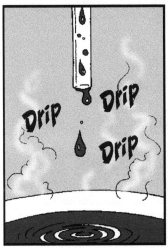

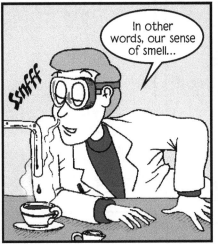

In other words, our sense of smell...

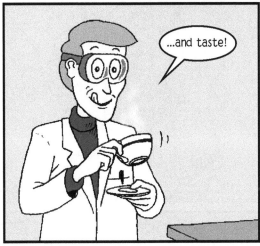

...and taste!

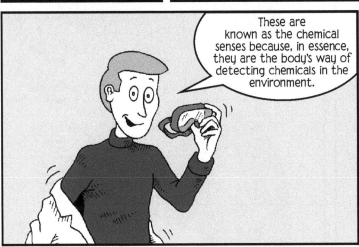

These are known as the chemical senses because, in essence, they are the body's way of detecting chemicals in the environment.

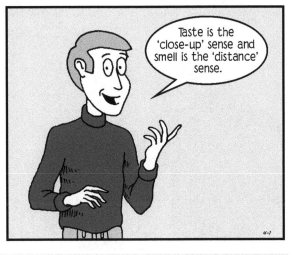

Taste is the 'close-up' sense and smell is the 'distance' sense.

4-1

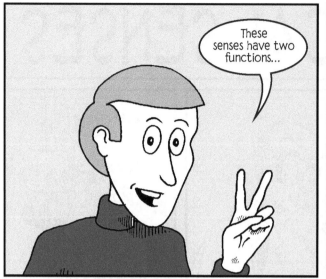

These senses have two functions...

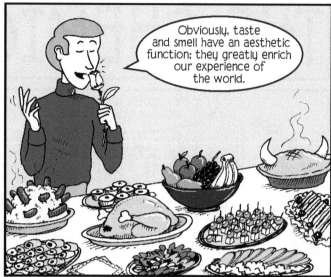

Obviously, taste and smell have an aesthetic function; they greatly enrich our experience of the world.

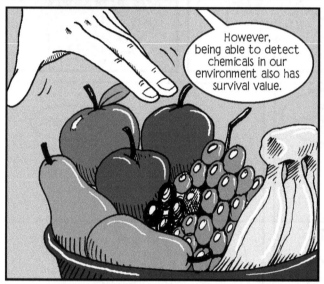

However, being able to detect chemicals in our environment also has survival value.

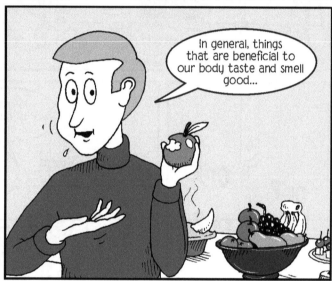

In general, things that are beneficial to our body taste and smell good...

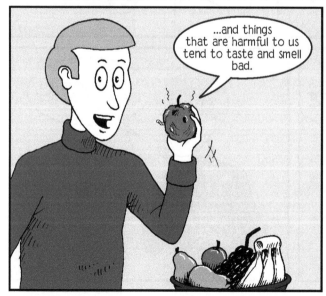

...and things that are harmful to us tend to taste and smell bad.

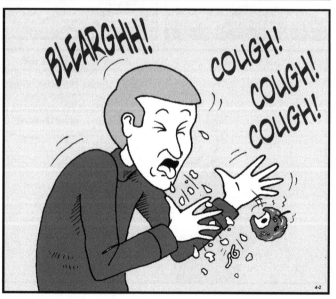

BLEARGHH!

COUGH! COUGH! COUGH!

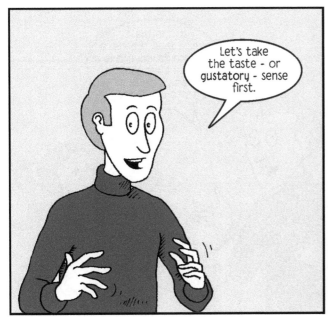

Let's take the taste - or gustatory - sense first.

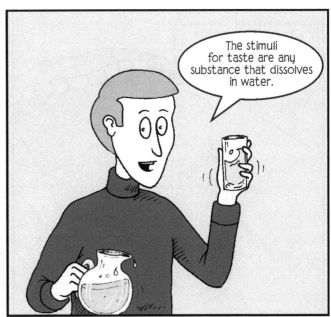

The stimuli for taste are any substance that dissolves in water.

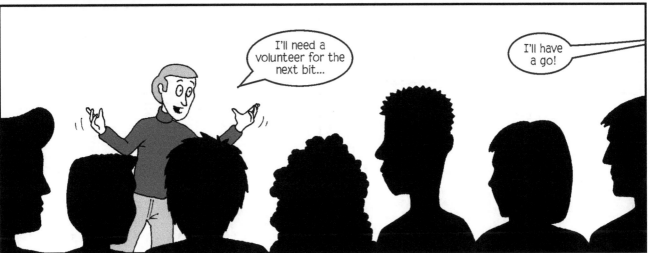

I'll need a volunteer for the next bit...

I'll have a go!

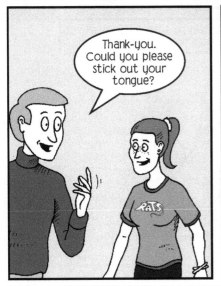

Thank-you. Could you please stick out your tongue?

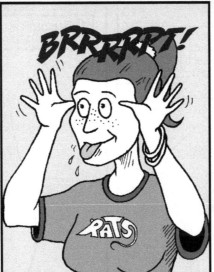

BRRRRRT!

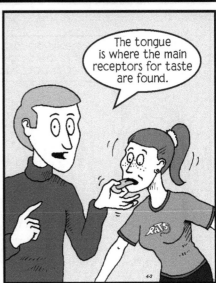

The tongue is where the main receptors for taste are found.

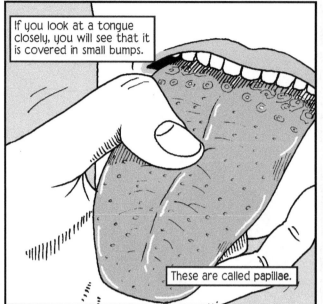

If you look at a tongue closely, you will see that it is covered in small bumps.

These are called papillae.

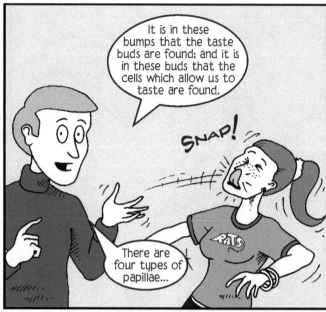

It is in these bumps that the taste buds are found; and it is in these buds that the cells which allow us to taste are found.

SNAP!

There are four types of papillae...

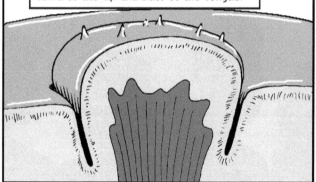

Fungiform papillae are the most numerous and look like mushrooms. These usually only have one taste bud each and are found towards the tip and sides of the tongue.

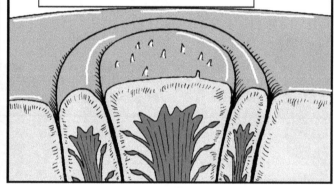

Circumvallate papillae look like flattened hills with a trench around them. These contain several taste buds each and are found towards the back of the tongue.

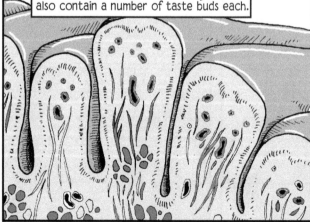

Foliate papillae are shaped like folds along the sides at the rear of the tongue and also contain a number of taste buds each.

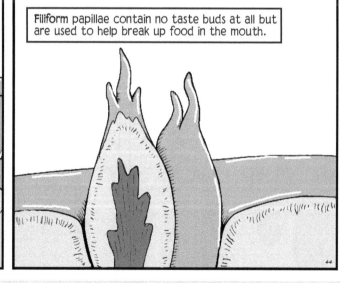

Filiform papillae contain no taste buds at all but are used to help break up food in the mouth.

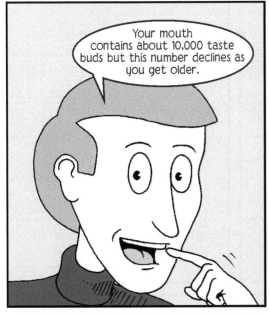

Your mouth contains about 10,000 taste buds but this number declines as you get older.

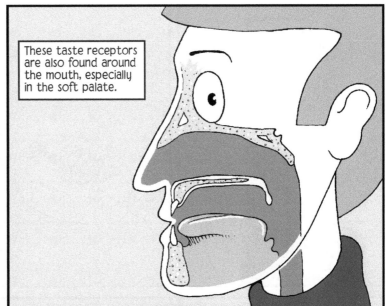

These taste receptors are also found around the mouth, especially in the soft palate.

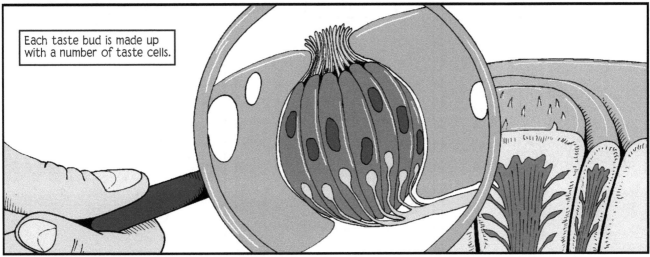

Each taste bud is made up with a number of taste cells.

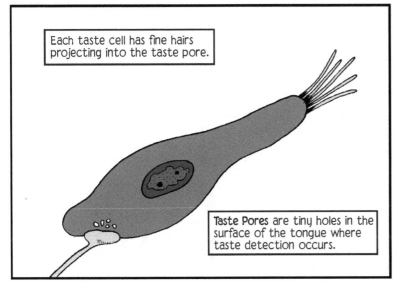

Each taste cell has fine hairs projecting into the taste pore.

Taste Pores are tiny holes in the surface of the tongue where taste detection occurs.

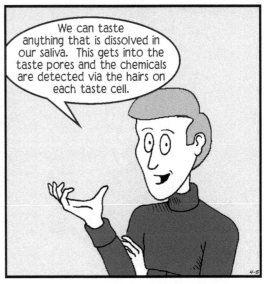

We can taste anything that is dissolved in our saliva. This gets into the taste pores and the chemicals are detected via the hairs on each taste cell.

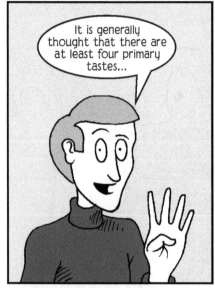

It is generally thought that there are at least four primary tastes...

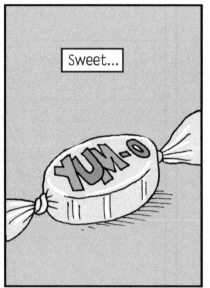

Sweet...

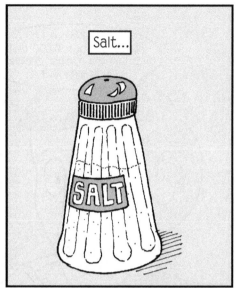

Salt...

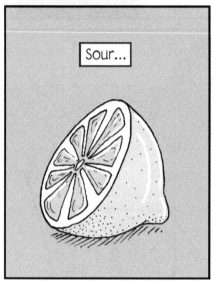

Sour...

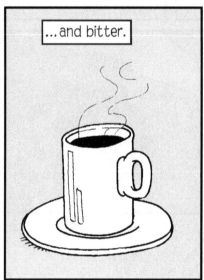

...and bitter.

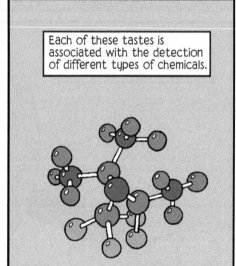

Each of these tastes is associated with the detection of different types of chemicals.

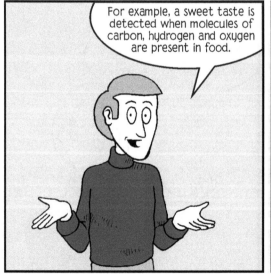

For example, a sweet taste is detected when molecules of carbon, hydrogen and oxygen are present in food.

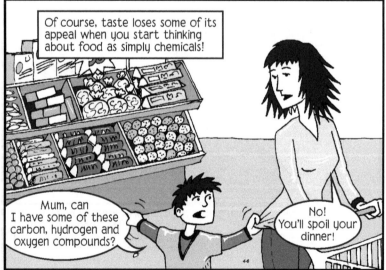

Of course, taste loses some of its appeal when you start thinking about food as simply chemicals!

Mum, can I have some of these carbon, hydrogen and oxygen compounds?

No! You'll spoil your dinner!

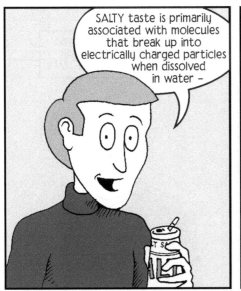

SALTY taste is primarily associated with molecules that break up into electrically charged particles when dissolved in water –

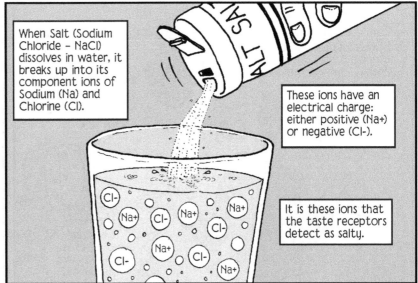

When Salt (Sodium Chloride – NaCl) dissolves in water, it breaks up into its component ions of Sodium (Na) and Chlorine (Cl).

These ions have an electrical charge: either positive (Na+) or negative (Cl-).

It is these ions that the taste receptors detect as salty.

Cl- Na+ Cl- Na+ Na+ Cl- Na+ Cl- Na+ Cl- Na+

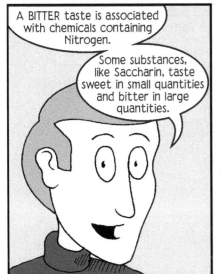

A BITTER taste is associated with chemicals containing Nitrogen.

Some substances, like Saccharin, taste sweet in small quantities and bitter in large quantities.

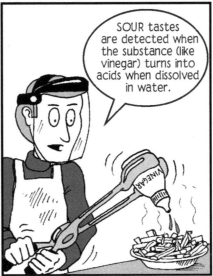

SOUR tastes are detected when the substance (like vinegar) turns into acids when dissolved in water.

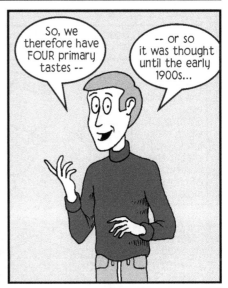

So, we therefore have FOUR primary tastes --

-- or so it was thought until the early 1900s...

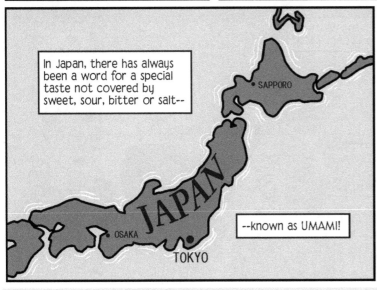

In Japan, there has always been a word for a special taste not covered by sweet, sour, bitter or salt--

SAPPORO

OSAKA

TOKYO

--known as UMAMI!

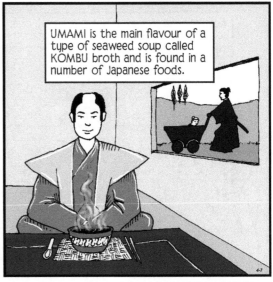

UMAMI is the main flavour of a type of seaweed soup called KOMBU broth and is found in a number of Japanese foods.

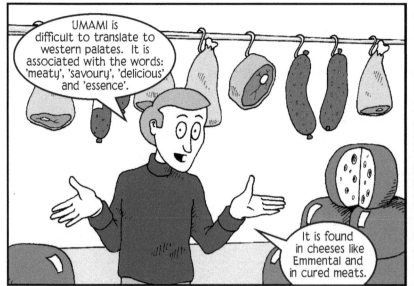

UMAMI is difficult to translate to western palates. It is associated with the words: 'meaty', 'savoury', 'delicious' and 'essence'.

It is found in cheeses like Emmental and in cured meats.

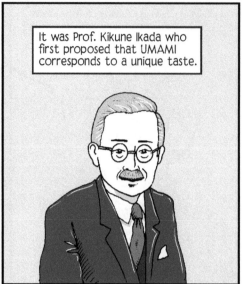

It was Prof. Kikune Ikada who first proposed that UMAMI corresponds to a unique taste.

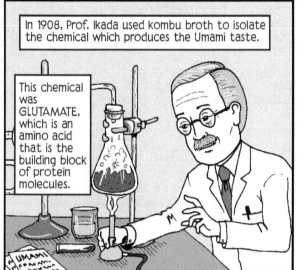

In 1908, Prof. Ikada used kombu broth to isolate the chemical which produces the Umami taste.

This chemical was GLUTAMATE, which is an amino acid that is the building block of protein molecules.

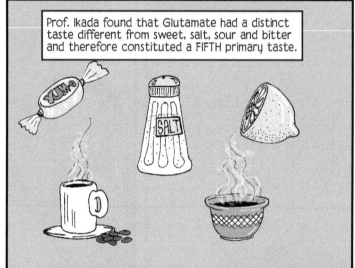

Prof. Ikada found that Glutamate had a distinct taste different from sweet, salt, sour and bitter and therefore constituted a FIFTH primary taste.

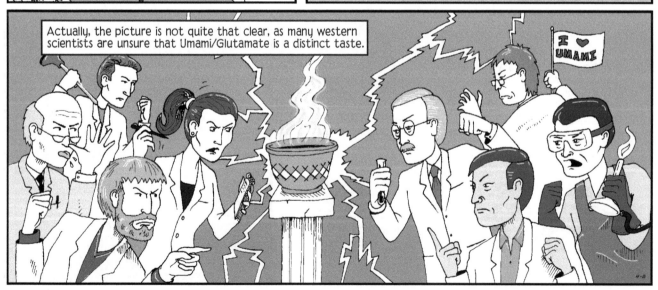

Actually, the picture is not quite that clear, as many western scientists are unsure that Umami/Glutamate is a distinct taste.

Once the chemical is detected by the taste receptors, the nerve impulse is carried to the brain along three large cranial nerves.

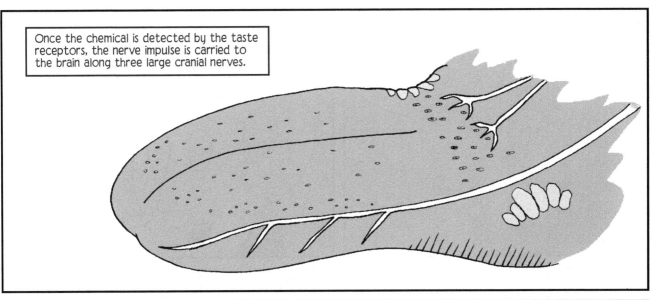

The taste information goes firstly to sub-cortical structures: the Medulla, then to the pons, the thalamus and the amygdala.

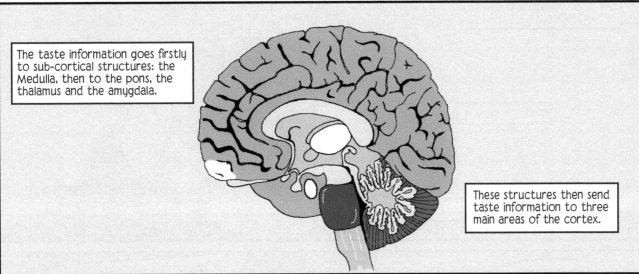

These structures then send taste information to three main areas of the cortex.

This information from the taste receptors, is added to information from the COMMON CHEMICAL SENSE.

The Common Chemical Sense is separate from the Taste sense—

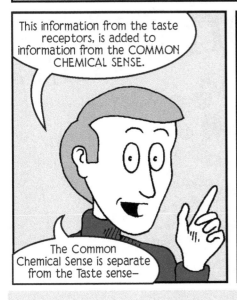

– it consists mostly of the TRIGEMINAL nerve of the head and free nerve endings in the mouth and nasal cavity.

This system is sensitive to a wide variety of different stimuli – in humans this includes spices like ginger and chilli!

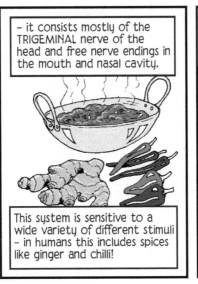

If you remember back to Chapter 2 when we talked about coding, it seems likely that the information for the sense of taste is coded in an across-fibre pattern although the exact mechanism is not fully understood.

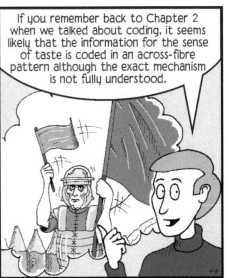

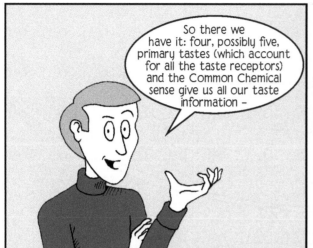

So there we have it: four, possibly five, primary tastes (which account for all the taste receptors) and the Common Chemical sense give us all our taste information –

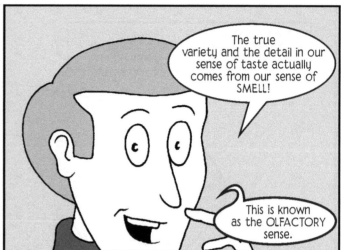

The true variety and the detail in our sense of taste actually comes from our sense of SMELL!

This is known as the OLFACTORY sense.

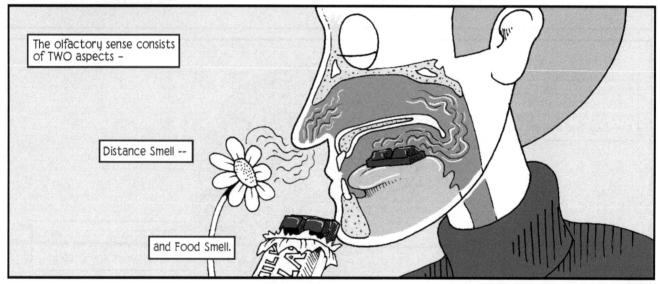

The olfactory sense consists of TWO aspects –

Distance Smell --

and Food Smell.

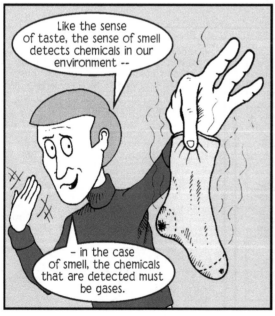

Like the sense of taste, the sense of smell detects chemicals in our environment --

- in the case of smell, the chemicals that are detected must be gases.

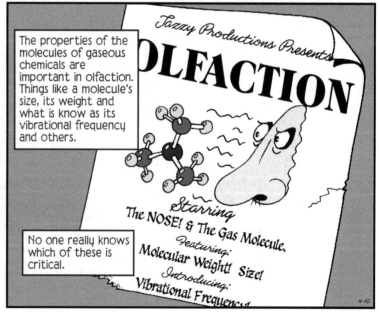

The properties of the molecules of gaseous chemicals are important in olfaction. Things like a molecule's size, its weight and what is know as its vibrational frequency and others.

No one really knows which of these is critical.

Jazzy Productions Presents

OLFACTION

Starring
The NOSE! & The Gas Molecule.
Featuring:
Molecular Weight! Size!
Introducing:
Vibrational Frequency

4-10

The receptors for smell are found in a small patch of the upper nasal passages known as the Olfactory Epithelium –

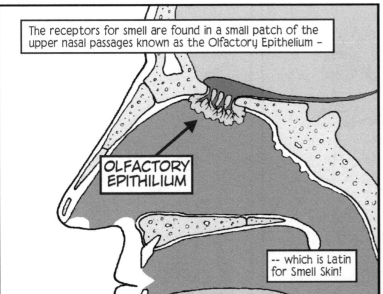

OLFACTORY EPITHILIUM

-- which is Latin for Smell Skin!

Each oval shaped receptor cell has a long extension to the surface of the Olfactory Epithelium called the OLFACTORY ROD.

OLFACTORY ROD

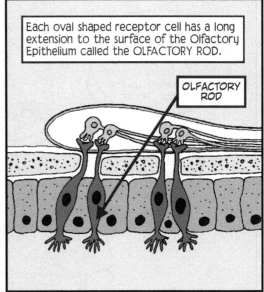

Each Olfactory receptor functions for only six to eight weeks before deteriorating. New receptor cells are constantly being produced to replace these.

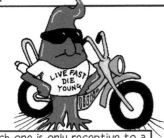

LIVE FAST DIE YOUNG

Each one is only receptive to a very narrow range of chemicals.

At the end of the olfactory rod there are very fine hair-like structures embedded in watery mucus. These are known as Olfactory Cilia.

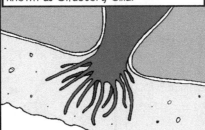

This mucus contains a special chemical called Olfactory Binding protein.

The purpose of which is to attract chemicals that are not normally attracted to water.

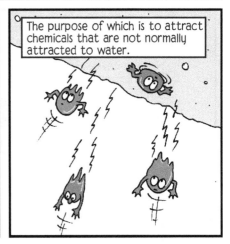

The olfactory cilia contain the actual receptor molecules which make contact with the smell stimulus.

The more cilia an animal has per receptor cell, the greater the smell sensitivity of that animal.

Humans are at the lower end of the smell sensitivity range with only approximately 10 million olfactory receptors and about 6-8 cilia per receptors.

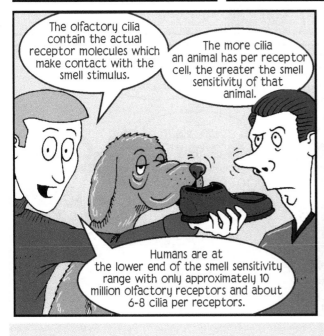

Dogs, on the other hand, have around 200 million olfactory receptors with around 100-150 cilia each.

so their noses are much more sensitive.

He was 6 foot tall, wears a dark suit, tie, bowler hat and lives at 52 Festive Road.

er... is it a shoe?

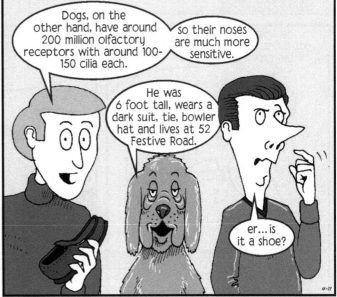

4-11

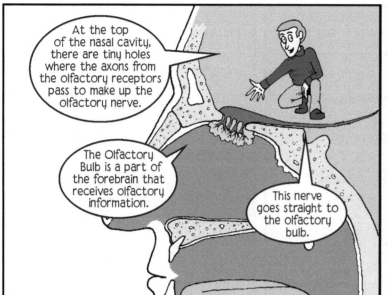

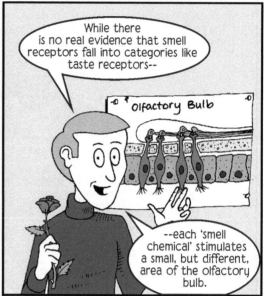

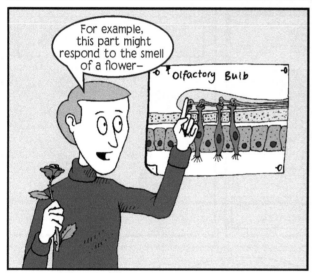

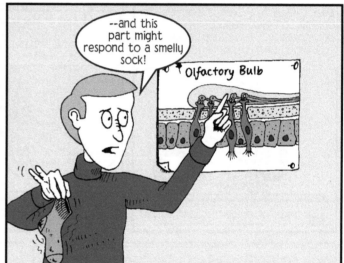

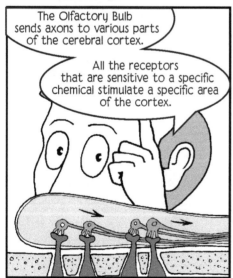

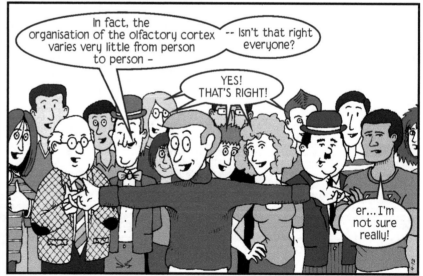

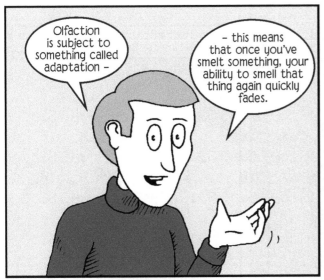

Olfaction is subject to something called adaptation –

– this means that once you've smelt something, your ability to smell that thing again quickly fades.

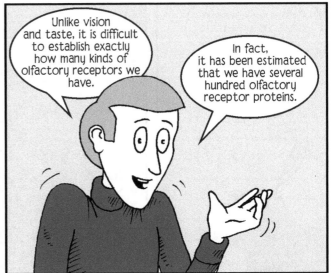

Unlike vision and taste, it is difficult to establish exactly how many kinds of olfactory receptors we have.

In fact, it has been estimated that we have several hundred olfactory receptor proteins.

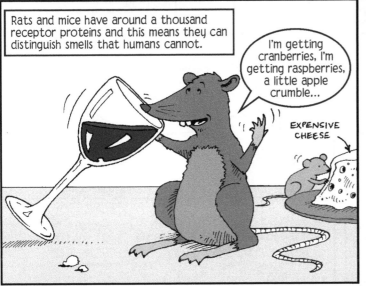

Rats and mice have around a thousand receptor proteins and this means they can distinguish smells that humans cannot.

I'm getting cranberries, I'm getting raspberries, a little apple crumble...

EXPENSIVE CHEESE

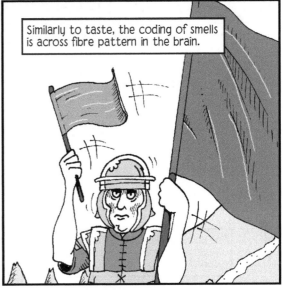

Similarly to taste, the coding of smells is across fibre pattern in the brain.

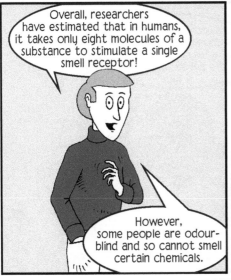

Overall, researchers have estimated that in humans, it takes only eight molecules of a substance to stimulate a single smell receptor!

However, some people are odour-blind and so cannot smell certain chemicals.

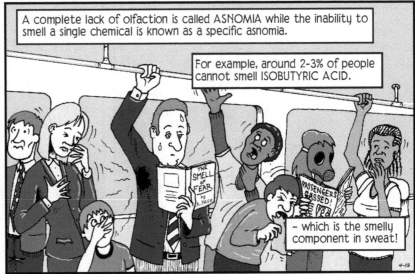

A complete lack of olfaction is called ASNOMIA while the inability to smell a single chemical is known as a specific asnomia.

For example, around 2-3% of people cannot smell ISOBUTYRIC ACID.

THE SMELL OF FEAR by A. Nose

PASSENGERS GASSED!

– which is the smelly component in sweat!

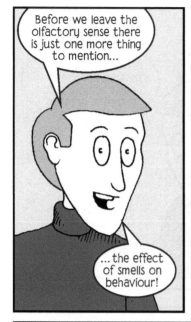

Before we leave the olfactory sense there is just one more thing to mention...

...the effect of smells on behaviour!

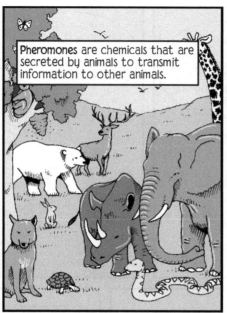

Pheromones are chemicals that are secreted by animals to transmit information to other animals.

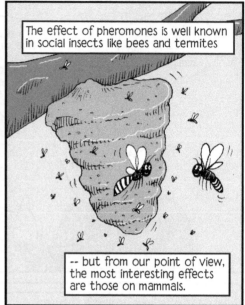

The effect of pheromones is well known in social insects like bees and termites

-- but from our point of view, the most interesting effects are those on mammals.

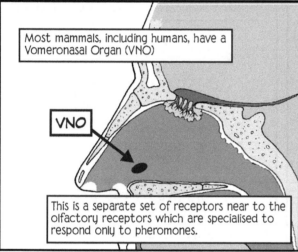

Most mammals, including humans, have a Vomeronasal Organ (VNO)

VNO

This is a separate set of receptors near to the olfactory receptors which are specialised to respond only to pheromones.

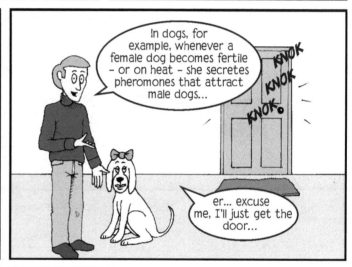

In dogs, for example, whenever a female dog becomes fertile - or on heat - she secretes pheromones that attract male dogs...

KNOK KNOK KNOK

er... excuse me, I'll just get the door...

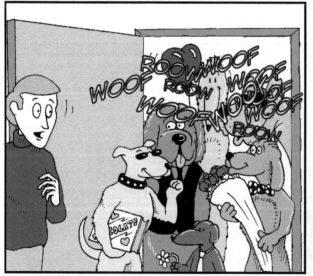

WOOOWOOF WOOF ROOW WOOF WOOF WOOF WOOF ROOW

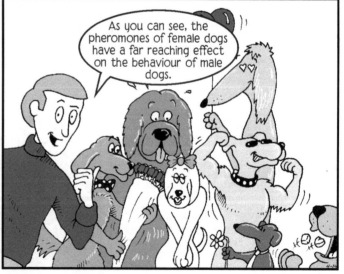

As you can see, the pheromones of female dogs have a far reaching effect on the behaviour of male dogs.

It must be pointed out that pheromone influences in mammals are subtle when compared to those in insects.

Mammals are complex creatures and their behaviour is affected by a number of different influences - one of which is pheromones.

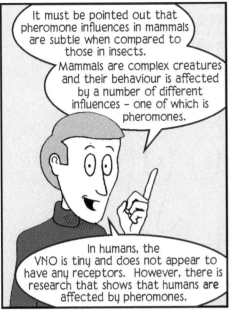

In humans, the VNO is tiny and does not appear to have any receptors. However, there is research that shows that humans **are** affected by pheromones.

A pheromone called Alpha Androstenol is present in a boar's saliva.

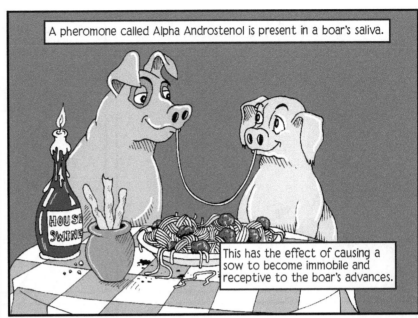

This has the effect of causing a sow to become immobile and receptive to the boar's advances.

This pheromone is also found in human armpit secretions.

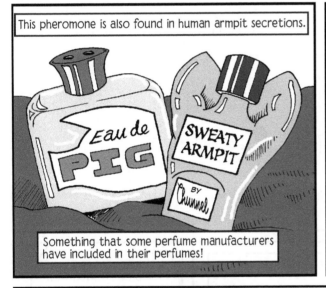

Something that some perfume manufacturers have included in their perfumes!

One study found that people wearing surgical masks impregnated with alpha androstenol rated photos of women as more attractive than those wearing masks without the chemical.

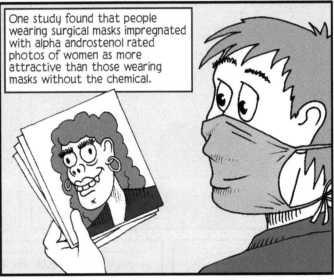

Several studies have also found that chemicals in our skin which we would describe as 'odourless' are capable of altering our skin temperature, sweating and other autonomic responses.

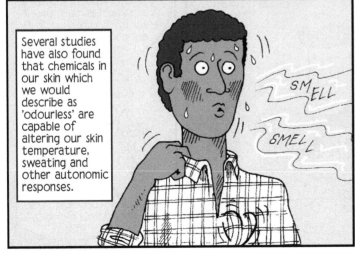

These and other studies have shown that there are human bodily secretions that act as pheromones but...

...their effects are much more subtle than in other mammals.

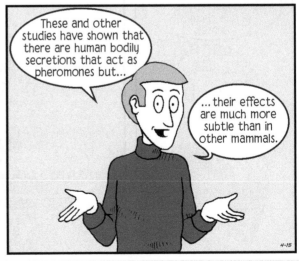

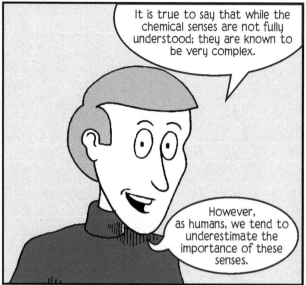

It is true to say that while the chemical senses are not fully understood; they are known to be very complex.

However, as humans, we tend to underestimate the importance of these senses.

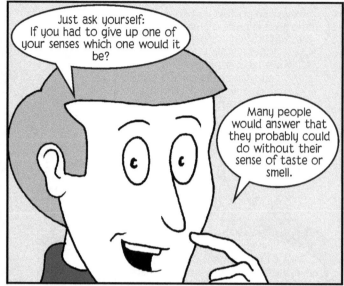

Just ask yourself: If you had to give up one of your senses which one would it be?

Many people would answer that they probably could do without their sense of taste or smell.

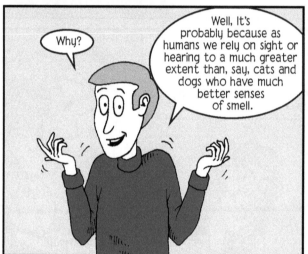

Why?

Well, It's probably because as humans we rely on sight or hearing to a much greater extent than, say, cats and dogs who have much better senses of smell.

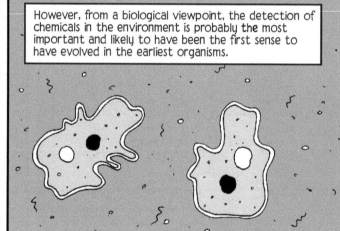

However, from a biological viewpoint, the detection of chemicals in the environment is probably **the** most important and likely to have been the first sense to have evolved in the earliest organisms.

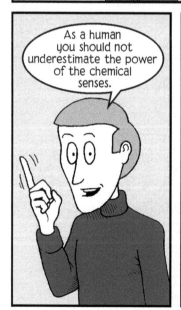

As a human you should not underestimate the power of the chemical senses.

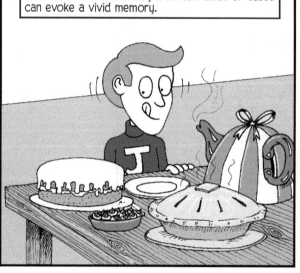

Just think about the way a certain smell or taste can evoke a vivid memory.

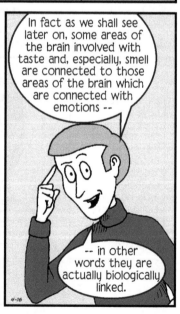

In fact as we shall see later on, some areas of the brain involved with taste and, especially, smell are connected to those areas of the brain which are connected with emotions --

-- in other words they are actually biologically linked.

The chemical senses

► **PAGE 79**

The chemical senses are the sense of taste (known as *gustation* or the *gustatory* sense) and smell (known as *olfaction* or the *olfactory* sense). They are both there for the detection of chemicals in the environment. These senses have *chemoreceptors* that detect chemicals (McBurney, 1984) although there are also other chemoreceptors inside the body.

The chemical senses are believed to be the oldest senses in evolutionary terms. Scott (1990) estimated that they have a history of around 500 million years.

► **PAGE 80**

Panel 3

The senses of taste and smell have related functions and while they are usually discussed separately, they act together when it comes to eating potentially harmful substances. What we perceive as the flavour of food comes from a combination of the taste and smell senses. When we have a cold and our nose is blocked, preventing us from smelling things, the flavour of food tends to be more bland.

Most of the cases of people complaining that they have lost the 'taste' of food (more accurately described as losing the *flavour* of food) are found to have an impaired sense of smell.

► **PAGE 82**

Panel 1

The chemoreceptors for taste are found in the taste buds that are found in the papillae on the tongue. Each papilla contains up to about ten taste buds and each taste bud can have up to fifty receptors.

► **PAGE 83**

Panel 1

In the tongue of an adult human the taste buds are located mainly around the outside edge. There are very few taste buds in the middle of the tongue.

Panel 4

The taste cells are the receptor cells for taste. These are the chemoreceptors for the gustatory sense. Unlike other senses, the receptors for taste are not neurons. They are modified skin cells. Like neurons, the taste cells have membranes that can create an action potential and they release neurotransmitters that affect neurons nearby. However, like skin cells they also periodically die, drop off and are replaced by a new taste cell.

▶ **PAGE 84**

Panels 1 to 5

Each of these primary tastes represents a different taste receptor. So there are sweet receptors, salt receptors, sour receptors and bitter receptors.

However, the taste of food is not constant. If you eat too much of one particular taste (boiled sweets for example) any subsequent similarly flavoured foods (sweet foods in this example) are likely to not taste of that flavour at all. In this case you would not be able to taste any other sweet foods for a while. This is called *adaptation* and it suggests that the particular taste receptors (sweet ones in this case) are fatigued. However, other tastes (salt, sour or bitter) will taste the same as normal. This means that there is little *cross-adaptation* of the primary tastes and is also evidence that there are different types of receptor, one type for each primary taste.

▶ **PAGE 84 (Panels 7 and 8) and PAGE 85 (Panels 1 to 4)**

The transduction of taste is similar to what occurs at a synapse. The food substance binds with a receptor site on the taste cell which causes a change in the cell's membrane and results in an action potential. Different substances bind with different types of taste cell and result in the different taste sensations.

Salt Receptors

To experience a salty taste we must have a substance that turns into ions when dissolved in water (see Chapter 1 notes regarding ions and the action potential). Table salt (Sodium Chloride, $NaCl$) is the best at evoking a salty taste but 'salts' that contain a metal and a small other molecule also elicit a salty taste. These include for example Potassium Chloride (KCl). When sodium ions are present in saliva, they enter the taste receptor and depolarise its resting potential causing an action potential (see Chapter 1 notes). This then causes the taste receptor to release a neurotransmitter that cause the firing of nearby neurons (Avenet & Lindemann, 1989; Kinnamon & Cummings, 1992).

Sour Receptors

Sour receptors respond to hydrogen ions present in acidic solutions. Kinnamon, Dionne and Beam (1988) have suggested that the hydrogen ions bind to potassium sites on the surface of the receptor's membrane. This stops potassium ions exiting the cell and this causes the depolarisation of the cell resulting in an action potential. However, the sourness of a substance is not just dependent on the number of hydrogen ions present so something else about the acid solution must also be detected.

Bitter and Sweet Receptors

Bitter and sweet receptors are more difficult to explain and they seem to be connected. Wong, Gannon and Margolskee (1996) used genetic engineering to prevent mice from tasting bitter substances and found that they were also unable to taste sweet foods.

Bitter receptors typically respond to substances containing plant alkoloids (such as quinine). Sweet receptors respond to sugar molecules like fructose (the sweet substance found in fruits). However, some sugars can elicit both a sweet and a bitter taste. An example of this is glycoside, which is a sugar molecule found on the skin of Seville oranges. However, glycoside tastes extremely bitter. In addition, artificial sweeteners like aspartame elicit a sweet taste in small amounts and bitterness in large amounts.

Both sweet and bitter (and indeed Umami) receptors operate in a similar manner. They are a bit like a metabotropic synapse (see Chapter 1 notes). When the correct ion molecule comes along, this binds onto the receptor site on the membrane. This then activates a G-Protein that causes the release of another chemical in the cell that activates the action potential (Lindeman, 1996).

There is some evidence that we have 40 to 80 different bitter receptors (Adler *et al.*, 2000; Matsunami, Montmayeur & Buck, 2000). This accounts for the myriad of substances that we taste as bitter. In chemical terms, these substances are not related. The only thing connecting them is that they tend to be toxic. Therefore, we have a large number of different receptors to ensure that we don't eat anything that could be harmful.

▶ **PAGE 86**

Panel 5

Whether Umami constitutes a separate taste quality or not is quite controversial. Chaudari, Landin and Roper (2000) proposed a fifth type of glutamate receptor that detects Umami or the taste of Monosodium Glutamate. This substance is often used as a flavour enhancer, especially in Asian cuisine (Kurihara, 1987; Scott & Plate-Salaman, 1991). However, some researchers don't accept that there are specific glutamate receptors in humans despite good evidence for their presence in other animal species.

There may also be a sixth 'primary' taste. It has been suggested that we also have specific taste receptors for fats (Fukuwatari *et al.*, 1997; Gilbertson *et al.*, 1997; Lohse *et al.*, 1997). Before these suggestions it was felt that fats were detected by feel in the mouth.

▶ **PAGE 87**

Panel 5

Taste Coding in the Brain

The four primary tastes of sweet, salt, sour and bitter imply that the brain codes information in a labelled-line fashion. In other words, a particular taste of sweet, for example, is sent to the brain intact so that all messages from that sweet receptor are interpreted by the brain as a sweet taste. However, the coding of taste information in the brain appears to be much more complicated (Hettinger & Frank, 1992). The taste receptors firing is combined in cells next along in the system. These cells respond mainly to one taste but a little to others as well. Therefore the taste interpretation by the brain depends on the analysis of a pattern of responses from a number of different taste receptors. In other words taste is in an across-pattern fibre coding (Erickson, DiLorenzo & Woodbury, 1994).

▶ **PAGE 88**

Panel 4

Chemicals that exist in their gaseous state are called *volatile*.

Panel 5

Almost all chemicals that have a smell can dissolve in fats and are organic compounds (contain a complex mixture of carbon, hydrogen and oxygen). However, there are a number of chemicals that have these characteristics that are completely odourless.

▶ **PAGE 89**

Panel 1

The *olfactory epithelium* consists of two patches of mucus membrane, each about 6.5 square centimetres in size. This is found at the top of the nasal cavities. We need to sniff in order for air to reach the olfactory epithelium. Normally only approximately 10 per cent of the air that enters our nose actually reaches the olfactory epithelium.

Panel 3

The chemoreceptors for olfaction are the olfactory cells. They are modified neurons that lie embedded in the olfactory mucus that lines the olfactory epithelium. There are many types of receptor each responding to different chemicals. It has proved very difficult to categorise these into classes like with taste receptors (Bartoshuk & Beauchamp, 1994). There may be hundreds of different types of receptor, each responsible for a particular smell (Toates, 2001).

Panels 6 and 7

It is actually quite difficult to estimate the number of olfactory cells that humans have in their nose. Figures vary from 10 million to around 50 million.

▶ **PAGE 90**

Panel 1

The olfactory epithelium lies on the *cribiform plate*. This is a bony part of the skull that lies just below the base of the front part of the brain.

Olfaction is unique when it comes to the senses because the axons from the receptors do not go to the thalamus first. This has led to suggestions that the direct connections to the olfactory bulb means that the sense of smell could influence the structures in the brain that control emotions. This may be the reason certain smells can be very evocative of memories.

Panel 2

There have been some attempts to categorise smells. Probably the most accepted form suggests we have seven types of odours that humans respond to (Green, 1994):

- Camphorous (that smells like mothballs)
- Musky (in some aftershaves)
- Floral (in flowers like roses)
- Putrid (like bad eggs)
- Ethereal ('clinical' like in ether)
- Pungent (like vinegar)
- Peppermint (obviously like mint!).

However, more modern research has suggested that it is very difficult to accept such a categorisation in its entirety.

Panels 3 and 4

This is an issue of coding. Olfaction is coded in terms of which area of the olfactory bulb is stimulated. Similar smells stimulate the same or a very similar area of the olfactory bulb while smells that are different to each other excite different areas of the olfactory bulb (Uchida, Takahashi & Mori, 2000).

▶ **PAGE 91**

Panel 1

Adaptation to a smell is quite fast (Kurahashi, Lowe & Gold, 1994).

Panel 6

Along with isobutyric acid, Amoore (1977) identified five other smells that are specific asnomias: fishy, musky, urinous, spermous and malty. He also identified another twenty-six, although the evidence for these is less convincing.

There cannot be many people who would complain that they cannot detect the smell of isobutyric acid!

These specific asnomias suggest that there may be individual receptor cells for each of these smells.

▶ **PAGE 92**

Panel 4

The vomeronasal organ (VNO) in adult humans is very small (Monti-Bloch, Jennings-White, Dolberg & Berliner, 1994) and does not appear to have any receptors (Keverne, 1999). However, there is evidence that it can influence the activity of the autonomic nervous system and hence be working at a non-conscious level (Bartoshok & Beauchamp, 1994; Monti-Bloch, Jennings-White, Dolberg & Berliner, 1994).

There is some evidence that human pheromones can influence the menstrual cycle in women (Stern & McClintock, 1998).

► **PAGE 93**

Panel 4

Kirk-Smith, Booth *et al.* (1978).

Panel 5

This refers to the study by Monti-Bloch, Jennings-White, Dolberg and Berliner (1994).

► **PAGE 94**

Panel 3

Olfaction can be seen as a very different experience when compared to the other senses. In some ways it is like vision since we can identify different separate smells like that of strong onions or cigar smoke. However, when two or three smells are mixed we can still identify the individual components. In this case it is more like the sense of hearing that analyses the components of a sound.

Additionally, we often find it very difficult to describe smells except to say that one smell is like another. This suggests that the olfactory system is there to detect things and not for analysing the particular qualities in a smell.

Nevertheless, probably because of the direct connections to the olfactory bulb in the brain, smells have the greatest ability to evoke vivid and often nostalgic memories.

CHAPTER 5
THE CONTROL OF MOVEMENT

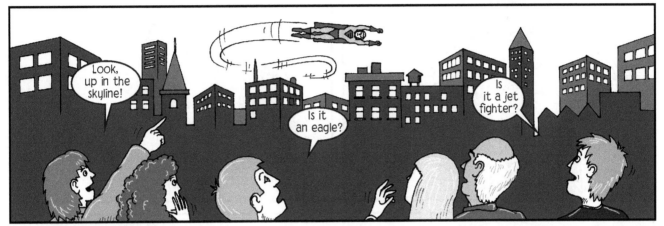

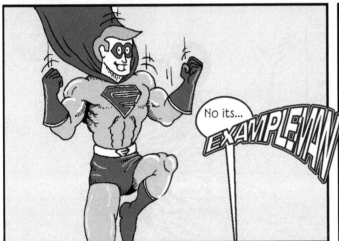

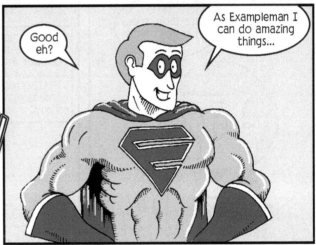

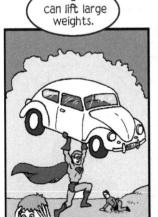

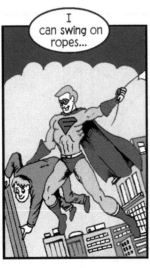

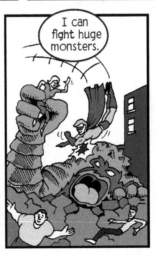

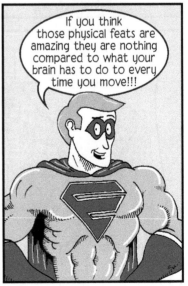

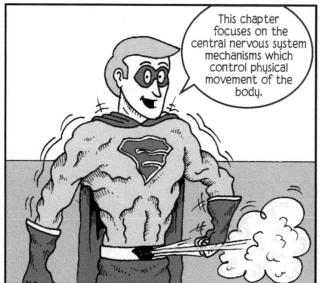

This chapter focuses on the central nervous system mechanisms which control physical movement of the body.

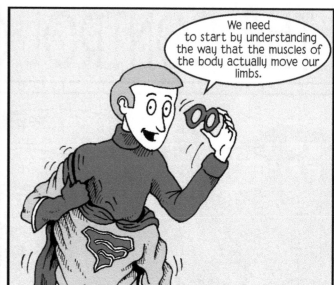

We need to start by understanding the way that the muscles of the body actually move our limbs.

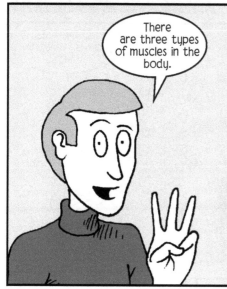

There are three types of muscles in the body.

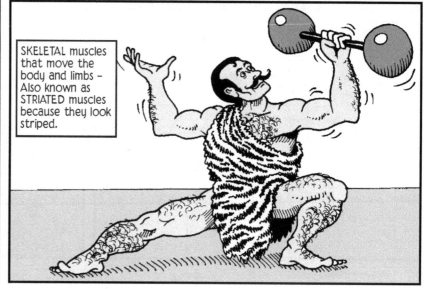

SKELETAL muscles that move the body and limbs – Also known as STRIATED muscles because they look striped.

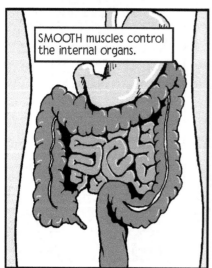

SMOOTH muscles control the internal organs.

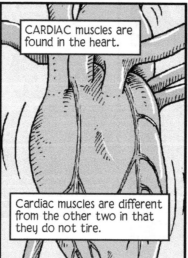

CARDIAC muscles are found in the heart.

Cardiac muscles are different from the other two in that they do not tire.

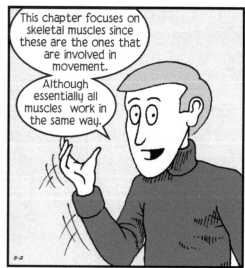

This chapter focuses on skeletal muscles since these are the ones that are involved in movement.

Although essentially all muscles work in the same way.

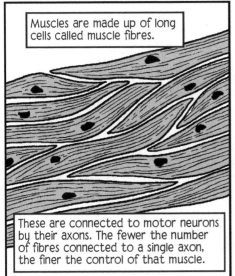

Muscles are made up of long cells called muscle fibres.

These are connected to motor neurons by their axons. The fewer the number of fibres connected to a single axon, the finer the control of that muscle.

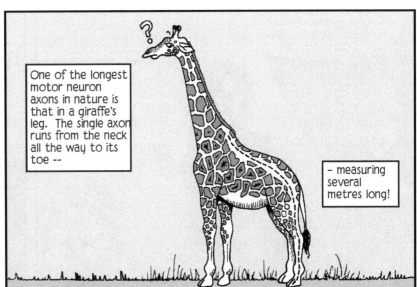

One of the longest motor neuron axons in nature is that in a giraffe's leg. The single axon runs from the neck all the way to its toe --

- measuring several metres long!

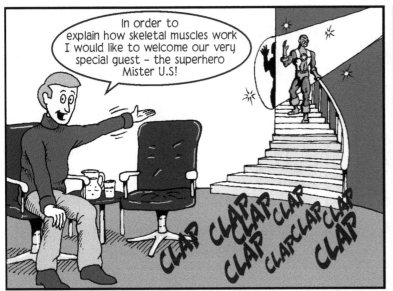

In order to explain how skeletal muscles work I would like to welcome our very special guest - the superhero Mister U.S!

CLAP CLAP CLAP CLAP CLAP CLAPCLAP CLAP CLAP

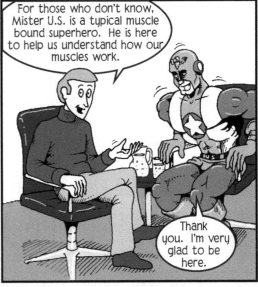

For those who don't know, Mister U.S. is a typical muscle bound superhero. He is here to help us understand how our muscles work.

Thank you. I'm very glad to be here.

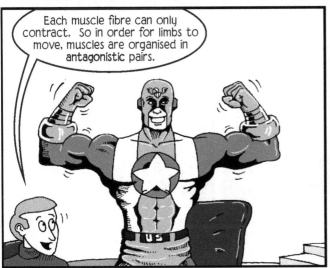

Each muscle fibre can only contract. So in order for limbs to move, muscles are organised in antagonistic pairs.

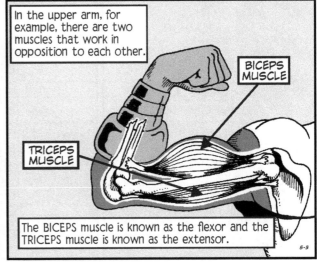

In the upper arm, for example, there are two muscles that work in opposition to each other.

BICEPS MUSCLE

TRICEPS MUSCLE

The BICEPS muscle is known as the flexor and the TRICEPS muscle is known as the extensor.

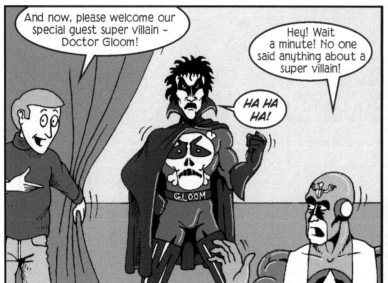

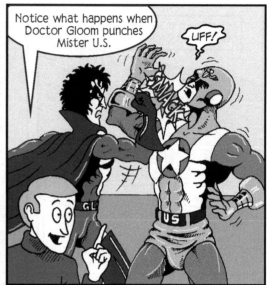

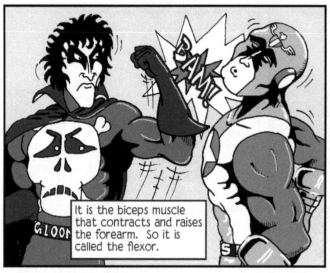

It is the biceps muscle that contracts and raises the forearm. So it is called the flexor.

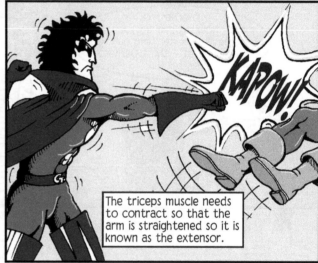

The triceps muscle needs to contract so that the arm is straightened so it is known as the extensor.

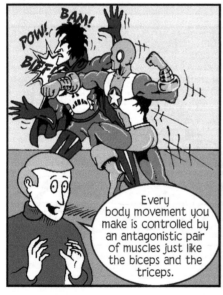

Every body movement you make is controlled by an antagonistic pair of muscles just like the biceps and the triceps.

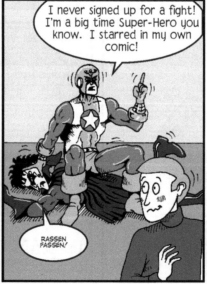

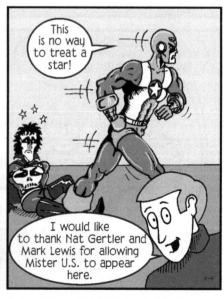

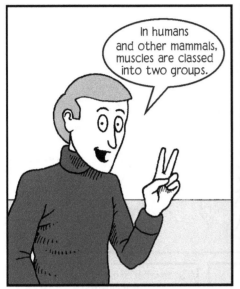

In humans and other mammals, muscles are classed into two groups.

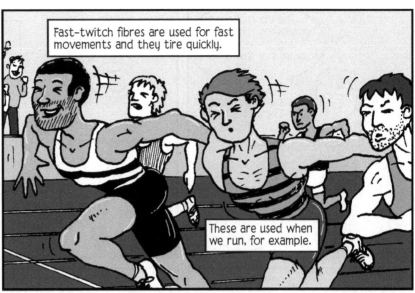

Fast-twitch fibres are used for fast movements and they tire quickly.

These are used when we run, for example.

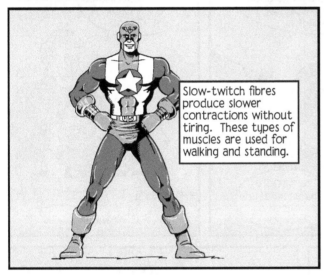

Slow-twitch fibres produce slower contractions without tiring. These types of muscles are used for walking and standing.

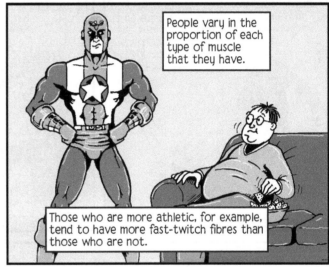

People vary in the proportion of each type of muscle that they have.

Those who are more athletic, for example, tend to have more fast-twitch fibres than those who are not.

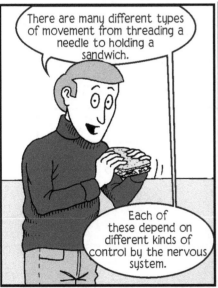

There are many different types of movement from threading a needle to holding a sandwich.

Each of these depend on different kinds of control by the nervous system.

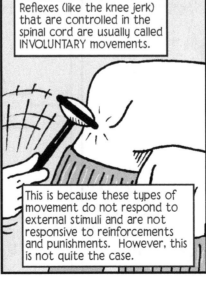

Reflexes (like the knee jerk) that are controlled in the spinal cord are usually called INVOLUNTARY movements.

This is because these types of movement do not respond to external stimuli and are not responsive to reinforcements and punishments. However, this is not quite the case.

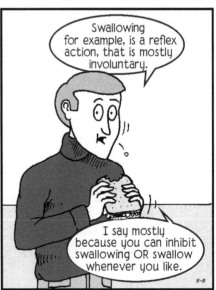

Swallowing for example, is a reflex action, that is mostly involuntary.

I say mostly because you can inhibit swallowing OR swallow whenever you like.

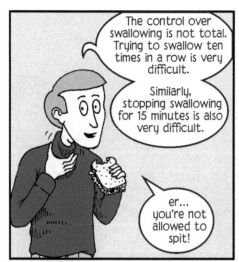

The control over swallowing is not total. Trying to swallow ten times in a row is very difficult.

Similarly, stopping swallowing for 15 minutes is also very difficult.

er... you're not allowed to spit!

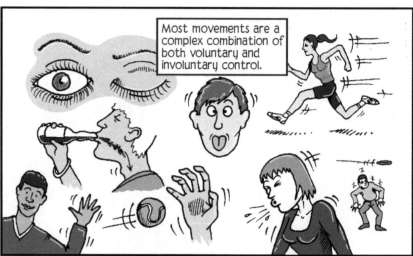

Most movements are a complex combination of both voluntary and involuntary control.

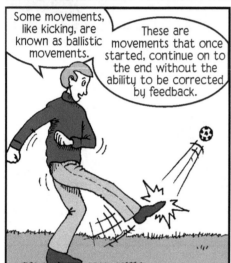

Some movements, like kicking, are known as ballistic movements.

These are movements that once started, continue on to the end without the ability to be corrected by feedback.

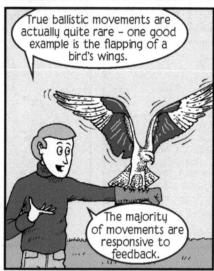

True ballistic movements are actually quite rare - one good example is the flapping of a bird's wings.

The majority of movements are responsive to feedback.

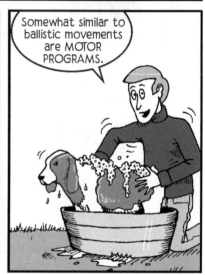

Somewhat similar to ballistic movements are MOTOR PROGRAMS.

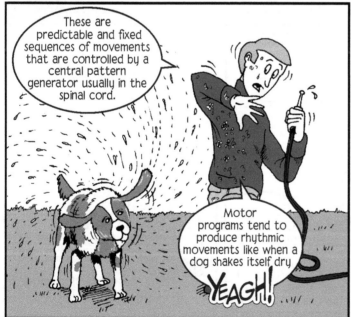

These are predictable and fixed sequences of movements that are controlled by a central pattern generator usually in the spinal cord.

Motor programs tend to produce rhythmic movements like when a dog shakes itself dry

YEAGH!

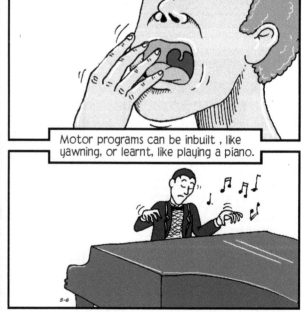

Motor programs can be inbuilt, like yawning, or learnt, like playing a piano.

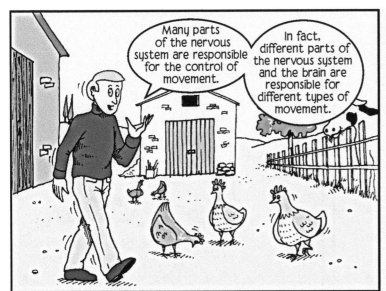

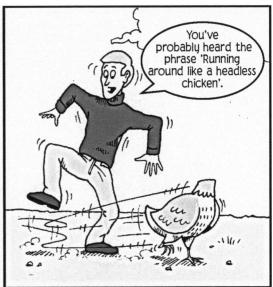

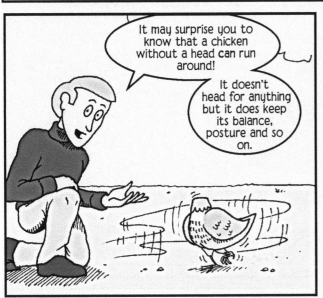

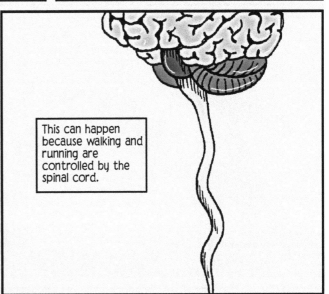

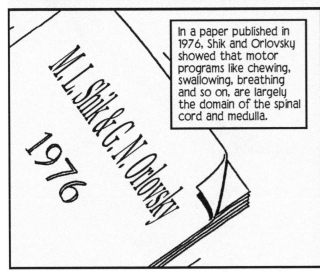

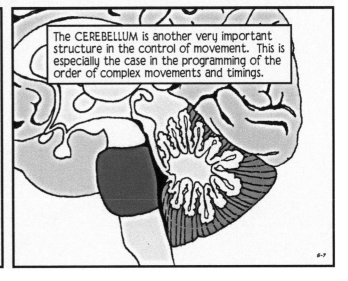

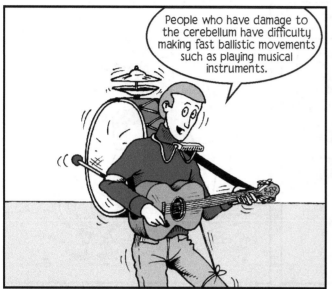

People who have damage to the cerebellum have difficulty making fast ballistic movements such as playing musical instruments.

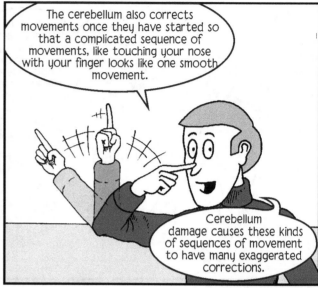

The cerebellum also corrects movements once they have started so that a complicated sequence of movements, like touching your nose with your finger looks like one smooth movement.

Cerebellum damage causes these kinds of sequences of movement to have many exaggerated corrections.

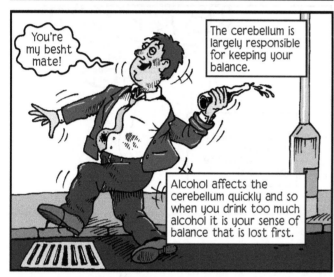

You're my besht mate!

The cerebellum is largely responsible for keeping your balance.

Alcohol affects the cerebellum quickly and so when you drink too much alcohol it is your sense of balance that is lost first.

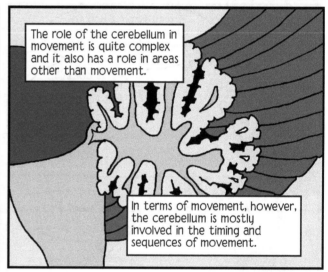

The role of the cerebellum in movement is quite complex and it also has a role in areas other than movement.

In terms of movement, however, the cerebellum is mostly involved in the timing and sequences of movement.

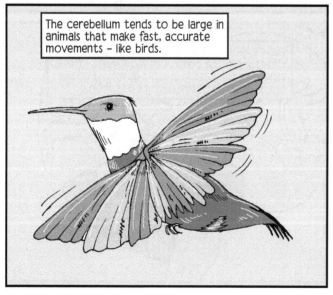

The cerebellum tends to be large in animals that make fast, accurate movements – like birds.

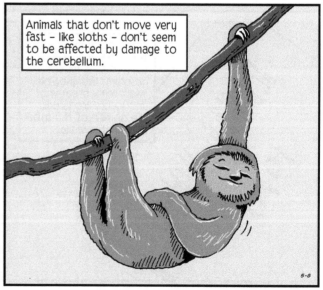

Animals that don't move very fast – like sloths – don't seem to be affected by damage to the cerebellum.

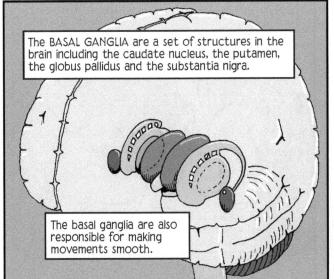

The BASAL GANGLIA are a set of structures in the brain including the caudate nucleus, the putamen, the globus pallidus and the substantia nigra.

The basal ganglia are also responsible for making movements smooth.

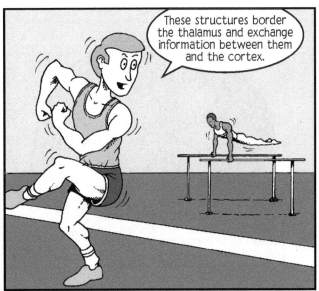

These structures border the thalamus and exchange information between them and the cortex.

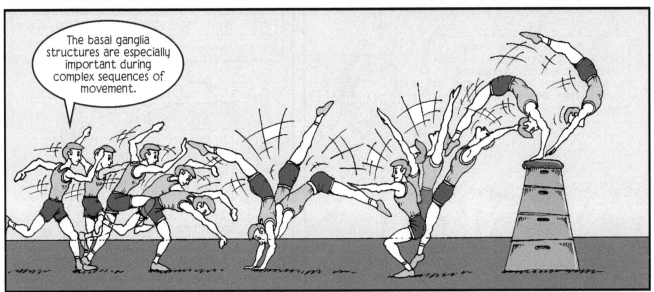

The basal ganglia structures are especially important during complex sequences of movement.

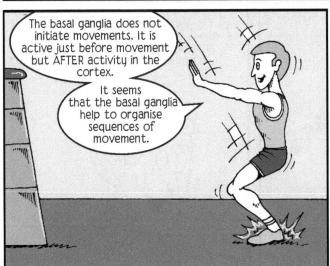

The basal ganglia does not initiate movements. It is active just before movement but AFTER activity in the cortex.

It seems that the basal ganglia help to organise sequences of movement.

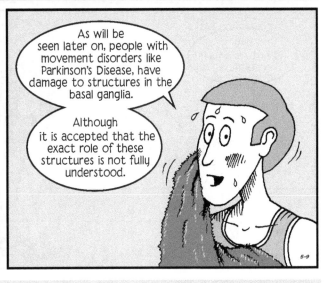

As will be seen later on, people with movement disorders like Parkinson's Disease, have damage to structures in the basal ganglia.

Although it is accepted that the exact role of these structures is not fully understood.

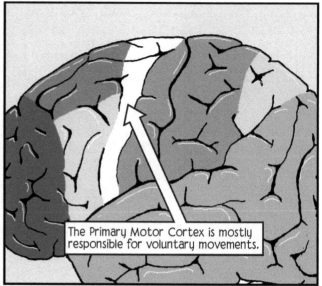

There are a number of different areas of the cortex involved in the control of movement.

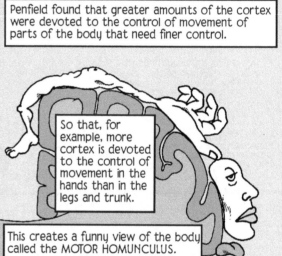

The Primary Motor Cortex is mostly responsible for voluntary movements.

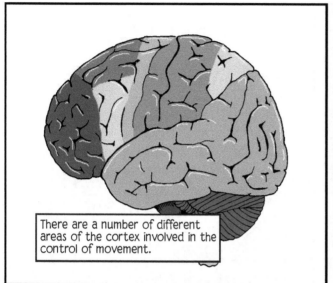

In 1937, Neurologist Wilder Penfield mapped the primary motor cortex by stimulating areas of the brain whilst his patients were undergoing brain surgery under local anaesthesia.

Penfield found that greater amounts of the cortex were devoted to the control of movement of parts of the body that need finer control.

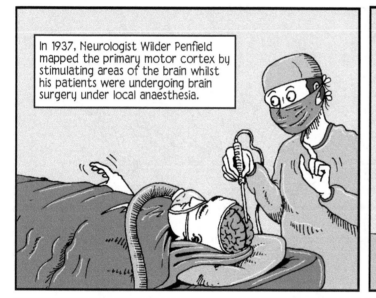

So that, for example, more cortex is devoted to the control of movement in the hands than in the legs and trunk.

This creates a funny view of the body called the MOTOR HOMUNCULUS.

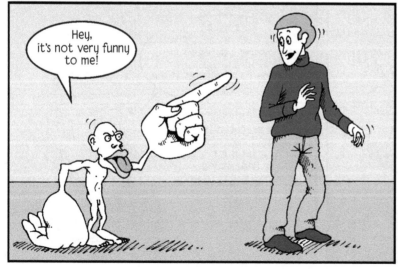

Hey, it's not very funny to me!

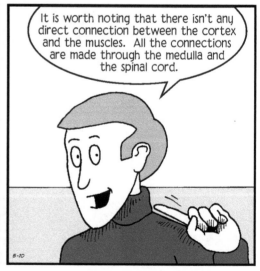

It is worth noting that there isn't any direct connection between the cortex and the muscles. All the connections are made through the medulla and the spinal cord.

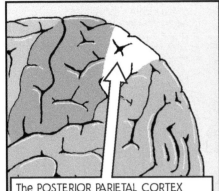

The POSTERIOR PARIETAL CORTEX contains neurons that respond mainly to visual or somatosensory stimuli and some that respond to current or movements in the future and some that respond to a complex mixture of stimuli and responses.

The PRIMARY SOMATOSENSORY CORTEX is involved with touch (see chapter 3) and is active especially when our hands hold something.

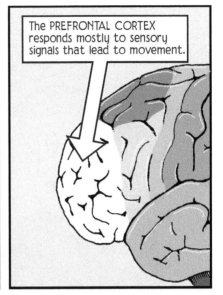

The PREFRONTAL CORTEX responds mostly to sensory signals that lead to movement.

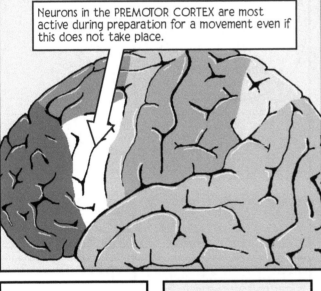

Neurons in the PREMOTOR CORTEX are most active during preparation for a movement even if this does not take place.

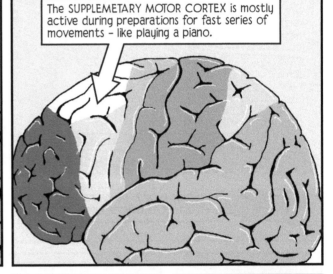

The SUPPLEMETARY MOTOR CORTEX is mostly active during preparations for fast series of movements – like playing a piano.

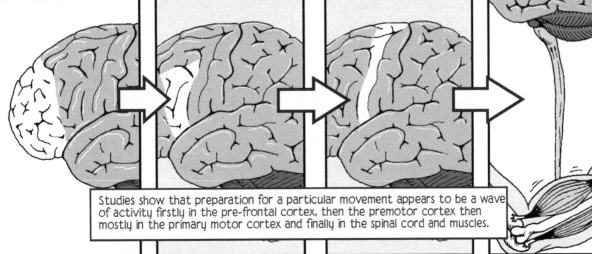

Studies show that preparation for a particular movement appears to be a wave of activity firstly in the pre-frontal cortex, then the premotor cortex then mostly in the primary motor cortex and finally in the spinal cord and muscles.

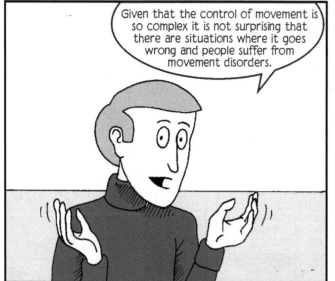

Given that the control of movement is so complex it is not surprising that there are situations where it goes wrong and people suffer from movement disorders.

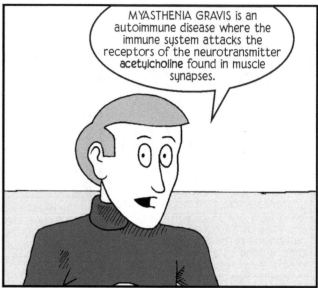

MYASTHENIA GRAVIS is an autoimmune disease where the immune system attacks the receptors of the neurotransmitter **acetylcholine** found in muscle synapses.

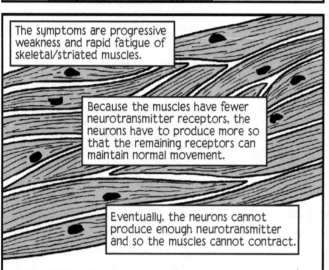

The symptoms are progressive weakness and rapid fatigue of skeletal/striated muscles.

Because the muscles have fewer neurotransmitter receptors, the neurons have to produce more so that the remaining receptors can maintain normal movement.

Eventually, the neurons cannot produce enough neurotransmitter and so the muscles cannot contract.

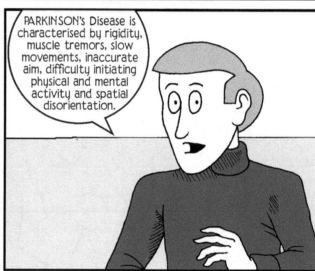

PARKINSON's Disease is characterised by rigidity, muscle tremors, slow movements, inaccurate aim, difficulty initiating physical and mental activity and spatial disorientation.

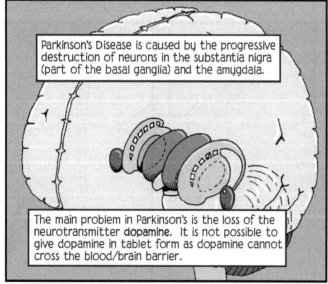

Parkinson's Disease is caused by the progressive destruction of neurons in the substantia nigra (part of the basal ganglia) and the amygdala.

The main problem in Parkinson's is the loss of the neurotransmitter **dopamine**. It is not possible to give dopamine in tablet form as dopamine cannot cross the blood/brain barrier.

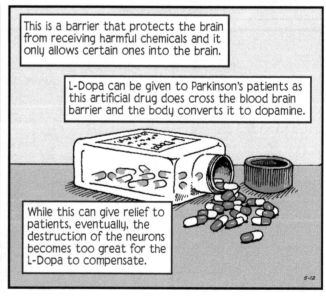

This is a barrier that protects the brain from receiving harmful chemicals and it only allows certain ones into the brain.

L-Dopa can be given to Parkinson's patients as this artificial drug does cross the blood brain barrier and the body converts it to dopamine.

While this can give relief to patients, eventually, the destruction of the neurons becomes too great for the L-Dopa to compensate.

5-12

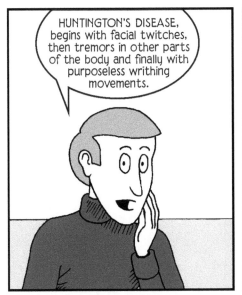

HUNTINGTON'S DISEASE, begins with facial twitches, then tremors in other parts of the body and finally with purposeless writhing movements.

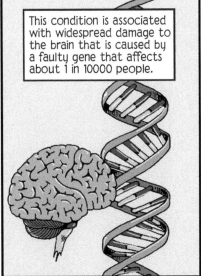

This condition is associated with widespread damage to the brain that is caused by a faulty gene that affects about 1 in 10000 people.

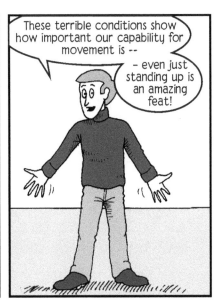

These terrible conditions show how important our capability for movement is --

– even just standing up is an amazing feat!

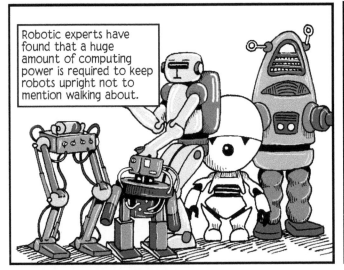

Robotic experts have found that a huge amount of computing power is required to keep robots upright not to mention walking about.

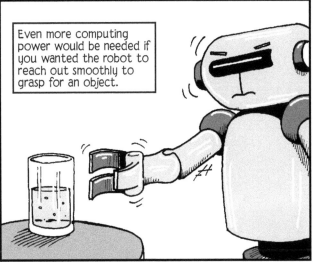

Even more computing power would be needed if you wanted the robot to reach out smoothly to grasp for an object.

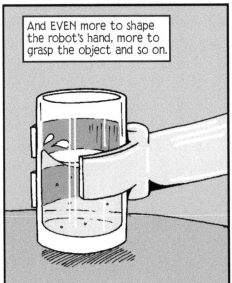

And EVEN more to shape the robot's hand, more to grasp the object and so on.

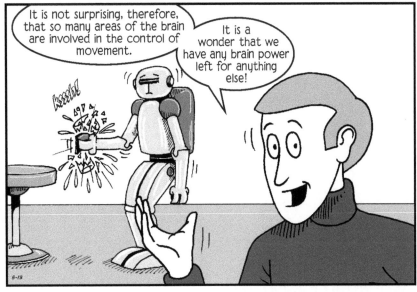

It is not surprising, therefore, that so many areas of the brain are involved in the control of movement.

It is a wonder that we have any brain power left for anything else!

The control of movement

► **PAGE 102**

Panel 1

Movement is the expression of behaviour by the brain. In fact, brains only exist in organisms that have complex movements. Plants don't need brains at all and neither do animals that don't move at all, like sponges. The sea squirt only moves as an infant. When it settles down on the sea bed as an adult it stops moving and doesn't need its brain any more and so digests it! (Kalat, 2004). A huge amount of the brain is used to control movement and Carlson (2001) describes this function as the 'ultimate function of the nervous system' (p.243).

Panel 5

Our autonomic nervous system controls two types of smooth muscle. The first type are *multiunit* smooth muscles found in large arteries, around hair follicles and in the eye (where they control the dilation of the pupil). The second type are *single-unit* smooth muscles found in the gut, the uterus and in small blood vessels.

Panel 6

The heart is made up of cardiac muscles that look striated and hence appear very similar to skeletal muscles. However, cardiac muscles behave like single-unit smooth muscles not like skeletal muscles. Both cardiac and single-unit smooth muscles contract in a rhythmical manner regardless of whether a nerve impulse has been sent to them or not. The rate of this contraction is controlled by the autonomic nervous system.

► **PAGE 103**

Panel 1

Skeletal muscles are made up of two types of muscle fibres: *extrafusal muscle fibres,* found on the outside of the muscle and *intrafusal muscle fibres,* found in the inner core of the muscles. Intrafusal fibres also act as receptors for stretching that are detected in proprioception (see Chapter 3).

The muscle fibres or cells are controlled by motor neurons connected to them at a point called the *neuromuscular junction.*

The biceps muscle has approximately a hundred muscle fibres to each motor neuron controlling it, whereas eye muscles have about three fibres to one neuron. This means that the brain control of the biceps muscle is much less precise than that of eye movements. So our eyes can move much more accurately than our arms.

Panel 3

Mister U.S. is Copyright and TM 1997 Nat Gertler and Mark Lewis and is used here by their kind permission.

Panel 6

Skeletal muscles are the muscles that move us around and thus are responsible for our behaviour. They are usually attached to bones at both ends so that the bones move when the muscles contract. They are attached to the bones via strong bands of connective tissue called *tendons*.

The movement described in this and subsequent panels is called *flexion* and *extension*. There are other types of movement (such as the movement of the eyes) that do not involve these actions.

▶ PAGE 104

Panels 3 to 5

Sometimes people refer to the 'flexing' of their muscles. However, it needs to be pointed out that in fact muscles *contract* and limbs flex!

Panel 6

Mister U.S. is not kidding! He first appeared in 'Big Bang Comics' Volume 2 number 8 published by Image Comics in 1997. Although one comic book appearance hardly makes him a 'big time super-hero'!

▶ PAGE 105

Panels 2 and 3

The work on fast and slow twitch fibres was conducted by Hennig and Lømo (1985).

In mammals (including humans) there is in fact a **range** of fibre types from the slow-twitch fibres to the fast-twitch fibres.

We rely on slow-twitch and intermediate fibres for non-strenuous movements such as talking and walking. Fast-twitch fibres are used for vigorous movements like running. The reason slow-twitch fibres do not tire is that they use oxygen during their movement. Slow-twitch muscle fibres are therefore called *aerobic*. Fast-twitch fires move without using oxygen and are called *anaerobic*. Fast twitch fibres tire quickly because eventually oxygen needs to be used to recover the muscles. The anaerobic reaction also produces chemicals including lactate and phosphate that accumulate in the muscles and cause muscle fatigue. It is these chemicals that give you the experience of tired muscles after you have run.

Panel 4

This refers to work by Andersen, Klitgaard and Saltin (1994). Additionally, work by Sjöström, Friden and Ekblom (1987) showed that a marathon runner built up more slow-twitch fibres than normal.

Panel 6

The knee-jerk reflex is completely controlled by the spinal cord. When the hammer hits the patella tendon (that connects the lower leg muscle – the quadriceps muscle to be precise – to the lower leg bone) the muscle stretches. This is detected by the intrafusal fibres (also called spindles) and sent to the spinal cord. This is connected to sensory neurons in the spinal cord that send a message to the quadriceps muscle to contract.

Why does it do this? Well, the stretch reflex (of which the knee jerk is one of many) allows the muscles to quickly compensate for the movement of its antagonistic pair. In the knee jerk reflex this allows the muscle to ensure that the leg remains straight and that your leg does not suddenly collapse from under you!

▶ **PAGE 106**

Panel 6

A central pattern generator is a set of neurons both in the spinal cord and in other areas that controls rhythmic movements like the flapping of a bird's wing or the shaking in a wet dog. However, in addition to central pattern generators, there are also other mechanisms that control motor programs.

▶ **PAGE 108**

Panel 1

Refers to work by Daum *et al.* (1993).

Panel 2

The role of the cerebellum in the control of movement is complex. However, it does not have what is referred to as an *executive* function. In other words it does not initiate movement. It appears to be responsible for adjusting movements based on previous experience and in relating movement feedback to other areas of the brain.

Panel 6

It was Murphy and O'Leary (1973) who found that damage to a sloth's cerebellum did not appear to result in any problems with movement.

▶ **PAGE 109**

Panel 1

There are several theories that attempt to explain the role of the basal ganglia structures in movement control (Mink, 1999; Prescott *et al.*, 1999 and Reiner, Medina & Veeman, 1998). Marsden (1987) stated that the basal ganglia 'deliver instructions, based on a read-out of ongoing activity in the sensorimotor cortex, to premotor areas in such a way as to set up the correct motor programs required for the next motor action' (p.294). In other words, the basal ganglia 'find' the correct motor program in readiness for it being used.

▶ **PAGE 110**

Panels 4 and 5

The diagram shown in panel 4 is based on the ideas of Penfield and Rasmussen (1950).

While the motor homunculus is being discussed it is worth noting the *homunculus fallacy* (Ramachandran, 1992; Zeki, 1993). This fallacy exists when someone explains the brain's control of behaviour by reference to a smaller 'man' inside the head that does the controlling. When attempting to understand how the brain moves a limb that has been pricked by a pin, for example, one way is to think of a little man in the 'head' who reacts to the pin and pulls a lever to move the limb. However, if this were really the case the little man would also need another little man in his head and so on.

While this may seem like an amusing aside, there are variations on this that are not as easy to ridicule. For example, some people think of the eyes as projecting an image in the brain onto some kind of inner 'screen'. In reality, however, images in the retina are just represented in terms of action potentials in the neurons of the brain.

Similarly, to refer to the motor homunculus is not to suggest that this creature really exists somewhere in the brain. It is simply a representation of the amount of cortical area devoted to movement in the brain.

▶ **PAGE 113**

Panel 1

Huntington's disease causes uncontrollable and jerky movements. As a result of these movements, which have been likened to a dance, this condition was known as Huntington's chorea because the word chorea derives from the Greek word 'Khoros', meaning dance.

This is a hereditary condition caused by a single dominant gene. This means that a person who has this gene will develop the condition and will pass it on to half of their children. The gene responsible has now been identified and genetic testing is available to the family members of sufferers.

One of the most famous cases of Huntington's disease was Woody Guthrie, who was a folk singer in the 1930s and 1940s. He is most notable for influencing a number of modern musicians, especially during the folk revival of the 1960s, including Bob Dylan. He died of the disease in 1967 at the age of 55. His wife was later to help found what is now the Huntington's Disease Society of America which is dedicated to finding a cure for the condition.

CHAPTER 6
TEMPERATURE REGULATION HUNGER AND THIRST

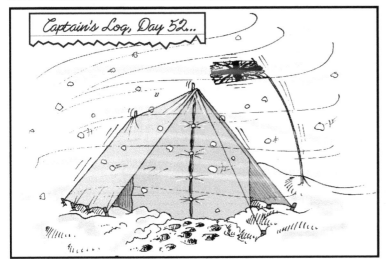

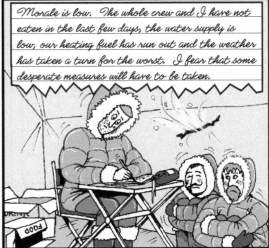

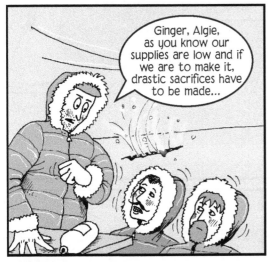

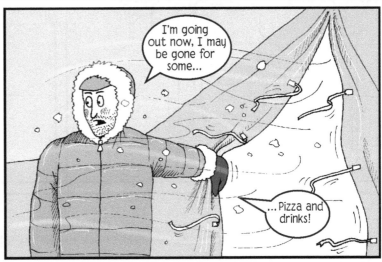

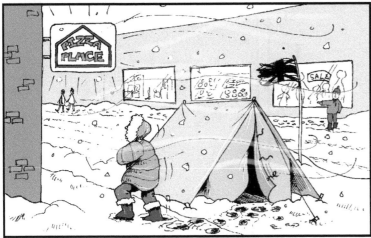

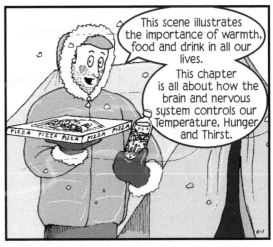

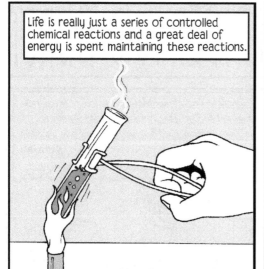

Life is really just a series of controlled chemical reactions and a great deal of energy is spent maintaining these reactions.

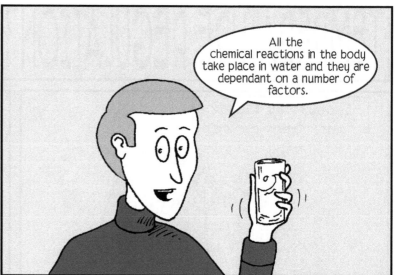

All the chemical reactions in the body take place in water and they are dependant on a number of factors.

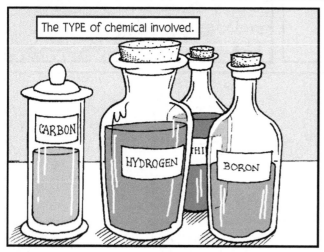

The TYPE of chemical involved.

CARBON

HYDROGEN

BORON

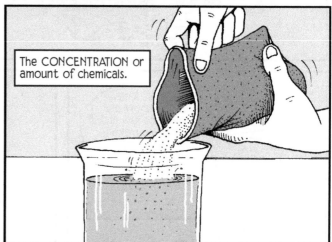

The CONCENTRATION or amount of chemicals.

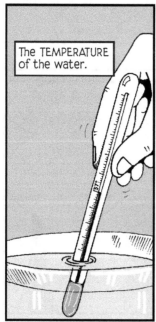

The TEMPERATURE of the water.

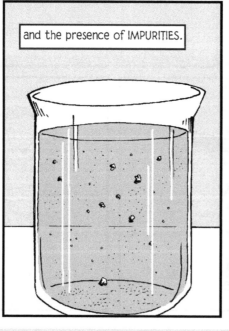

and the presence of IMPURITIES.

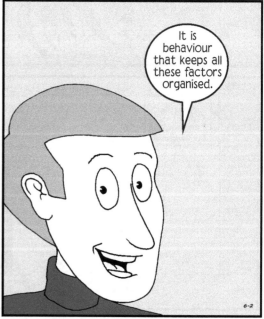

It is behaviour that keeps all these factors organised.

6-2

In 1929, Walter Cannon suggested the concept of HOMEOSTASIS.

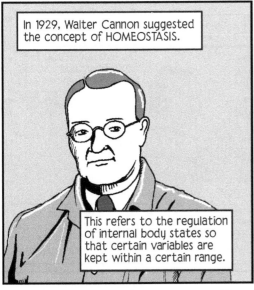

This refers to the regulation of internal body states so that certain variables are kept within a certain range.

So, for example, as the external environmental temperature increases, the body attempts to reduce the internal temperature by sweating.

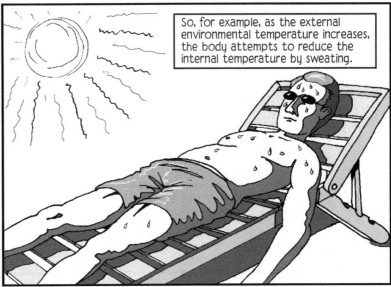

Homeostatic mechanisms cause physiological and behavioural activities that keep variables such as temperature, water and chemicals in a set range.

In fact, some ranges are so narrow that they are known as a SET POINT.

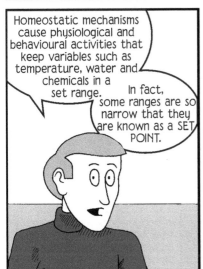

For example, if the amount of calcium in the blood drops below 0.16 grams per litre, then the calcium storage deposits in the bones will release more calcium into the bloodstream.

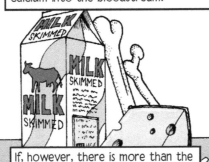

If, however, there is more than the set point of 0.16 grams per litre then calcium is stored or excreted.

Similar mechanisms exist to maintain constant blood levels of water, oxygen, glucose, salt, protein and acidity.

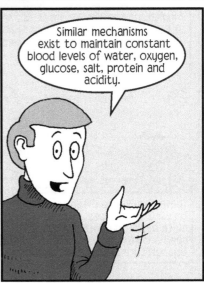

In mammals, temperature control, thirst and hunger are **nearly** homeostatic because they also anticipate future needs.

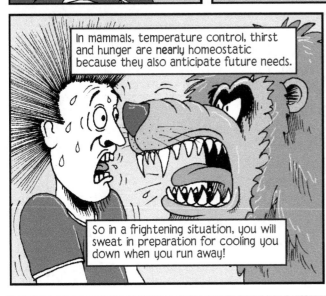

So in a frightening situation, you will sweat in preparation for cooling you down when you run away!

Some set points vary with the time of day, time of year and other conditions.

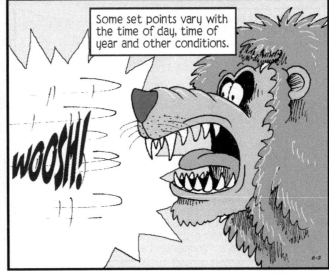

WOOSH!

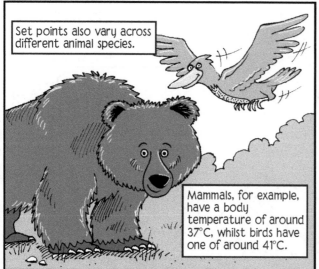

Set points also vary across different animal species.

Mammals, for example, have a body temperature of around 37°C, whilst birds have one of around 41°C.

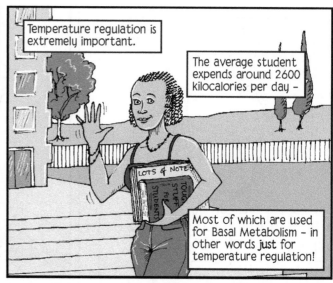

Temperature regulation is extremely important.

The average student expends around 2600 kilocalories per day –

Most of which are used for Basal Metabolism – in other words just for temperature regulation!

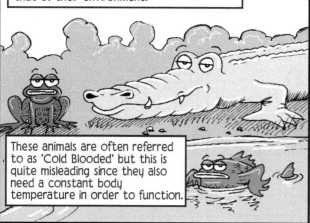

Amphibians, reptiles and most fish are known as POIKILOTHERMIC. This means that their body temperature is always the same as that of their environment.

These animals are often referred to as 'Cold Blooded' but this is quite misleading since they also need a constant body temperature in order to function.

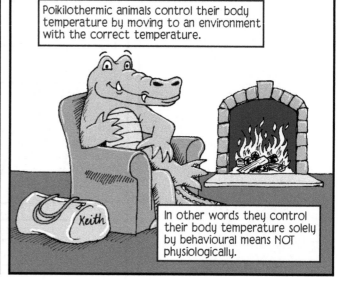

Poikilothermic animals control their body temperature by moving to an environment with the correct temperature.

In other words they control their body temperature solely by behavioural means NOT physiologically.

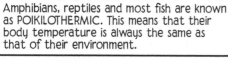

Mammals and birds are known as HOMEOTHERMIC.

This means that they have physiological mechanisms to keep their body temperature constant despite variations in the environmental temperature.

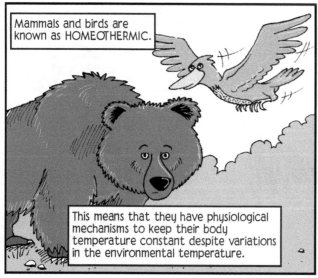

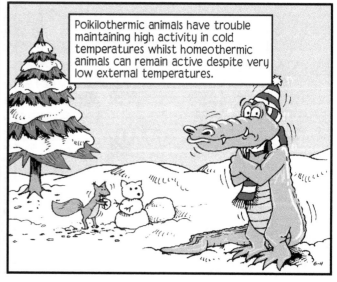

Poikilothermic animals have trouble maintaining high activity in cold temperatures whilst homeothermic animals can remain active despite very low external temperatures.

The reason mammals have an internal temperature of 37°C is due to a 'trade-off' amongst many factors.

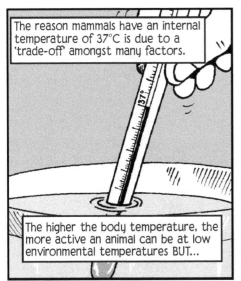

The higher the body temperature, the more active an animal can be at low environmental temperatures BUT...

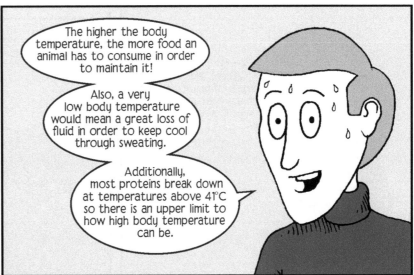

The higher the body temperature, the more food an animal has to consume in order to maintain it!

Also, a very low body temperature would mean a great loss of fluid in order to keep cool through sweating.

Additionally, most proteins break down at temperatures above 41°C so there is an upper limit to how high body temperature can be.

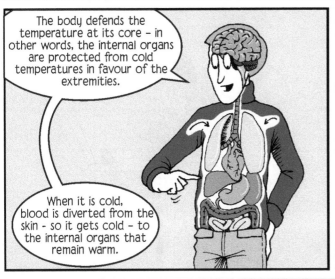

The body defends the temperature at its core – in other words, the internal organs are protected from cold temperatures in favour of the extremities.

When it is cold, blood is diverted from the skin - so it gets cold - to the internal organs that remain warm.

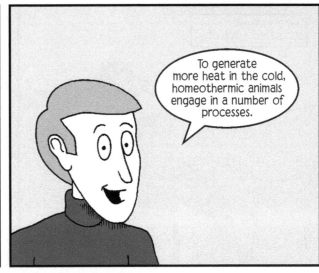

To generate more heat in the cold, homeothermic animals engage in a number of processes.

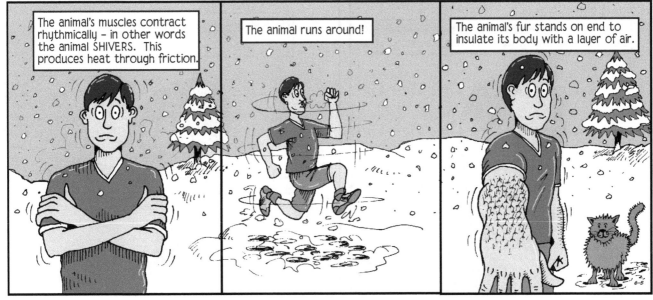

The animal's muscles contract rhythmically – in other words the animal SHIVERS. This produces heat through friction.

The animal runs around!

The animal's fur stands on end to insulate its body with a layer of air.

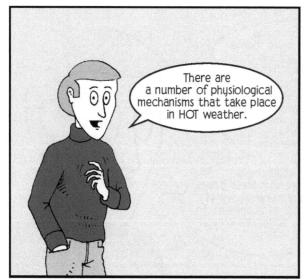

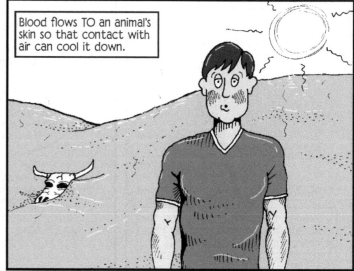

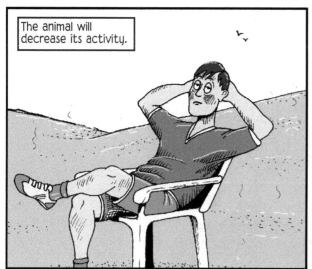

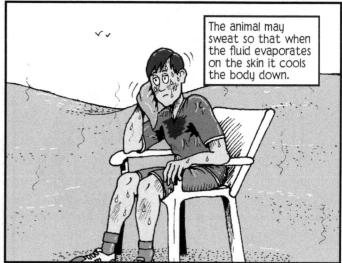

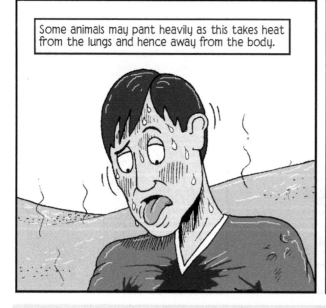

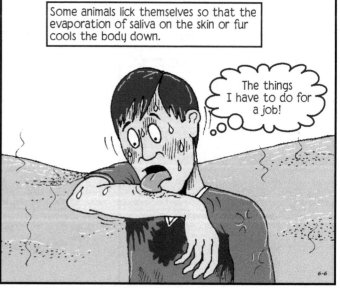

These physiological changes are mostly controlled by certain areas in the hypothalamus.

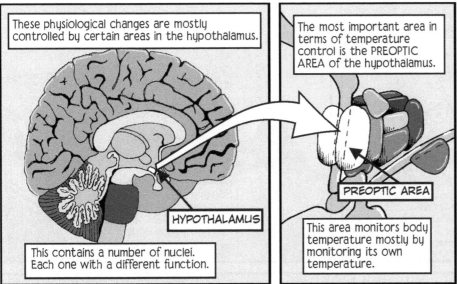

HYPOTHALAMUS

This contains a number of nuclei. Each one with a different function.

The most important area in terms of temperature control is the PREOPTIC AREA of the hypothalamus.

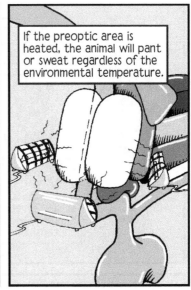

PREOPTIC AREA

This area monitors body temperature mostly by monitoring its own temperature.

If the preoptic area is heated, the animal will pant or sweat regardless of the environmental temperature.

Like reptiles and other poikilothermic animals, mammals and birds will also move to warmer or cooler areas in order to control body temperature.

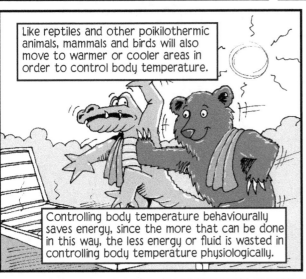

Controlling body temperature behaviourally saves energy, since the more that can be done in this way, the less energy or fluid is wasted in controlling body temperature physiologically.

Temperature control is especially important when we are ill.

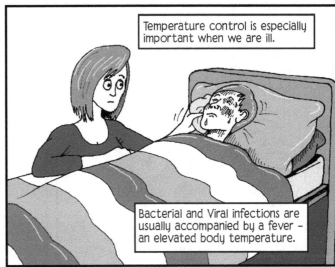

Bacterial and Viral infections are usually accompanied by a fever – an elevated body temperature.

You probably assumed that it is the virus or bacteria that causes the high temperature.

Actually, a fever is part of the body's defense AGAINST the virus or bacteria.

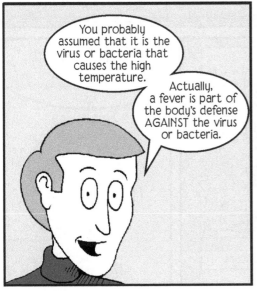

Newborn rabbits are unable to shiver in response to infections but they will move to a hotter place – so that they develop a fever by behavioural means.

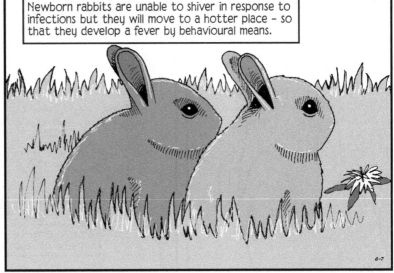

6-7

125

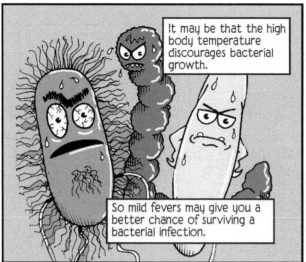

It may be that the high body temperature discourages bacterial growth.

So mild fevers may give you a better chance of surviving a bacterial infection.

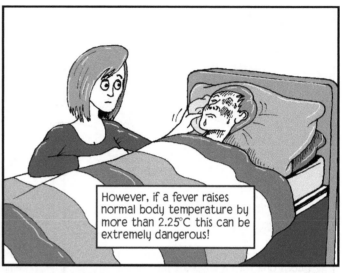

However, if a fever raises normal body temperature by more than 2.25°C this can be extremely dangerous!

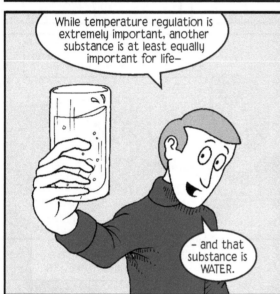

While temperature regulation is extremely important, another substance is at least equally important for life—

– and that substance is WATER.

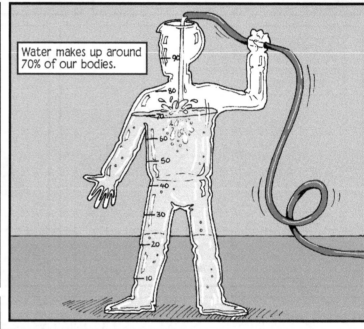

Water makes up around 70% of our bodies.

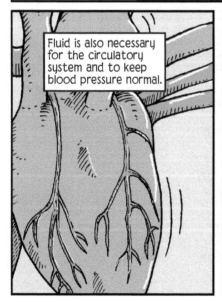

Fluid is also necessary for the circulatory system and to keep blood pressure normal.

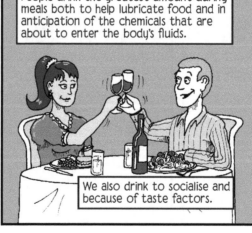

People drink the greatest amount during meals both to help lubricate food and in anticipation of the chemicals that are about to enter the body's fluids.

We also drink to socialise and because of taste factors.

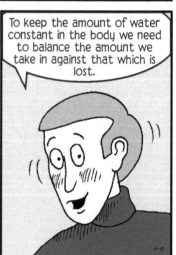

To keep the amount of water constant in the body we need to balance the amount we take in against that which is lost.

We lose water in a variety of ways...

Obviously by sweating, urination and defecation.

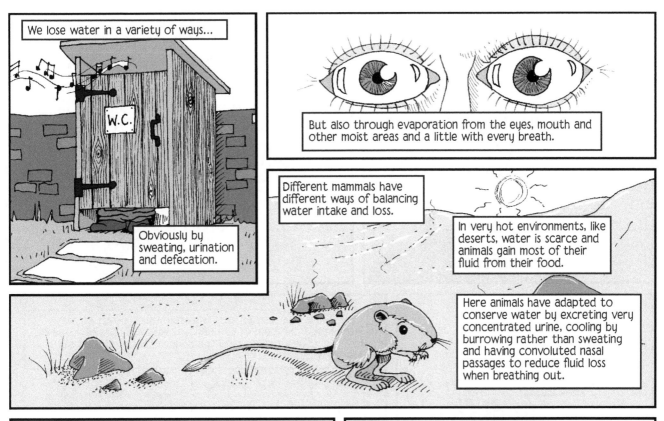

But also through evaporation from the eyes, mouth and other moist areas and a little with every breath.

Different mammals have different ways of balancing water intake and loss.

In very hot environments, like deserts, water is scarce and animals gain most of their fluid from their food.

Here animals have adapted to conserve water by excreting very concentrated urine, cooling by burrowing rather than sweating and having convoluted nasal passages to reduce fluid loss when breathing out.

Mammals living in or near water however, have very different survival strategies that are unconcerned with gaining or losing water since fluid is all around them.

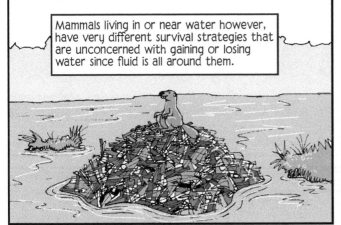

Humans are able to change their water conservation strategy according to their circumstances.

So when water is plentiful, people consume and excrete plentifully!

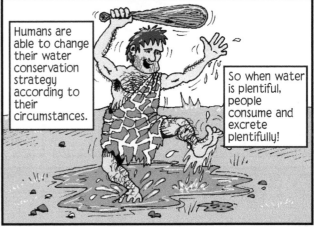

In hot, dry environments, people conserve water by excreting less water through their urine.

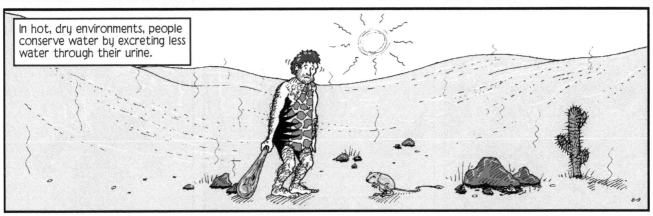

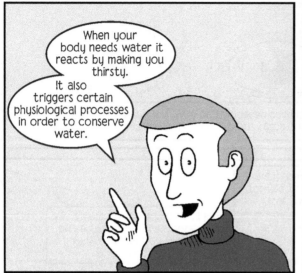

When your body needs water it reacts by making you thirsty.

It also triggers certain physiological processes in order to conserve water.

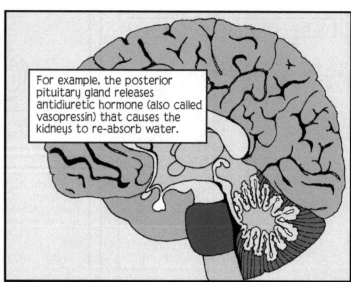

For example, the posterior pituitary gland releases antidiuretic hormone (also called vasopressin) that causes the kidneys to re-absorb water.

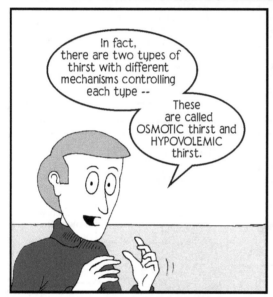

In fact, there are two types of thirst with different mechanisms controlling each type --

These are called OSMOTIC thirst and HYPOVOLEMIC thirst.

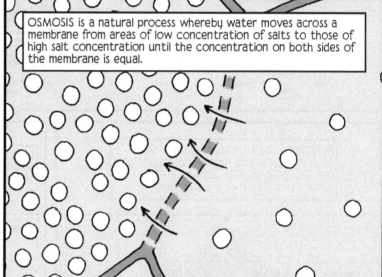

OSMOSIS is a natural process whereby water moves across a membrane from areas of low concentration of salts to those of high salt concentration until the concentration on both sides of the membrane is equal.

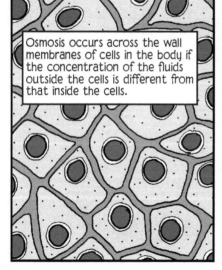

Osmosis occurs across the wall membranes of cells in the body if the concentration of the fluids outside the cells is different from that inside the cells.

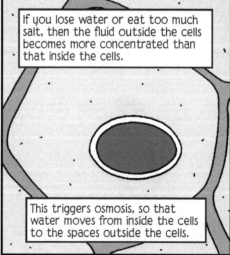

If you lose water or eat too much salt, then the fluid outside the cells becomes more concentrated than that inside the cells.

This triggers osmosis, so that water moves from inside the cells to the spaces outside the cells.

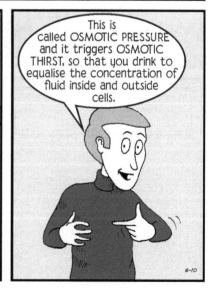

This is called OSMOTIC PRESSURE and it triggers OSMOTIC THIRST, so that you drink to equalise the concentration of fluid inside and outside cells.

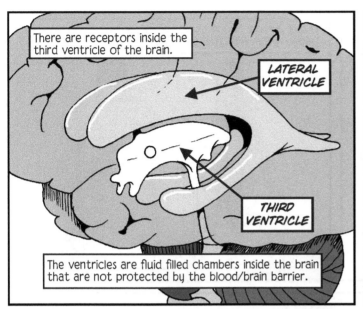

There are receptors inside the third ventricle of the brain.

LATERAL VENTRICLE

THIRD VENTRICLE

The ventricles are fluid filled chambers inside the brain that are not protected by the blood/brain barrier.

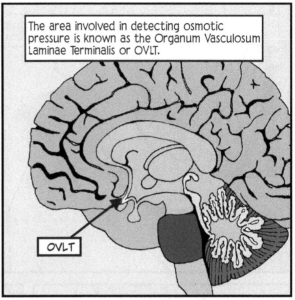

The area involved in detecting osmotic pressure is known as the Organum Vasculosum Laminae Terminalis or OVLT.

OVLT

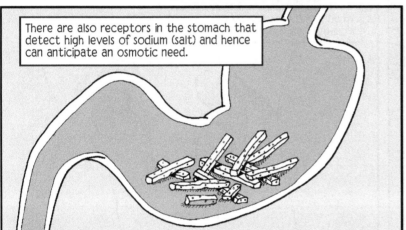

There are also receptors in the stomach that detect high levels of sodium (salt) and hence can anticipate an osmotic need.

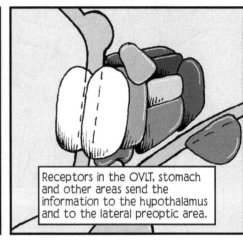

Receptors in the OVLT, stomach and other areas send the information to the hypothalamus and to the lateral preoptic area.

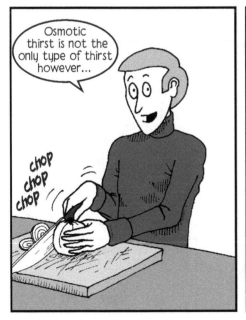

Osmotic thirst is not the only type of thirst however...

chop chop chop

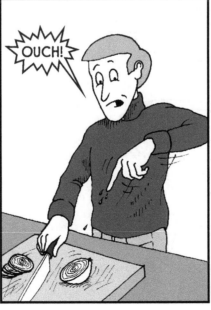

OUCH!

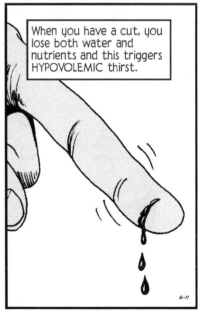

When you have a cut, you lose both water and nutrients and this triggers HYPOVOLEMIC thirst.

6-11

HYPOVOLEMIC thirst is triggered when there is a drop in blood pressure, which is usually a result of a deep cut.

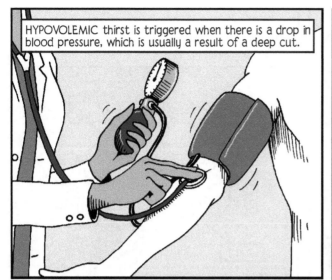

After a reduction in blood volume, an animal will drink more water with salts and impurities than pure water.

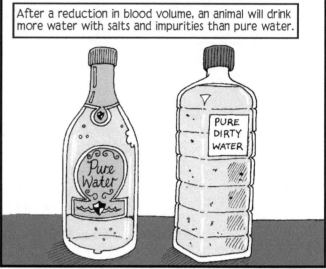

Baroreceptors in large veins detect the pressure of blood returning to the heart.

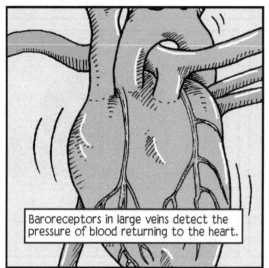

When blood pressure drops, the kidneys release the hormone RENIN.

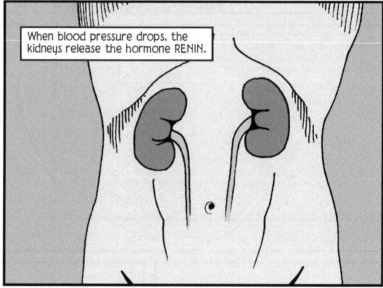

Renin causes a chain reaction of hormone release that results in the stimulation of the SUBFORNICAL ORGAN that adjoins the 3rd ventricle.

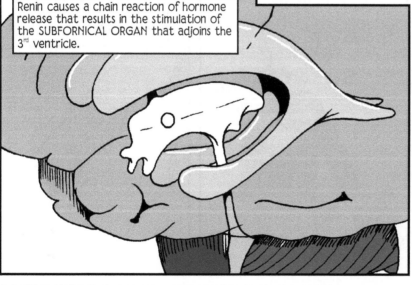

This then stimulates the preoptic area of the hypothalamus that directs drinking.

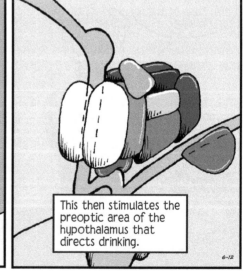

6-12

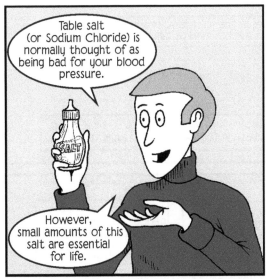

Table salt (or Sodium Chloride) is normally thought of as being bad for your blood pressure.

However, small amounts of this salt are essential for life.

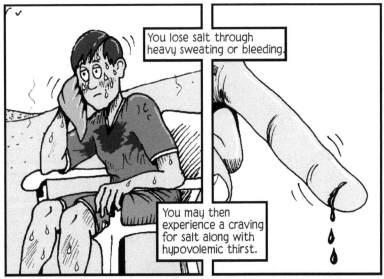

You lose salt through heavy sweating or bleeding.

You may then experience a craving for salt along with hypovolemic thirst.

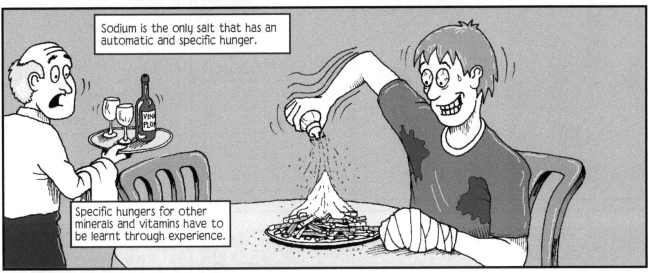

Sodium is the only salt that has an automatic and specific hunger.

Specific hungers for other minerals and vitamins have to be learnt through experience.

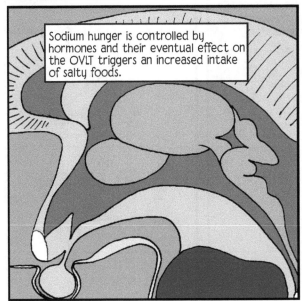

Sodium hunger is controlled by hormones and their eventual effect on the OVLT triggers an increased intake of salty foods.

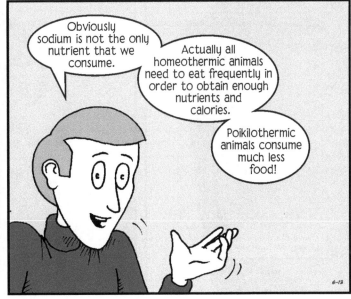

Obviously sodium is not the only nutrient that we consume.

Actually all homeothermic animals need to eat frequently in order to obtain enough nutrients and calories.

Poikilothermic animals consume much less food!

6-13

The function of the digestive system is to break down food into smaller chemicals that our cells can use.

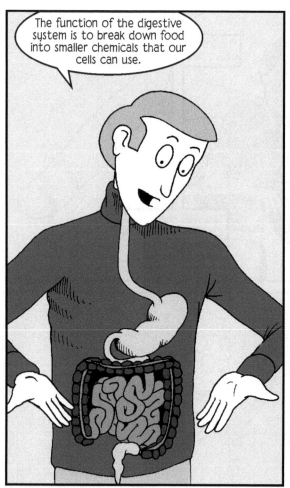

Digestion begins in the mouth, where food is broken down and mixed with saliva.

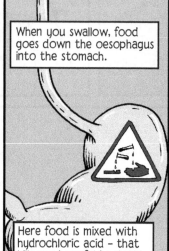

Saliva contains enzymes that start to beak down carbohydrate in food into smaller sugar molecules.

When you swallow, food goes down the oesophagus into the stomach.

Here food is mixed with hydrochloric acid - that kills any harmful bacteria - and enzymes that further break down the food.

A round sphincter muscle periodically opens at the end of the stomach and releases food into the small intestines.

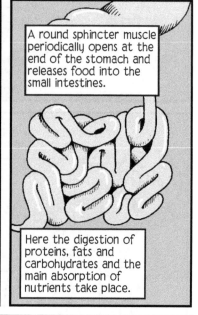

Here the digestion of proteins, fats and carbohydrates and the main absorption of nutrients take place.

In the large intestines, water and minerals are absorbed.

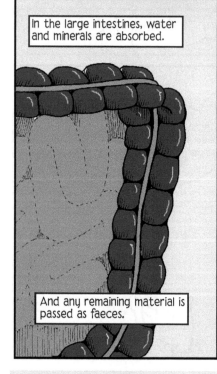

And any remaining material is passed as faeces.

The nutrient molecules from food are absorbed into the bloodstream and carried to body cells to use and store.

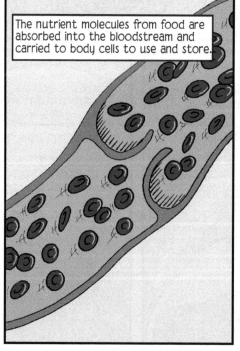

These stores are later converted to glucose which is the body's primary fuel.

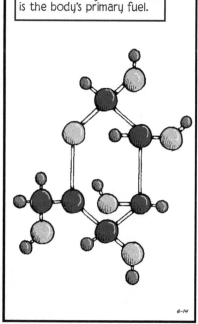

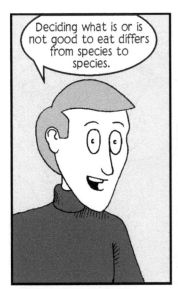

Deciding what is or is not good to eat differs from species to species.

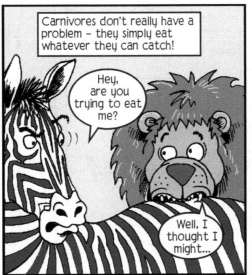

Carnivores don't really have a problem - they simply eat whatever they can catch!

Hey, are you trying to eat me?

Well, I thought I might...

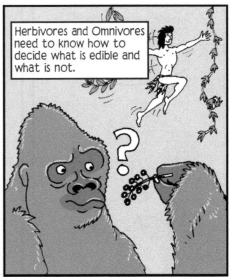

Herbivores and Omnivores need to know how to decide what is edible and what is not.

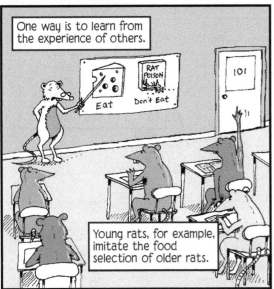

One way is to learn from the experience of others.

EAT

RAT POISON

Eat   Don't Eat

101

Young rats, for example, imitate the food selection of older rats.

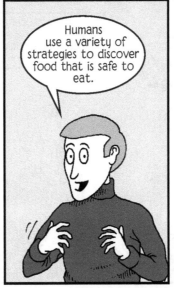

Humans use a variety of strategies to discover food that is safe to eat.

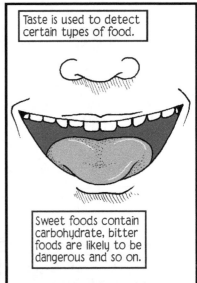

Taste is used to detect certain types of food.

Sweet foods contain carbohydrate, bitter foods are likely to be dangerous and so on.

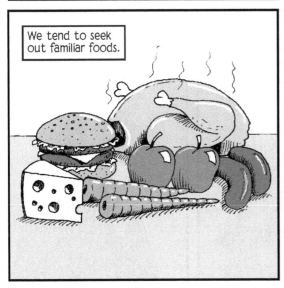

We tend to seek out familiar foods.

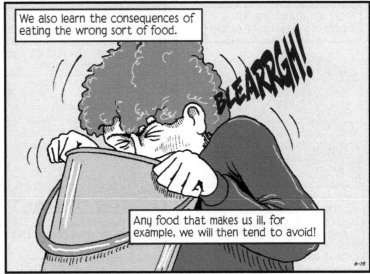

We also learn the consequences of eating the wrong sort of food.

BLEARRGH!

Any food that makes us ill, for example, we will then tend to avoid!

6-15

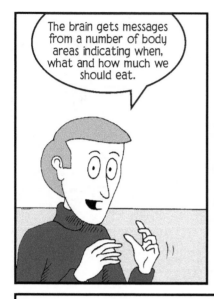

The brain gets messages from a number of body areas indicating when, what and how much we should eat.

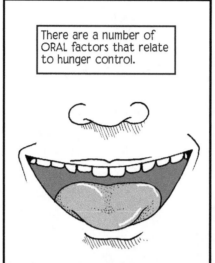

There are a number of ORAL factors that relate to hunger control.

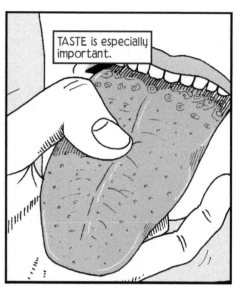

TASTE is especially important.

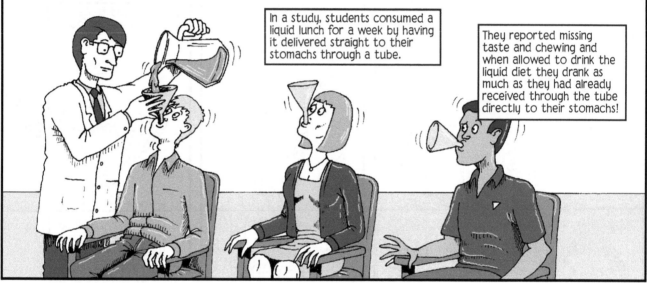

In a study, students consumed a liquid lunch for a week by having it delivered straight to their stomachs through a tube.

They reported missing taste and chewing and when allowed to drink the liquid diet they drank as much as they had already received through the tube directly to their stomachs!

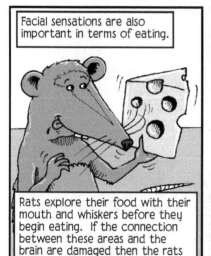

Facial sensations are also important in terms of eating.

Rats explore their food with their mouth and whiskers before they begin eating. If the connection between these areas and the brain are damaged then the rats cannot eat properly.

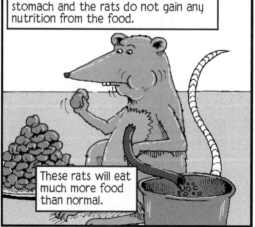

In SHAM FEEDING studies, rats have a tube fitted whereby they can eat and swallow but the food cannot reach the stomach and the rats do not gain any nutrition from the food.

These rats will eat much more food than normal.

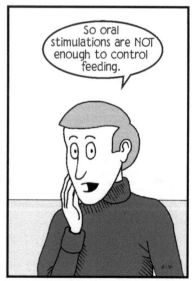

So oral stimulations are NOT enough to control feeding.

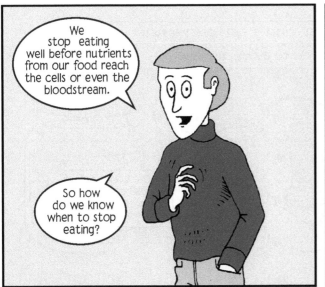

We stop eating well before nutrients from our food reach the cells or even the bloodstream.

So how do we know when to stop eating?

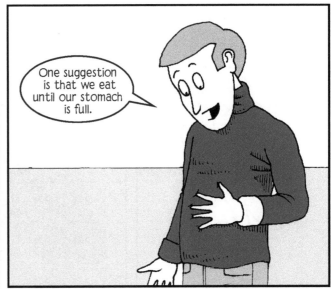

One suggestion is that we eat until our stomach is full.

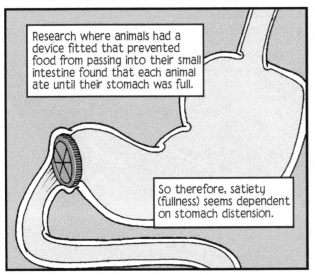

Research where animals had a device fitted that prevented food from passing into their small intestine found that each animal ate until their stomach was full.

So therefore, satiety (fullness) seems dependent on stomach distension.

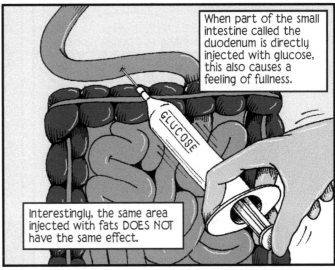

When part of the small intestine called the duodenum is directly injected with glucose, this also causes a feeling of fullness.

Interestingly, the same area injected with fats DOES NOT have the same effect.

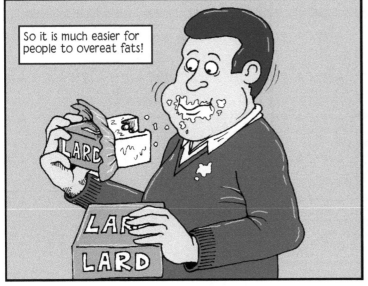

So it is much easier for people to overeat fats!

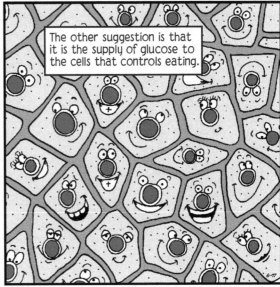

The other suggestion is that it is the supply of glucose to the cells that controls eating.

In fact, research HAS found glucose receptors in the hypothalamus.

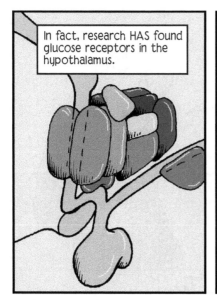

However, fruit sugar (fructose) also suppresses hunger and this cannot be converted to glucose or get through the blood/brain barrier to the hypothalamus.

So the availability of glucose cannot be the only mechanism to suppress hunger.

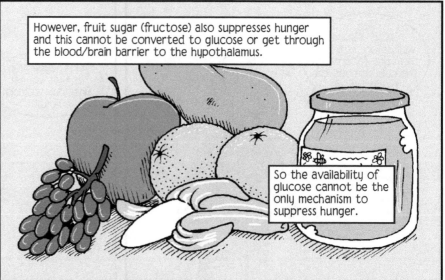

It is worth pointing out that it is not the amount of glucose in the blood that affects hunger since this hardly varies at all.

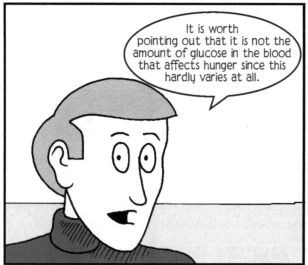

The availability of glucose to cells DOES vary according to two hormones produced by the pancreas.

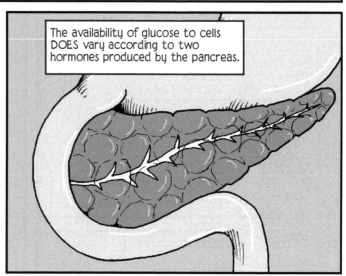

Insulin facilitates the entry of glucose into cells.

Glucagon has the reverse effect, so that liver cells convert stored glycogen to glucose and thus raising blood glucose levels.

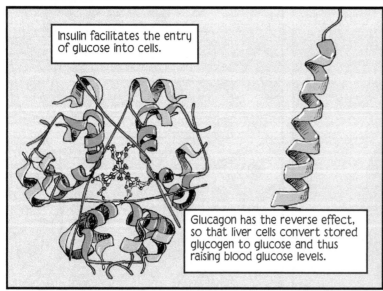

Basically, when insulin levels are high, hunger is low since the blood is supplying cells with glucose.

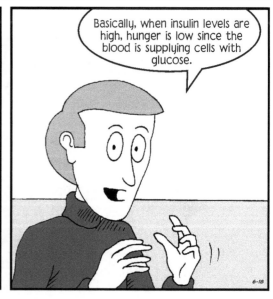

6-18

The Hypothalamus seems to be the most important area of the brain in terms of controlling eating.

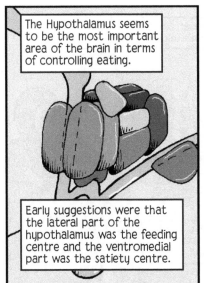

Early suggestions were that the lateral part of the hypothalamus was the feeding centre and the ventromedial part was the satiety centre.

Modern research has shown that this as a little too simplistic.

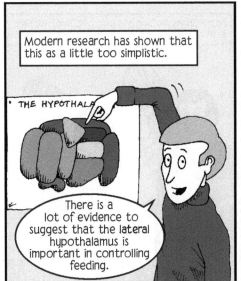

THE HYPOTHALA

There is a lot of evidence to suggest that the lateral hypothalamus is important in controlling feeding.

Damage to the lateral hypothalamus causes animals to stop eating and drinking.

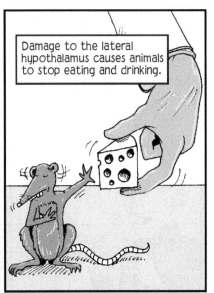

While stimulation of this area causes an animal to eat and engage in food seeking behaviour.

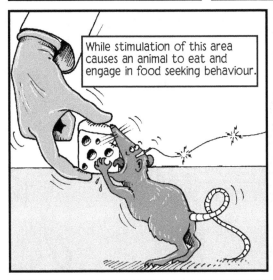

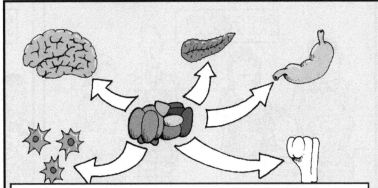

The hypothalamus is connected to the medulla where taste is processed, to dopamine nerve cells that reinforce learned behaviours, to the forebrain structures facilitating ingestion and swallowing of food and also to the pancreas to stimulate the release of insulin and stomach juices.

Damage to the ventromedial areas of the hypothalamus causes overeating.

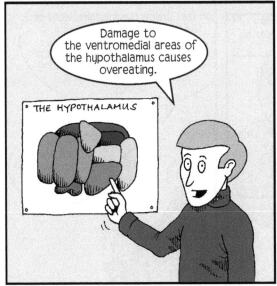

THE HYPOTHALAMUS

Rats with damage to the paraventricular nucleus of the hypothalamus eat much larger meals than normal.

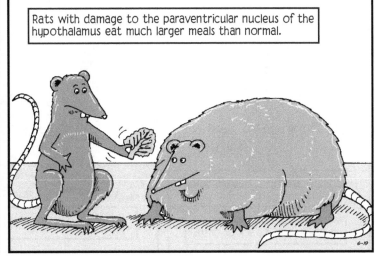

In terms of survival, animals need to make a decision about whether to either eat only what is needed at any one time or to eat as much as possible in one meal in case no more food is available for a while.

This depends on how difficult it is to find food and the consequences of carrying extra weight.

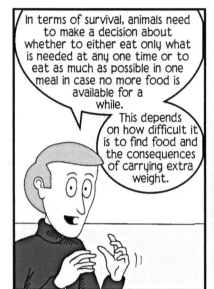

From an evolutionary perspective, humans appear to have developed a strategy of eating as much as they can when they find food.

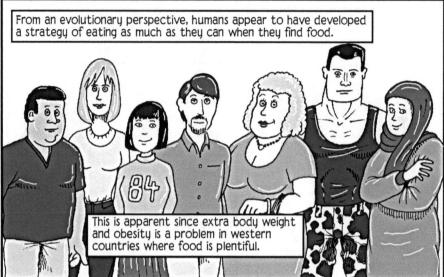

This is apparent since extra body weight and obesity is a problem in western countries where food is plentiful.

Genetics also play a role in body size.

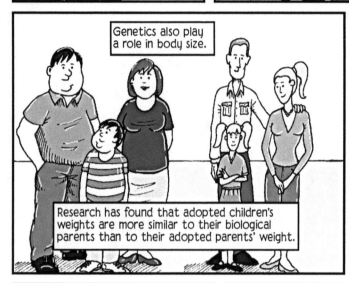

Research has found that adopted children's weights are more similar to their biological parents than to their adopted parents' weight.

People with high metabolic rates produce more heat and thus maintain their weight.

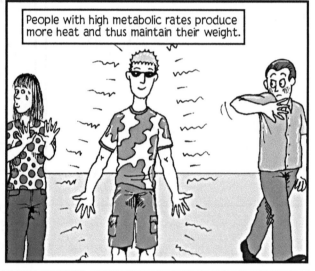

While exercise can increase your energy expenditure, since your muscles are quite efficient, it is difficult to lose a great deal of weight this way.

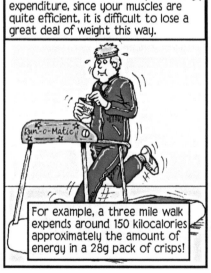

For example, a three mile walk expends around 150 kilocalories approximately the amount of energy in a 28g pack of crisps!

Similarly, if you reduce your intake of food by dieting, your body reacts by reducing your metabolic rate!

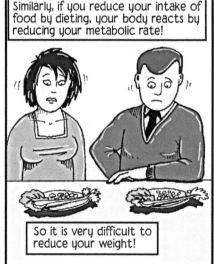

So it is very difficult to reduce your weight!

In fact, given the multiple areas of the brain that control eating, it seems more amazing that the majority of people DO eat a good balance of foods and that eating problems are not **more** widespread.

Anyway, all this talk of food has made me hungry – I'm off for a snack!

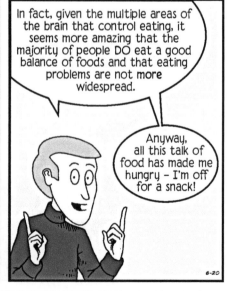

6-20

Temperature regulation hunger and thirst

▶ **PAGE 119**

Panel 6

There is a link connecting temperature regulation, hunger and thirst. These three areas are connected in explaining the *motivation* of animals and people. In other words, they explain why people do what they do. In psychological terms, motivation explains the factors that begin and maintain behaviour. Motivation expands the 'causes' of behaviour beyond just the outside stimuli to internal states like hunger and thirst. However, motivation is a concept not some kind of brain structure. There is no 'motivation centre' in the brain, for example.

There are three theories of motivation in psychology: *instincts, drive theory* and *arousal theory.*

Instincts

The ancient Greeks believed that animal and human behaviour was motivated by instincts. An instinct is an automatic, unlearned behaviour that happens in all members of a particular species. In animals, a good example of this is migration in birds. Early theorists (e.g. McDougall, 1908) also suggested that human motivation was determined by instincts in areas like aggression and maternal behaviour. In more modern times, however, the idea of human motivation being guided by instincts is less popular although instincts in animals are definitely accepted.

Drive Theory

Drive theory suggests that the body maintains certain factors in a balance called *homeostasis.* Any change from homeostasis causes a drive, which is an aroused condition (Hull, 1951). So, for example, if the temperature drops, the person or animal engages a drive that causes them to seek warmth. As the temperature rises the drive drops. The main criticism of drive theory is that much behaviour is difficult to associate with the maintenance of the physical aspects of the body. Students can be very motivated to get high marks in exams, for example, although this does not impact on their immediate bodily needs. This problem led to an expansion of drive theory to include *incentive* theory that allows for motivation by external stimuli (Bolles, 1975). In this case exam marks act as incentives.

Arousal Theory

Arousal theory is another modification of drive theory that states that motivation concerns the maintenance of an optimal level of physiological arousal (Fiske & Maddi, 1961). The optimal level varies from person to person.

More modern approaches to drive theory see drives as states of the brain (Stellar & Stellar, 1985).

▶ **PAGE 121**

Panel 1

The best analogy for homeostasis is a room thermostat. This is the device that ensures that the heating in a home keeps the room at a constant temperature. The thermostat monitors the temperature in the room and is set at a specific temperature, for example 20°C. If the room temperature drops below 20°C then the thermostat turns the heating on to raise the temperature. When the temperature reaches 20°C then the thermostat turns the heating off. Homeostasis has a similar principle, when a substance in the body drops below a certain level or range then the body engages physiological and behavioural mechanisms to obtain the substance until it reaches the required level.

Panel 6

There are other reasons that temperature regulation, hunger and thirst are not completely homeostatic. Firstly, as noted, they anticipate future needs (Appley, 1991). Secondly, set points for body temperature, body fat and other factors vary with time of day and time of year (Mrosovsky, 1990). Finally, with hunger people (and animals) will overeat in the presence of particularly tasty food meaning that there must also be non-homeostatic mechanisms at work (de Castro & Plunkett, 2002).

▶ **PAGE 122**

Panels 3 to 5

The distinction between *Homeothermic* (mammals and birds) and *Poikilothermic* (reptiles, amphibians and fish) animals used by Kalat (2004) is not used by all. Garrett (2003), for example, describes mammals and birds as *Endothermic* and reptiles, amphibians and fish as *Homeothermic*. Toates (2001), however, uses *Endothermic* to refer to animals that have an internal heat source (mammals and birds) and *Ectothermic* for those that have an external heat source (reptiles, amphibians and fish). In fact the distinction is relative rather than absolute and is quite a complex area.

In addition, it is a fallacy to refer to reptiles and amphibians by the term 'cold blooded'. These and other poikilothermic animals still need to keep their body temperature constant. The real difference between poikilothermic and homeothermic animals (mammals and birds) is that whilst homeothermic animals can generate their own body heat whilst poikilothermic animals control their body temperature by selecting different environmental locations.

The other difference is that homeothermic animals need to ingest many more calories in order to control their temperature. Poikilothermic animals need to eat much less food in comparison. Additionally, the smaller the homeothermic animal the more food they need to consume. Mice, for example, need to eat much more proportionally than an elephant. This is because small animals have a large surface area to their skin when compared to the mass of their body. This means that small animals lose a lot more heat from their body to the environment than larger animals. The smaller the surface area to body mass ratio, the more heat is lost and the more food needs to be consumed (comparatively speaking of course) in order to replace that body temperature.

Panel 6

Poikilothermic animals such as reptiles and fish are quite vulnerable to very cold weather. If the environmental temperature is below the freezing point of water there is a danger that the animal's blood will freeze. This causes ice crystals to form in the blood vessels. These ice crystals rupture the blood vessels and break the cell walls causing the animal to die. Some poikilothermic animals can survive in extremely cold environments by having antifreeze chemicals in their blood and having other mechanisms to reduce the damage done to blood vessels during a cold period.

▶ **PAGE 123**

Panel 1

Reproductive cells, like sperm and eggs, tend to need slightly lower temperatures than the rest of the body for their development.

Panel 7

Goose bumps are the result of an attempt to raise the hairs on our body. Since we don't have much 'fur' the raising of the hairs does not really help to increase the insulation of the body.

▶ **PAGE 124**

Panel 1

It is generally easier to heat up the body than to cool it down. Cooling down the body can create serious problems with dehydration since it involves using water from the body to evaporate at the surface.

Panel 4

Cats and dogs, for example, only sweat from the pads on their feet.

▶ **PAGE 125**

Panel 2

The preoptic area is so called because it is close to the Optic Chiasm (see Chapter 2 on Vision).

The other area of the hypothalamus that is important in temperature control is the *anterior hypothalamus*. The preoptic area and the anterior hypothalamus together are considered one area that is sometimes referred to as the POA/AH area. This area also receives information from receptors in the skin.

Nelson and Prosser (1981) reported the finding that this area monitors its own temperature.

Panel 3

If the preoptic area is cooled down the animal will also engage in behavioural activity to heat itself up (Santinoff, 1964).

Panel 4

See Refinetti and Carlisle (1986).

Panel 6

When you have an infection, the white blood cells in your blood fight the bacteria or virus causing the infection. These white cells are called *leukocytes* and they cause the release of chemicals called *prostaglandins*. It is the prostaglandins that stimulate the POA/AH to raise body temperature and therefore cause a fever.

Panel 7

The work on newborn rabbits was carried out by Satinoff, McEwan and Williams (1976).

▶ **PAGE 126**

Panel 1

The finding that moderate fevers increase your chances of survival was reported by Kluger (1991).

Panel 2

A fever of 41°C to 43°C can be fatal (Rommel, Pabst & McLellan, 1998).

Panel 3

Humans can survive for a few weeks without food but cannot go without water for more than a few days.

Panel 4

Most mammals are 70 per cent water.

▶ **PAGE 127**

Panel 1

The body has many different adaptations to prevent the loss of water. The nose, for example, is designed to reabsorb the water vapour in our breath.

Panel 6

The human ability to adapt to hot environments is dependent on the release of a hormone. *Vasopressin* is released when the body needs to conserve water. This causes the constriction of blood vessels and therefore compensates for a decrease in blood volume. Vasopressin is also known as *anti-diuretic hormone* because it causes the kidneys to reabsorb water from the urine and thus excrete more concentrated urine.

Bear in mind that these mechanisms can only compensate up to a point for human life in dry, hot environments. Desert mammals, like gerbils, are much better adapted for living in these environments than humans.

▶ **PAGE 128**

Panel 4

Osmosis is a natural occurrence where water molecules move from an area of low 'salt' concentration to an area of high 'salt' concentration across a semi-permeable membrane. As highlighted in the notes for Chapter 1, cell walls are considered 'semi-permeable' since they allow some substances through and not others. One of the things that the membrane allows 'free' passage to are water molecules. The spaces inside cells are called *intracellular* spaces and the spaces between cells is called *extracellular*. Both the intracellular and the extracellular spaces are filled with salts dissolved in water.

If the extracellular spaces are more concentrated with salts than the intracellular spaces, then osmosis causes water to move from the inside of cells to the outside of cells until the concentration of both fluids is the same. If this movement of water is extensive then this will cause the cells to shrink.

If the fluid inside cells is more concentrated with salts than that on the outside then osmosis causes water to move from the extracellular spaces to the intracellular spaces until the concentration of salts equalises.

The 'need' for the water to move from an area of low concentration to an area of high concentration is known as *osmotic pressure*. It is osmotic pressure that triggers osmotic thirst.

Panel 7

We actually stop drinking well before water reaches the cells. There are receptors in the stomach and other parts of the digestive system that detect how much water has been drunk that then stop drinking behaviour (Huang, Sved & Stricker, 2000).

▶ **PAGE 129**

Panel 1

The blood/brain barrier is not completely absent in the third ventricle. It is, however, the part of the barrier that allows most substances through (Simon, 2000).

Panel 7

Hypovolemic thirst means thirst caused by low volume.

▶ **PAGE 130**

Panel 1

Hypovolemic thirst can also be triggered through very heavy sweating and excessive diarrhoea.

Panel 2

See Stricker (1969).

Panels 3 to 4

The triggers for hypovolemic thirst are based on two different mechanisms. The first uses receptors attached to large veins to detect a drop in blood pressure (these receptors are called *baroreceptors*). The second mechanism depends on the detection of a drop in blood volume. This causes the release of hormones by the kidneys that cause the constriction of the blood vessels to compensate for the drop in blood volume.

▶ **PAGE 131**

Panel 4

See Leshem (1999) and Richter (1936).

Panel 5

The hormonal control of sodium hunger was reported by Schulkin (1991). The automatic hunger for sodium is also controlled by hormones. When a drop in salt in the body is detected, the adrenal glands produce *aldosterone* that causes the kidneys, the salivary and sweat glands to retain salt. This also causes an increase in the preference for salty foods.

Panel 6

While hunger is considered a homeostatic drive it has some notable differences from thirst and temperature control. Firstly, hunger concerns a number of different factors (in other words the different nutrients found in food) and not just one as in the case of thirst or temperature. Secondly, the set points of the nutrients required change (sometimes dramatically and quickly). In essence, hunger is a very complex drive that provides energy for body activity and fuel for maintaining body temperature.

▶ **PAGE 132**

Panel 1

The function of the digestive system is to break down food into small enough molecules that can be absorbed into the bloodstream and ultimately be used by the body's cells. The first aspect of this is to break the food down physically by chewing. The second aspect is to mix the food with chemicals that break the food down chemically. These chemicals are called *enzymes*. There are different enzymes that break down different foods.

Panel 3

The stomach has several functions. Firstly, the start of protein digestion happens in the stomach. Secondly, the stomach acts as a container for food. This storage is useful for protecting the body from absorbing anything harmful. The initial process is to kill any harmful bacteria with the acid that is part of the stomach juices. In addition, if the stomach lining is irritated then the stomach regurgitates its contents. However, if the toxic substance does not irritate the stomach lining and does get absorbed into the bloodstream then it is quickly detected in the *area postrema* of the brain. This is an area in the brain where the blood-brain barrier is weak so toxic substances can directly cause vomiting. The force of the vomiting can be an indicator of the toxicity of the ingested food.

Panel 6

Cells use glucose for energy. Excess nutrients are stored as glycogen (for later conversion to glucose); fats (these can also be used for energy later on); and proteins.

▶ **PAGE 133**

Panel 1

One of the more complex aspects of hunger for an animal is deciding what and how much to eat. Some animals, like some snakes, eat huge meals at one time and then can spend several weeks without eating. Other animals (like some small birds) tend to eat many small meals throughout the day.

Panel 4

Children tend to acquire cultural tastes as well as their parents' tastes. This is especially the case with regard to spicy food (Rozin, 1990).

The work on young rat food preference was reported by Galef (1992).

Panel 8

The avoidance of food following illness is called a *conditioned taste aversion*. This happens after only one pairing of food with illness. This is quite incredible, especially given that the illness will tend to happen several hours after the food is eaten. See Rozin and Kalat (1971) and Rozin and Zellner (1985).

▶ **PAGE 134**

Panel 4

See Jordan (1969) and Spiegel (1973).

Panel 6

See Smith (1998).

▶ **PAGE 135**

Panel 3

The study that showed that satiety was determined by stomach fullness was conducted by Deutsch, Young and Kalogeris (1978).

The stretching of the stomach walls is conveyed to the brain via the *vagus* nerve. Information about the nutrient content of the stomach is sent to the brain by the *splanchnic* nerve.

There is also evidence that the stretching of the walls of the small intestine (known as the duodenum) also causes a feeling of fullness (Seeley, Kaplan & Grill, 1995).

▶ PAGE 136

Panel 5

People produce more insulin when they eat and when they are getting ready to eat. This prepares the body for the entry of glucose into the cells.

Panel 6

Excessively high or low levels of insulin in the blood are both causes of overeating.

People with obesity tend to produce more insulin than people of normal weight (Johnson & Wildman, 1983).

▶ PAGE 137

Panel 2

Leibowitz and Hoebel (1998) compared the lateral hypothalamus to a large railway station. This is because it contains a large number of neuron groups and many axons, all of which control eating behaviour. They also summarised the lateral hypothalamus' contribution to feeding:

i)   It alters the taste sensation and salivation response to certain tastes.
ii) It is connected to the pituitary gland and causes it to release hormones that result in an increase of insulin secretion.
iii) It stimulates other areas of the brain, including the cortex, causing them to increase their response to the visual, taste, and smell aspects of food (Critchley & Rolls, 1996).
iv) Axons that pass through the lateral hypothalamus help to reinforce learned behaviours associated with certain foods.
v)   It stimulates areas of the spinal cord to begin autonomic responses like the secretion of digestive enzymes.

Stimulating the lateral hypothalamus in an animal causes it to eat and seek food. Damage to the lateral hypothalamus will cause an animal to refuse to eat or drink.

Panel 7

Damage to the paraventricular nucleus of the hypothalamus causes rats to eat larger meals not eat more frequently (Leibowitz, Hammer & Chang, 1981). More frequent eating is caused by damage to the ventromedial hypothalamus (Peters, Sensenig & Reich, 1973). Both situations cause rats to gain excessive amounts of weight.

▶ PAGE 138

Panel 6

The best way to lose weight is to use a combination of moderate exercise coupled with a decrease in food intake. Exercise also helps to lower blood pressure, lower blood cholesterol and generally improve levels of health (Campfield, Smith & Burn, 1998).

CHAPTER 7
EMOTIONS AND SEXUAL BEHAVIOUR

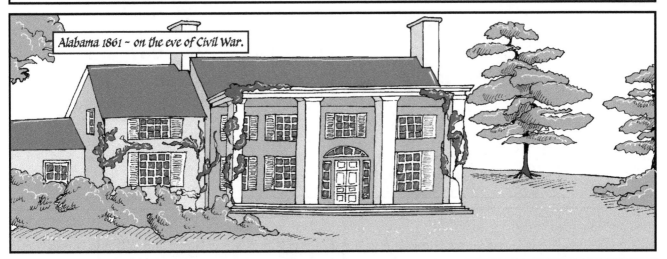

Alabama 1861 ~ on the eve of Civil War.

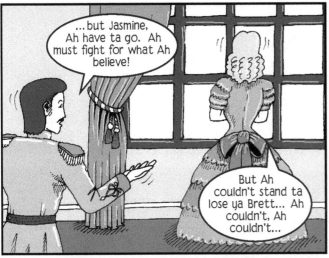

...but Jasmine, Ah have ta go. Ah must fight for what Ah believe!

But Ah couldn't stand ta lose ya Brett... Ah couldn't, Ah couldn't...

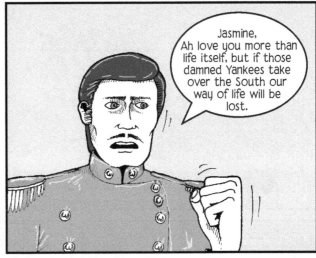

Jasmine, Ah love you more than life itself, but if those damned Yankees take over the South our way of life will be lost.

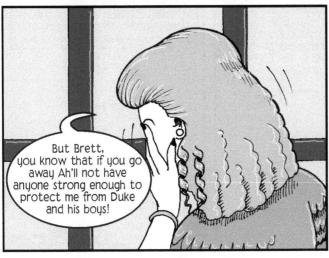

But Brett, you know that if you go away Ah'll not have anyone strong enough to protect me from Duke and his boys!

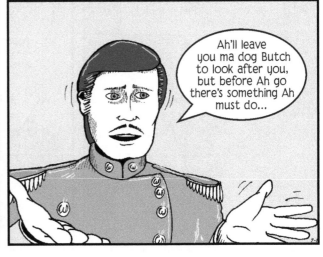

Ah'll leave you ma dog Butch to look after you, but before Ah go there's something Ah must do...

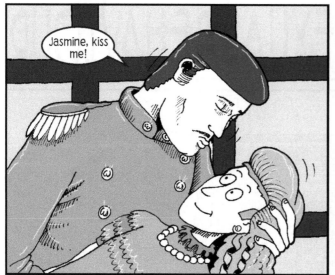

Jasmine, kiss me!

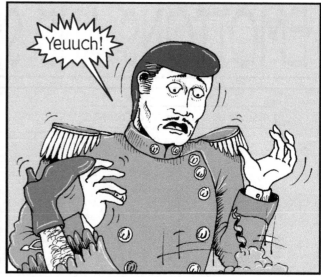

Yeuuch!

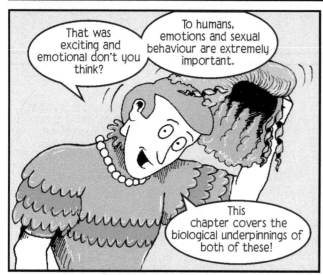

That was exciting and emotional don't you think?

To humans, emotions and sexual behaviour are extremely important.

This chapter covers the biological underpinnings of both of these!

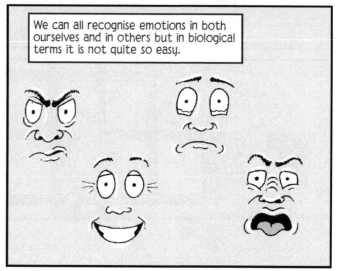

We can all recognise emotions in both ourselves and in others but in biological terms it is not quite so easy.

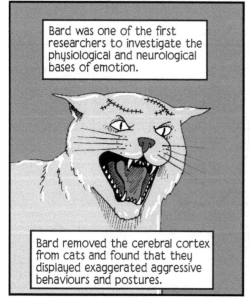

Bard was one of the first researchers to investigate the physiological and neurological bases of emotion.

Bard removed the cerebral cortex from cats and found that they displayed exaggerated aggressive behaviours and postures.

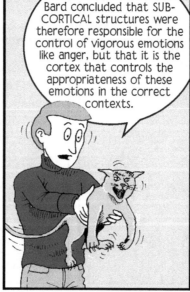

Bard concluded that SUB-CORTICAL structures were therefore responsible for the control of vigorous emotions like anger, but that it is the cortex that controls the appropriateness of these emotions in the correct contexts.

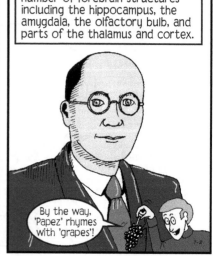

J. W. Papez suggested that emotional responses depend on a number of forebrain structures including the hippocampus, the amygdala, the olfactory bulb, and parts of the thalamus and cortex.

By the way, 'Papez' rhymes with 'grapes'!

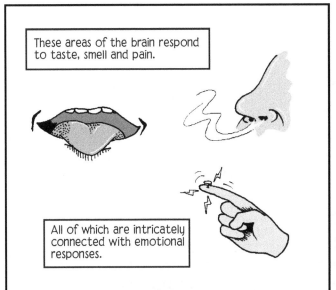

These areas of the brain respond to taste, smell and pain.

All of which are intricately connected with emotional responses.

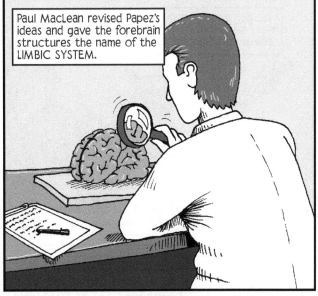

Paul MacLean revised Papez's ideas and gave the forebrain structures the name of the LIMBIC SYSTEM.

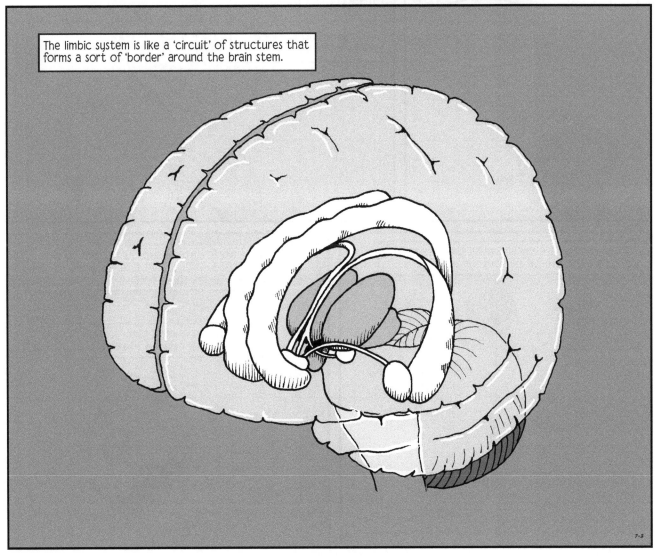

The limbic system is like a 'circuit' of structures that forms a sort of 'border' around the brain stem.

MacLean also noticed that the size of the limbic system varies little across mammals compared to the cerebral cortex.

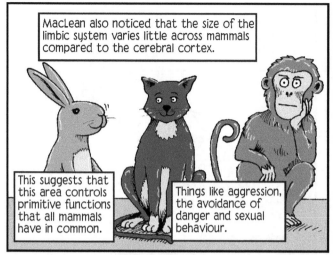

This suggests that this area controls primitive functions that all mammals have in common.

Things like aggression, the avoidance of danger and sexual behaviour.

Later research clarified the role of the limbic system.

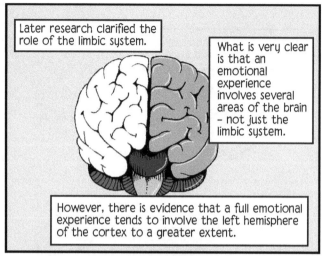

What is very clear is that an emotional experience involves several areas of the brain – not just the limbic system.

However, there is evidence that a full emotional experience tends to involve the left hemisphere of the cortex to a greater extent.

Emotions, however, are not just present in the Brain.

Emotions are often accompanied by physiological changes to the body.

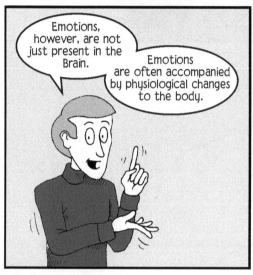

These changes are known as AUTONOMIC AROUSAL and include an increase in heart rate, perspiration, blood pressure and so on.

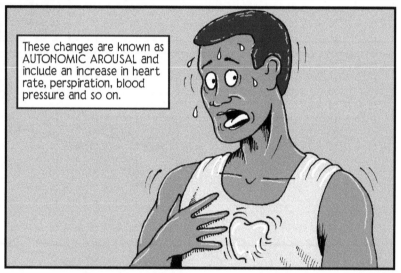

These changes are controlled by the sympathetic and parasympathetic nervous systems.

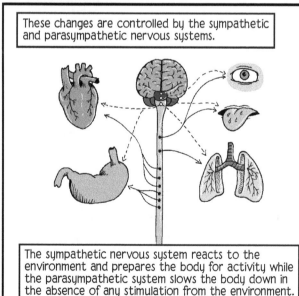

The sympathetic nervous system reacts to the environment and prepares the body for activity while the parasympathetic system slows the body down in the absence of any stimulation from the environment.

Neurons in the limbic system send their signals to the hindbrain structures – like the medulla and pons – which are then relayed to the spinal cord.

It is the spinal cord that controls the sympathetic nervous system.

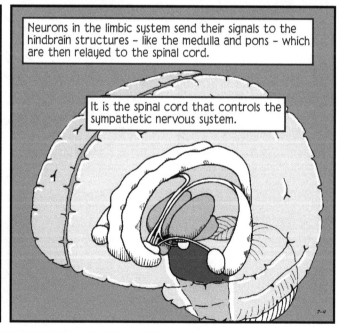

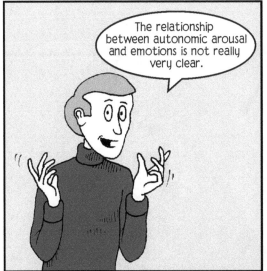

The relationship between autonomic arousal and emotions is not really very clear.

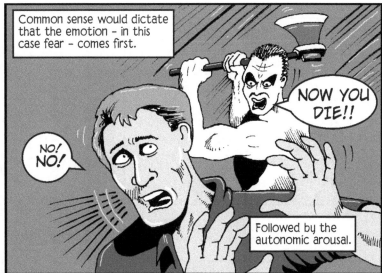

Common sense would dictate that the emotion - in this case fear - comes first.

NO! NO!

NOW YOU DIE!!

Followed by the autonomic arousal.

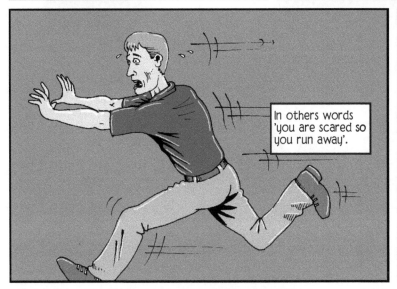

In others words 'you are scared so you run away'.

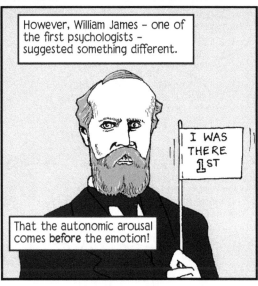

However, William James - one of the first psychologists - suggested something different.

I WAS THERE 1ST

That the autonomic arousal comes before the emotion!

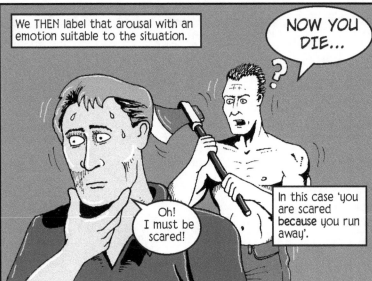

We THEN label that arousal with an emotion suitable to the situation.

NOW YOU DIE...

?

Oh! I must be scared!

In this case 'you are scared because you run away'.

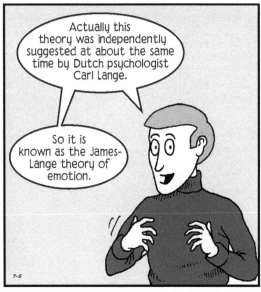

Actually this theory was independently suggested at about the same time by Dutch psychologist Carl Lange.

So it is known as the James-Lange theory of emotion.

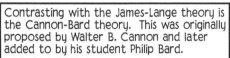

Contrasting with the James-Lange theory is the Cannon-Bard theory. This was originally proposed by Walter B. Cannon and later added to by his student Philip Bard.

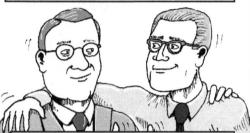

The Cannon-Bard theory suggests that emotion AND the autonomic arousal occur at the same time BUT independently from each other.

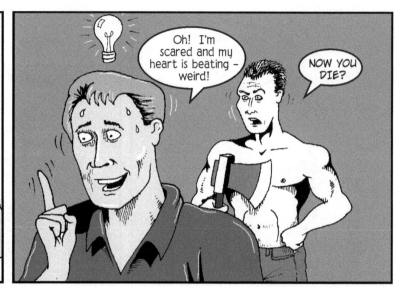

Oh! I'm scared and my heart is beating – weird!

NOW YOU DIE?

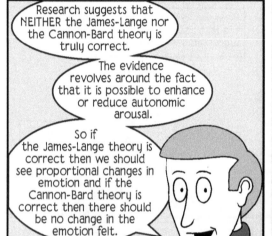

Research suggests that NEITHER the James-Lange nor the Cannon-Bard theory is truly correct.

The evidence revolves around the fact that it is possible to enhance or reduce autonomic arousal.

So if the James-Lange theory is correct then we should see proportional changes in emotion and if the Cannon-Bard theory is correct then there should be no change in the emotion felt.

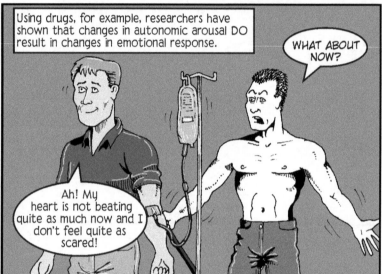

Using drugs, for example, researchers have shown that changes in autonomic arousal DO result in changes in emotional response.

WHAT ABOUT NOW?

Ah! My heart is not beating quite as much now and I don't feel quite as scared!

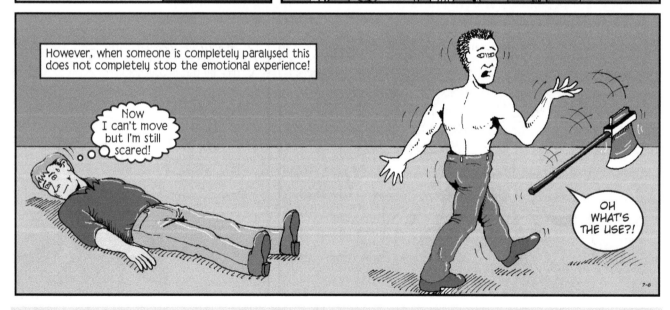

However, when someone is completely paralysed this does not completely stop the emotional experience!

Now I can't move but I'm still scared!

OH WHAT'S THE USE?!

7-6

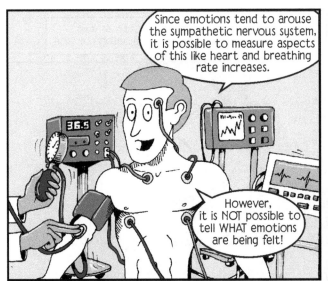

Since emotions tend to arouse the sympathetic nervous system, it is possible to measure aspects of this like heart and breathing rate increases.

However, it is NOT possible to tell WHAT emotions are being felt!

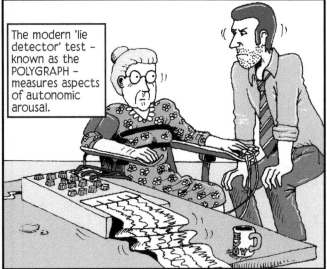

The modern 'lie detector' test – known as the POLYGRAPH – measures aspects of autonomic arousal.

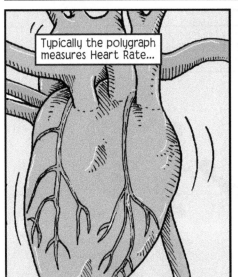

Typically the polygraph measures Heart Rate...

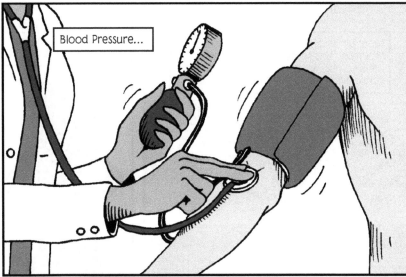

Blood Pressure...

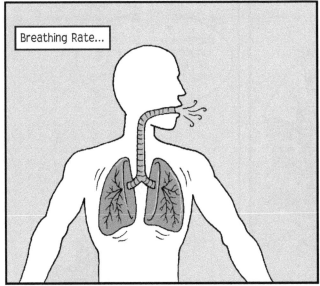

Breathing Rate...

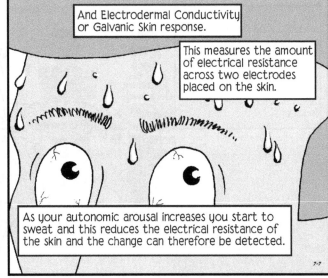

And Electrodermal Conductivity or Galvanic Skin response.

This measures the amount of electrical resistance across two electrodes placed on the skin.

As your autonomic arousal increases you start to sweat and this reduces the electrical resistance of the skin and the change can therefore be detected.

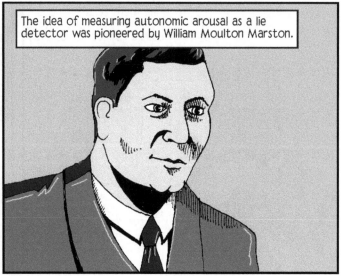

The theory behind the polygraph is that when someone lies, their nervousness increases and so their autonomic arousal increases and these changes can be measured.

The idea of measuring autonomic arousal as a lie detector was pioneered by William Moulton Marston.

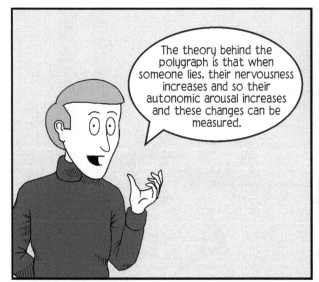

Later under the pen name of 'Charles Moulton', this respected psychologist also created and wrote the adventures of the comic book character 'Wonder Woman'.

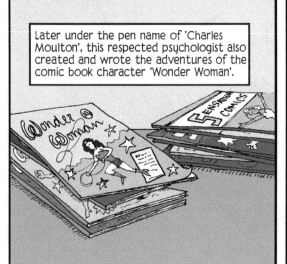

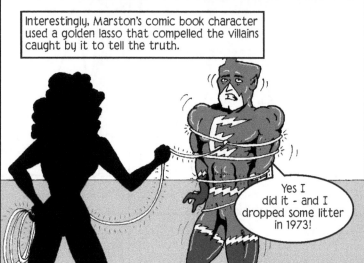

Interestingly, Marston's comic book character used a golden lasso that compelled the villains caught by it to tell the truth.

Yes I did it - and I dropped some litter in 1973!

The problem with the idea of measuring changes in autonomic arousal to detect lying is that some people can remain very calm whilst lying while others can be very nervous and yet be completely innocent.

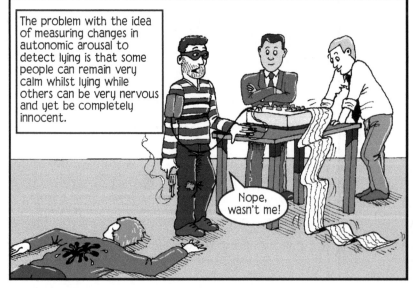

Nope, wasn't me!

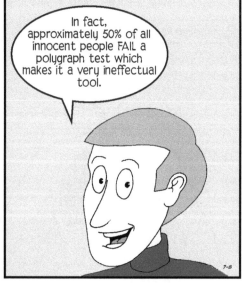

In fact, approximately 50% of all innocent people FAIL a polygraph test which makes it a very ineffectual tool.

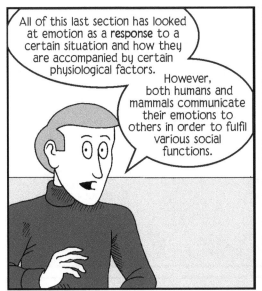

All of this last section has looked at emotion as a **response** to a certain situation and how they are accompanied by certain physiological factors. However, both humans and mammals communicate their emotions to others in order to fulfil various social functions.

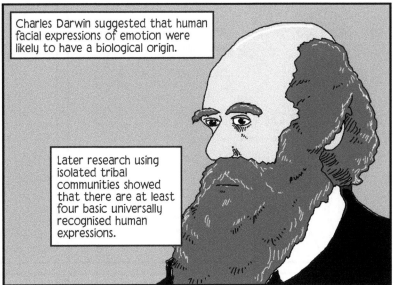

Charles Darwin suggested that human facial expressions of emotion were likely to have a biological origin.

Later research using isolated tribal communities showed that there are at least four basic universally recognised human expressions.

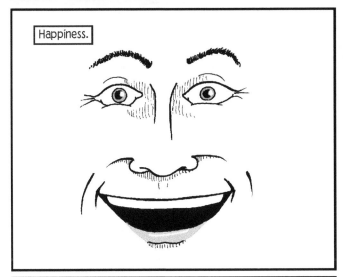

Happiness.

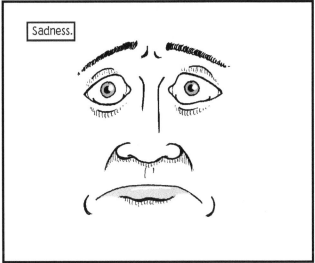

Sadness.

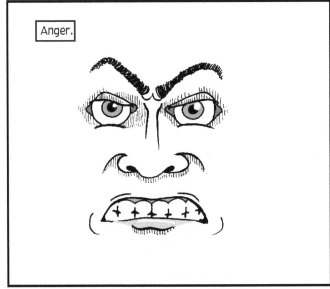

Anger.

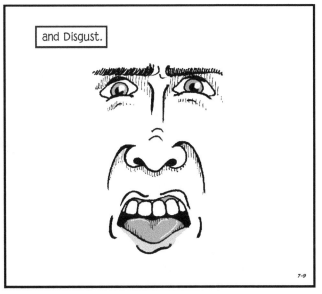

and Disgust.

7-9

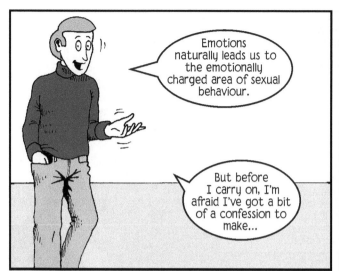

Emotions naturally leads us to the emotionally charged area of sexual behaviour.

But before I carry on, I'm afraid I've got a bit of a confession to make...

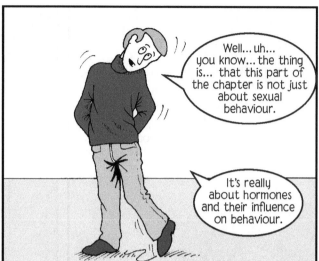

Well...uh... you know...the thing is... that this part of the chapter is not just about sexual behaviour.

It's really about hormones and their influence on behaviour.

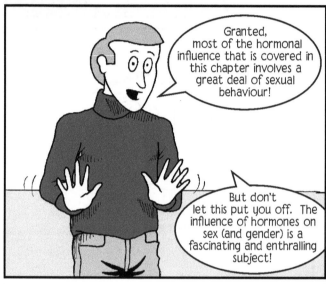

Granted, most of the hormonal influence that is covered in this chapter involves a great deal of sexual behaviour!

But don't let this put you off. The influence of hormones on sex (and gender) is a fascinating and enthralling subject!

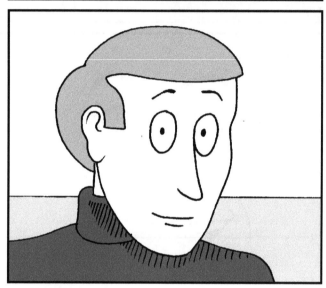

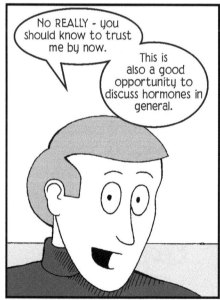

No REALLY - you should know to trust me by now.

This is also a good opportunity to discuss hormones in general.

However, I must warn you that there is some quite frank discussion from here on.

ADULTS ONLY

18

Suggested for Mature Readers

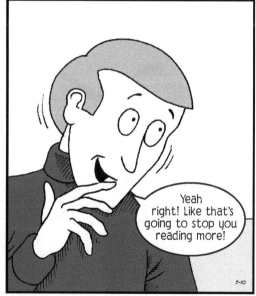

Yeah right! Like that's going to stop you reading more!

7-10

Hormones are chemicals that are secreted by a gland and sent by the bloodstream to the target.

Hormones control a large variety of human behaviour – especially sexual behaviour!

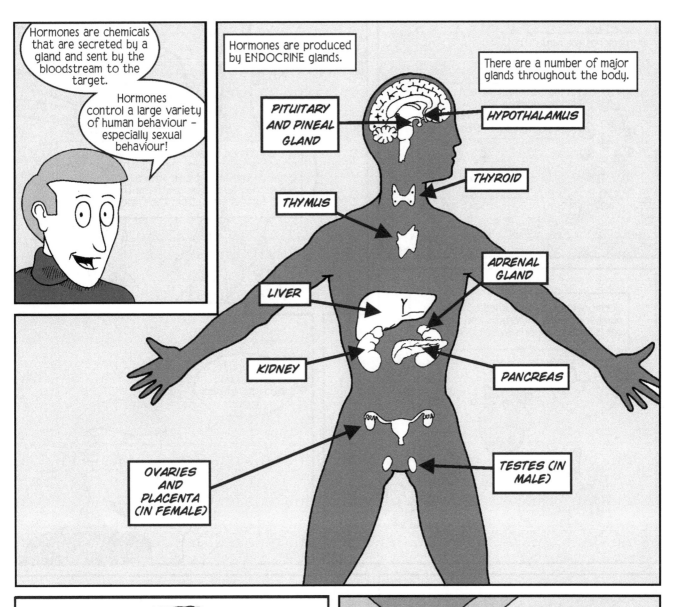

Hormones are produced by ENDOCRINE glands.

There are a number of major glands throughout the body.

PITUITARY AND PINEAL GLAND

HYPOTHALAMUS

THYROID

THYMUS

ADRENAL GLAND

LIVER

KIDNEY

PANCREAS

OVARIES AND PLACENTA (IN FEMALE)

TESTES (IN MALE)

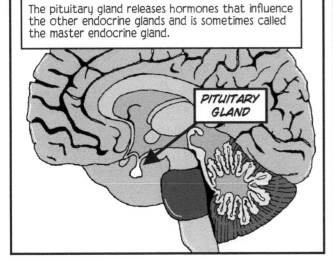

The pituitary gland releases hormones that influence the other endocrine glands and is sometimes called the master endocrine gland.

PITUITARY GLAND

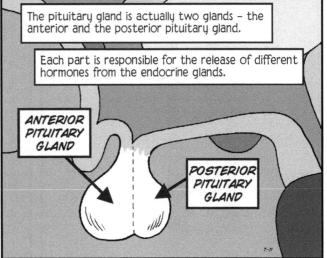

The pituitary gland is actually two glands – the anterior and the posterior pituitary gland.

Each part is responsible for the release of different hormones from the endocrine glands.

ANTERIOR PITUITARY GLAND

POSTERIOR PITUITARY GLAND

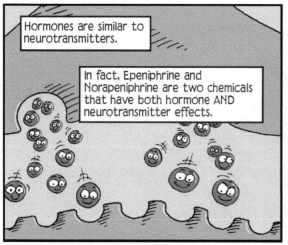

Hormones are similar to neurotransmitters.

In fact, Epeniphrine and Norapeniphrine are two chemicals that have both hormone AND neurotransmitter effects.

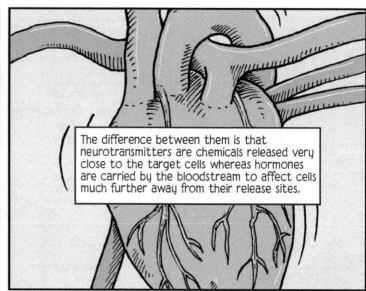

The difference between them is that neurotransmitters are chemicals released very close to the target cells whereas hormones are carried by the bloodstream to affect cells much further away from their release sites.

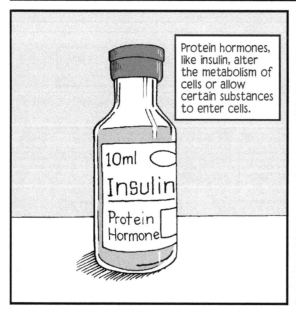

Hormones are also designed to affect a number of different organs and body parts to achieve one overall effect.

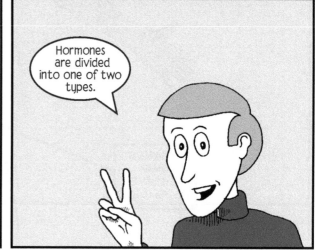

Hormones are divided into one of two types.

Protein hormones, like insulin, alter the metabolism of cells or allow certain substances to enter cells.

10ml Insulin Protein Hormone

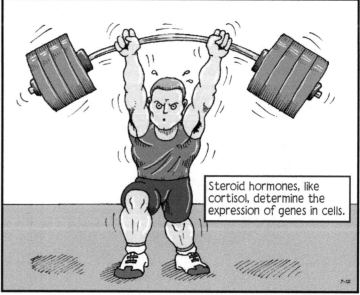

Steroid hormones, like cortisol, determine the expression of genes in cells.

7-12

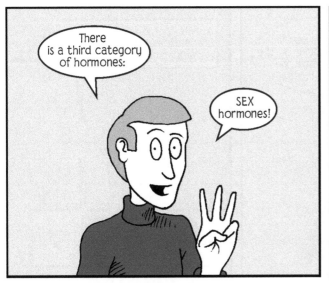

There is a third category of hormones:

SEX hormones!

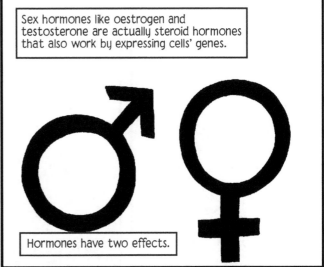

Sex hormones like oestrogen and testosterone are actually steroid hormones that also work by expressing cells' genes.

Hormones have two effects.

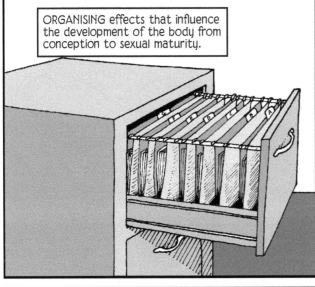

ORGANISING effects that influence the development of the body from conception to sexual maturity.

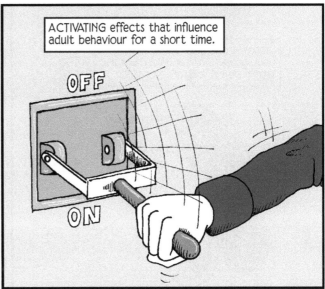

ACTIVATING effects that influence adult behaviour for a short time.

OFF

ON

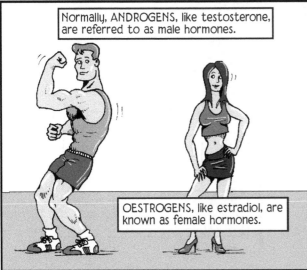

Normally, ANDROGENS, like testosterone, are referred to as male hormones.

OESTROGENS, like estradiol, are known as female hormones.

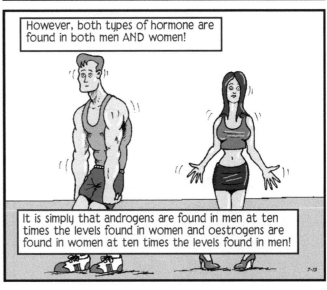

However, both types of hormone are found in both men AND women!

It is simply that androgens are found in men at ten times the levels found in women and oestrogens are found in women at ten times the levels found in men!

7-13

During early pre-natal development in mammals, the reproductive organs of a male and female foetus are identical.

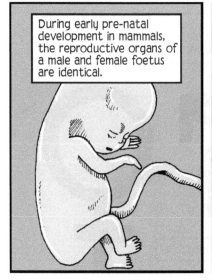

Whether these structures become male or female depend on the influence of testosterone in early development.

A male foetus has a Y chromosome that causes the development of testes.

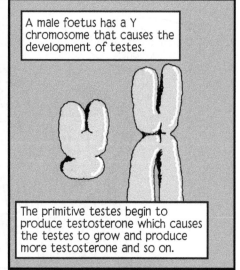

The primitive testes begin to produce testosterone which causes the testes to grow and produce more testosterone and so on.

Testosterone also causes the development of various structures into male reproductive organs.

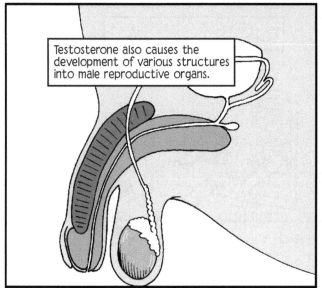

A female foetus does not develop testes and therefore does not get influenced by testosterone.

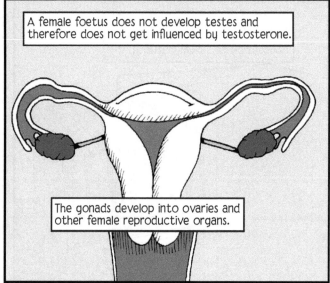

The gonads develop into ovaries and other female reproductive organs.

It is true, however, that a female foetus exposed to sufficient testosterone at a particular moment of development would develop male sexual organs!

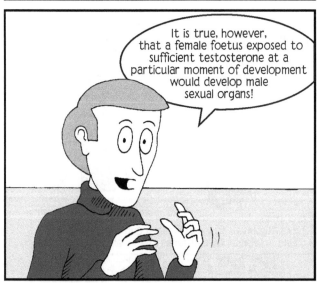

Changes in the foetus depend on the amount of testosterone it is exposed to during a SENSITIVE period in gestation.

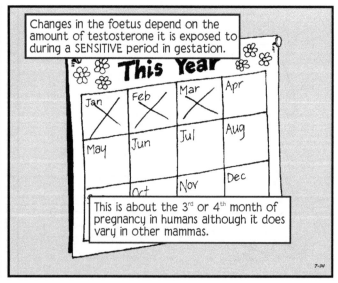

This is about the 3rd or 4th month of pregnancy in humans although it does vary in other mammas.

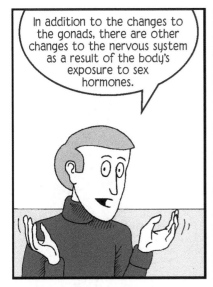

In addition to the changes to the gonads, there are other changes to the nervous system as a result of the body's exposure to sex hormones.

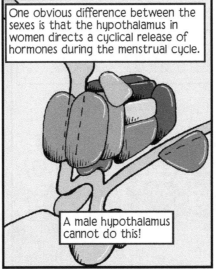

One obvious difference between the sexes is that the hypothalamus in women directs a cyclical release of hormones during the menstrual cycle.

A male hypothalamus cannot do this!

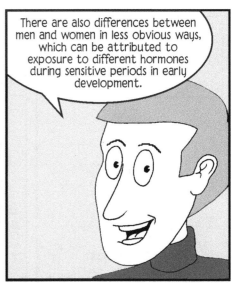

There are also differences between men and women in less obvious ways, which can be attributed to exposure to different hormones during sensitive periods in early development.

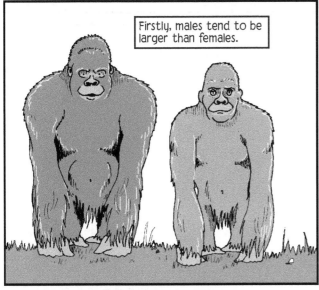

Firstly, males tend to be larger than females.

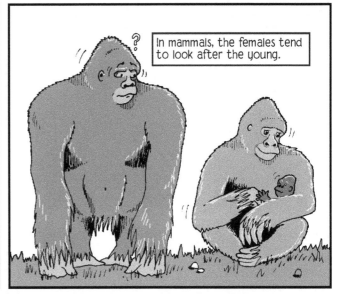

In mammals, the females tend to look after the young.

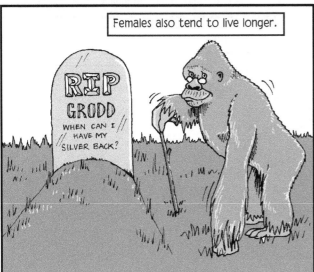

Females also tend to live longer.

RIP
GRODD
WHEN CAN I HAVE MY SILVER BACK?

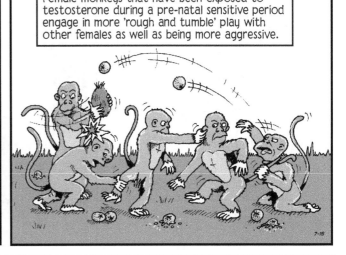

Female monkeys that have been exposed to testosterone during a pre-natal sensitive period engage in more 'rough and tumble' play with other females as well as being more aggressive.

There is some research evidence to suggest that girls who are exposed to male hormones in pre-natal development will engage in more boy-like behaviour like playing with boy's toys.

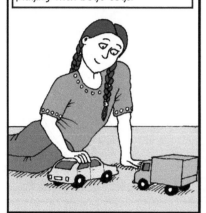

Of course, this finding is controversial and somewhat difficult to uphold since the girls involved had genetic abnormalities and tended to look more masculine.

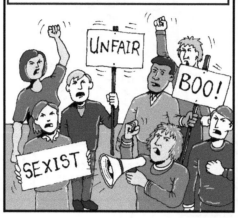

UNFAIR

BOO!

SEXIST

As mentioned earlier, hormones also have effects throughout life NOT just during a sensitive pre-natal period.

These are known as ACTIVATING effects.

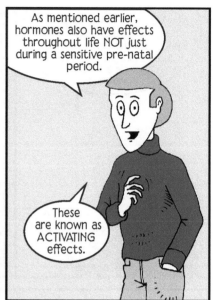

If the testes of a male rat are removed, then its interest in sexual activity decreases.

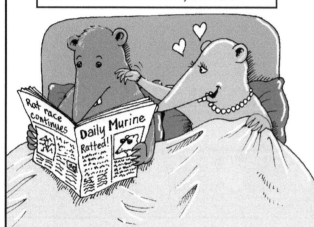

Rat race continues

Daily Murine

Ratted!

If the rat is then injected with testosterone its sexual interest returns.

Ooh Harold!

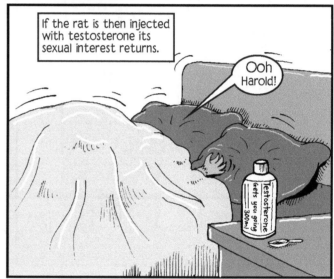

Testosterone (gets you going 300ml)

The same is true of female rats.

If their ovaries are removed, sexual behaviour decreases until female hormones are injected.

Certain behaviours can also **trigger** hormone release.

For example, dominance hierarchies in some monkey species causes the suppression of hormone release in the lower ranks.

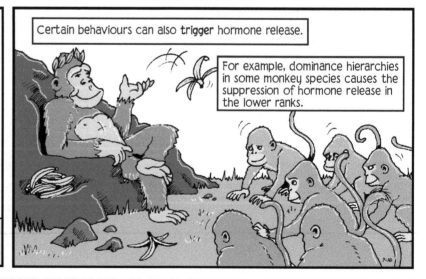

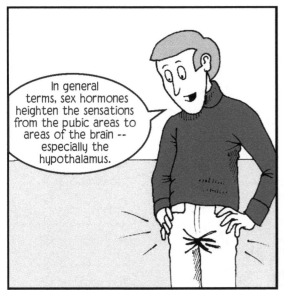

In general terms, sex hormones heighten the sensations from the pubic areas to areas of the brain -- especially the hypothalamus.

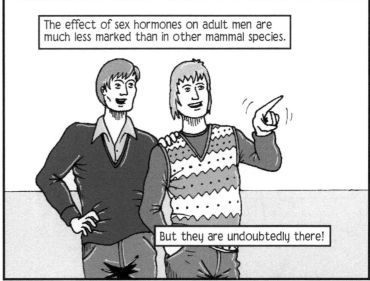

The effect of sex hormones on adult men are much less marked than in other mammal species.

But they are undoubtedly there!

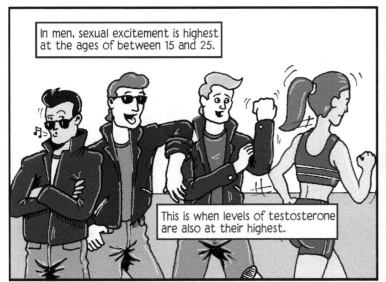

In men, sexual excitement is highest at the ages of between 15 and 25.

This is when levels of testosterone are also at their highest.

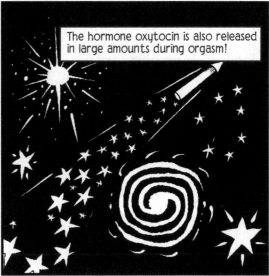

The hormone oxytocin is also released in large amounts during orgasm!

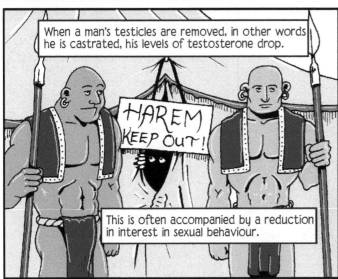

When a man's testicles are removed, in other words he is castrated, his levels of testosterone drop.

HAREM KEEP OUT!

This is often accompanied by a reduction in interest in sexual behaviour.

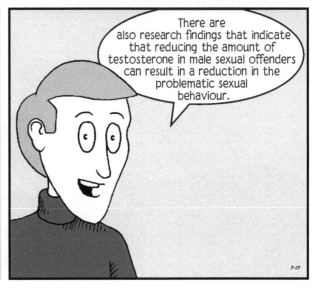

There are also research findings that indicate that reducing the amount of testosterone in male sexual offenders can result in a reduction in the problematic sexual behaviour.

7-17

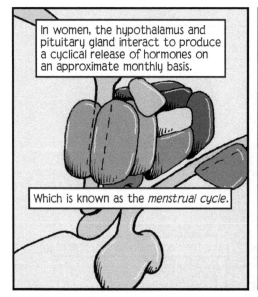

In women, the hypothalamus and pituitary gland interact to produce a cyclical release of hormones on an approximate monthly basis.

Which is known as the *menstrual cycle*.

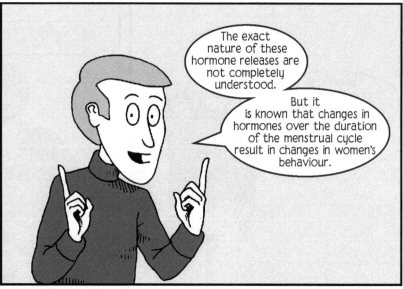

The exact nature of these hormone releases are not completely understood.

But it is known that changes in hormones over the duration of the menstrual cycle result in changes in women's behaviour.

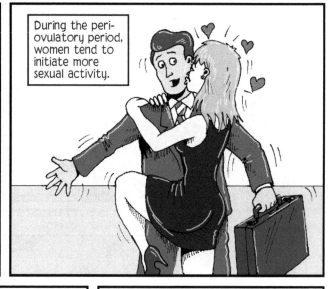

These changes in behaviour tend to occur around the moment just before ovulation - in other words just before the egg is released from the ovary - around the middle of the menstrual cycle.

This is known as the **peri-ovulatory** period and is the time of maximum fertility for a woman and is accompanied by high levels of estrogen.

During the peri-ovulatory period, women tend to initiate more sexual activity.

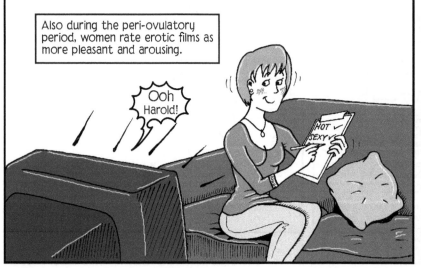

Also during the peri-ovulatory period, women rate erotic films as more pleasant and arousing.

Ooh Harold!

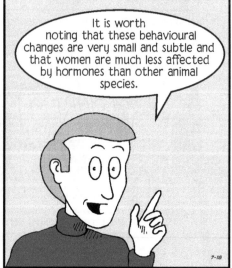

It is worth noting that these behavioural changes are very small and subtle and that women are much less affected by hormones than other animal species.

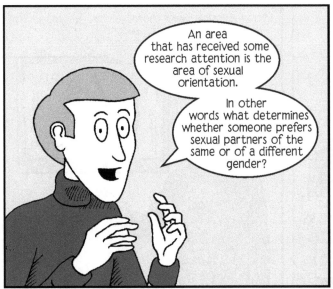

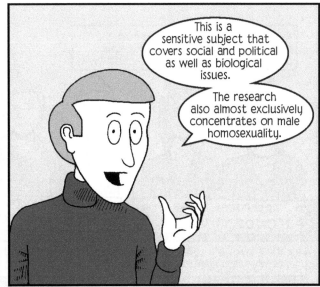

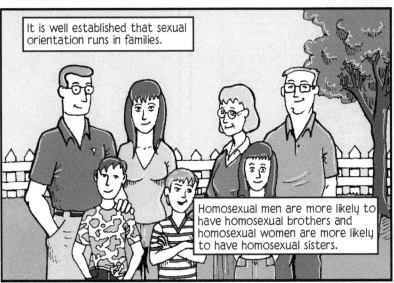

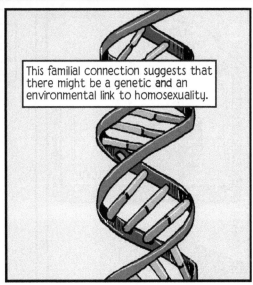

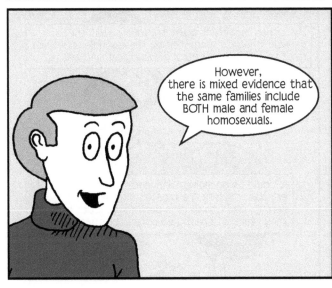

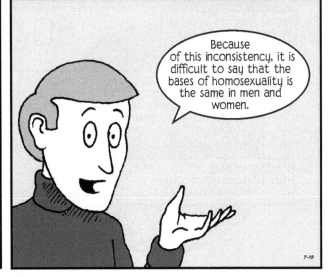

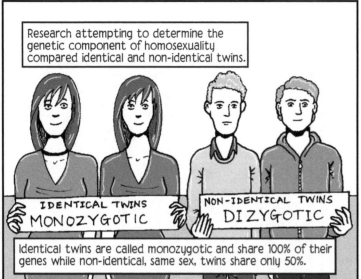

Research attempting to determine the genetic component of homosexuality compared identical and non-identical twins.

IDENTICAL TWINS MONOZYGOTIC

NON-IDENTICAL TWINS DIZYGOTIC

Identical twins are called monozygotic and share 100% of their genes while non-identical, same sex, twins share only 50%.

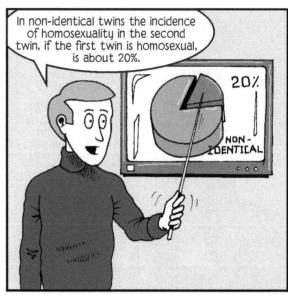

In non-identical twins the incidence of homosexuality in the second twin, if the first twin is homosexual, is about 20%.

20%

NON-IDENTICAL

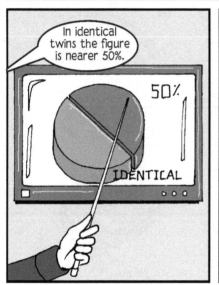

In identical twins the figure is nearer 50%.

50%

IDENTICAL

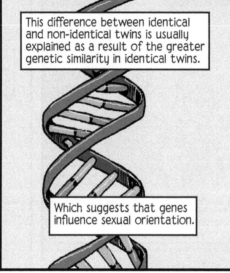

This difference between identical and non-identical twins is usually explained as a result of the greater genetic similarity in identical twins.

Which suggests that genes influence sexual orientation.

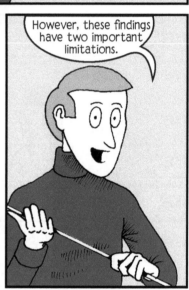

However, these findings have two important limitations.

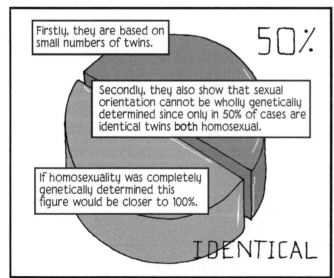

Firstly, they are based on small numbers of twins.

Secondly, they also show that sexual orientation cannot be wholly genetically determined since only in 50% of cases are identical twins both homosexual.

If homosexuality was completely genetically determined this figure would be closer to 100%.

50%

IDENTICAL

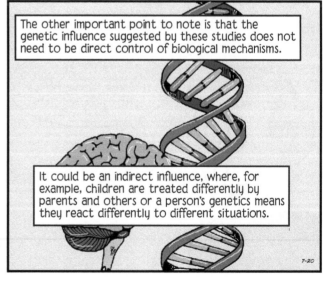

The other important point to note is that the genetic influence suggested by these studies does not need to be direct control of biological mechanisms.

It could be an indirect influence, where, for example, children are treated differently by parents and others or a person's genetics means they react differently to different situations.

7-20

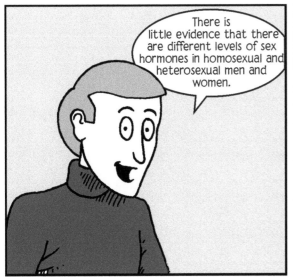

There is little evidence that there are different levels of sex hormones in homosexual and heterosexual men and women.

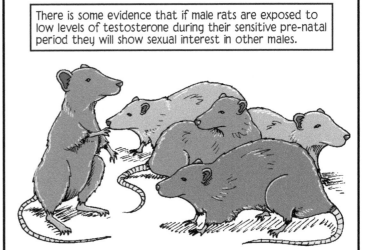

There is some evidence that if male rats are exposed to low levels of testosterone during their sensitive pre-natal period they will show sexual interest in other males.

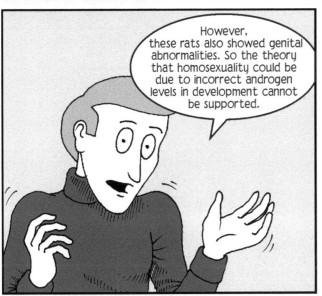

However, these rats also showed genital abnormalities. So the theory that homosexuality could be due to incorrect androgen levels in development cannot be supported.

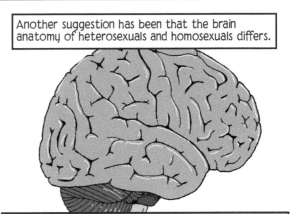

Another suggestion has been that the brain anatomy of heterosexuals and homosexuals differs.

However, only very small anatomical differences have ever been found between these two groups. Furthermore, even these small differences are to areas of the brain not known to have any sexual function.

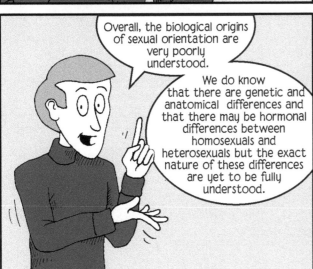

Overall, the biological origins of sexual orientation are very poorly understood.

We do know that there are genetic and anatomical differences and that there may be hormonal differences between homosexuals and heterosexuals but the exact nature of these differences are yet to be fully understood.

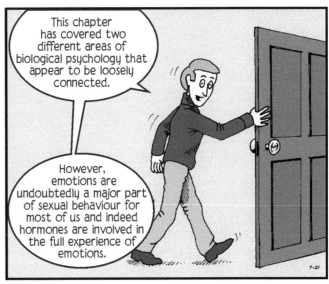

This chapter has covered two different areas of biological psychology that appear to be loosely connected.

However, emotions are undoubtedly a major part of sexual behaviour for most of us and indeed hormones are involved in the full experience of emotions.

7-21

Emotions and sexual behaviour

▶ **PAGE 148**

Panel 3

Like hunger and thirst, sexual behaviour can be seen as a motivation. However, the problem with seeing sex like this is that unlike hunger and thirst, it is difficult to connect sexual behaviour with a physiological need. Basically, unlike hunger, for example, where you will die if the need for food is not fulfilled, you can go without sex without any damage to your own body. As Garrett (2003) put it 'sex ensures the survival of the species, but not of the individual' (p.155).

Panel 4

The biggest problem with studying emotions is that emotion cannot be observed and is very difficult to infer from observed behaviour. This is even more difficult when you consider animal work. How can you infer an emotion in an animal if they cannot communicate? For this and other, similar, reasons Antonio Damasio (1999) concluded that emotions also require consciousness.

Panel 5

See Bard (1929, 1934).

Panel 7

See Papez (1937).

▶ **PAGE 149**

Panel 2

See MacLean (1949, 1958, 1970).

▶ **PAGE 150**

Panel 2

In addition to the structures that make up the limbic system, there are three other brain structures that are important in the control of emotion:

The Amygdala

This is the brain structure that is most involved in emotion. It receives information from all of the senses. The amygdala's most important emotional role concerns the creation and control of fear and anxiety. It is, however, involved in other emotions.

The Pre-frontal Cortex

Damage to the pre-frontal cortex causes emotional responses to be 'weaker' or 'blunted'. Its role appears to be in using emotional information for other purposes.

Right Hemisphere

Damage to the right hemisphere of the brain often causes difficulties in recognising emotions in others and also impairs emotions involved in autonomic nervous system responses.

▶ **PAGE 152**

Panel 1

There is also the Schacter-Singer theory which is also known as Cognitive-Arousal theory (Schacter & Singer, 1962). This suggests that you feel the arousal and then cognitively assign an emotion to it based on context and previous experience. If the arousal is due to being chased by a lion, for example, you are likely to label this as fear. If, on the other hand, the arousal is due to the effect of a roller coaster then you will be more likely to label this as excitement.

▶ **PAGE 154**

Panel 6

See Forman and McCauley (1986) and Patrick and Iacono (1989).

▶ **PAGE 155**

Panel 1

There is research evidence that different facial expressions are related to feeling actual emotions (Ekman, 1992; Izard, 1971).

Actually, the facial expression you make can influence the emotion you feel. Strack, Martin and Stepper (1988) found that people rated cartoons as funnier when they held a pen between their teeth than when they held the pen in their lips. In muscular terms, holding a pen in your teeth represents a smile while holding it in your lips prevents a smile. This idea has led some researchers to suggest that the face and its muscles are the source of emotion (see Tomkins, 1962, 1980).

Panel 2

This refers to work by Darwin (1872).

Panels 3 to 6

It was work by Ekman and Oster (1979) who demonstrated the culturally universal nature of these six facial expressions. In fact, Izard (1977) found that 'shame' and 'interest' may also be universal facial expressions.

Bear in mind that the influence of culture also comes to bear on facial expressions. These six (possibly eight) expressions may well be recognised by all cultures but facial expressions are also influenced by culture. Different cultures influence how someone controls their facial expression. Each culture (or subculture) has rules about which facial expressions can be made under what circumstances. These are called *display rules* (see Ekman & Friesen, 1975; and Ekman, Friesen & Ellsworth, 1982). Studies have shown that Japanese individuals, for example, will show less revulsion to an unpleasant film when they know they are being observed when compared to American individuals (Ekman, 1977). In general, Japanese culture allows much less emotional expression than western culture.

McCloud (2006) has some very interesting applications of the six universal expressions. He 'mixes' different expressions in order to show how more complex emotional expressions might arise.

▶ **PAGE 156**

Panel 2

Actually, hormones have a huge influence on our behaviour in general as well as on sexual behaviour. For example, there is evidence for the influence of, especially, testosterone on aggressive behaviour. Archer and Lloyd (1985) linked the action of testosterone to the greater aggression exhibited by males of many animal species. The effect of testosterone on aggression appears to be both during an animal's development and birth.

▶ **PAGE 157**

Panel 4

In an earlier chapter it was noted that the pituitary gland is not made up of neurons, it is an endocrine gland. Actually this is not quite true. The posterior pituitary is actually an extension of the hypothalamus and **is** made up of neurons. This part of the pituitary gland releases the hormones *oxytocin* and *vasopressin*, that are manufactured in the hypothalamus, into the bloodstream.

It is the *anterior* pituitary that is not made up of neurons. Like other hormone glands, it is made up of *glandular tissue*. The hypothalamus controls the release into the bloodstream of the six hormones manufactured by the anterior pituitary gland.

▶ **PAGE 158**

Panel 3

Hormones are also very good for causing long-lasting changes in various parts of the body. It is hormones that cause migratory birds to deposit fats that allow them to survive the migration for example.

▶ **PAGE 159**

Panel 1

Actually there are more categories of hormone. There are also *thyroid* hormones and *monoamines*. Thyroid hormones are those released by the thyroid gland and include thyroxine, while monoamines are hormones like dopamine and epinephrine. In addition, there are a number of other hormones that cannot be easily classified and some chemicals in the body that might be considered hormones, although researchers are currently uncertain about them.

Panel 2

Sex hormones have effects on the brain, the genitals and other organs.

Panel 6

Men and women differ in the manner in which they can be affected by sex hormones. There are certain genes in the body that are affected by sex hormones and are referred to as *sex-limited* genes. The effects of these are different in males and females. An example of this effect is when oestrogen activates the genes in females that cause the development and growth of breasts during adolescence.

Testosterone is sometimes referred to as an anabolic steroid. This refers to the fact that testosterone influences muscle growth. Anabolic steroids have received a poor reputation due to their association with drug abuse by athletes. Anabolic steroids can also be created by artificial means.

▶ **PAGE 161**

Panel 7

See Quadagno, Briscoe and Quadagno (1977) and Young, Goy and Phoenix (1964).

▶ **PAGE 162**

Panel 1

See Berenbaum (1999).

Panel 3

Please note that in humans the activating effects of hormones do not cause any behaviour to occur. The effects are on brain activity and sensitivity in pubic areas (Etgen *et al.*,1999).

Panels 5 and 6

See Baum and Vreeburg (1973) and Matuszewich, Lorrain and Hull (2000).

Panel 7

Eberhart, Keverne and Meller (1980) found that levels of the hormone testosterone changed with the social rank of male talapoin monkeys.

▶ **PAGE 163**

Panel 1

See Komisaruk, Addler and Hutchinson (1972).

Panel 4

See Murphy *et al.*, (1990).

Panel 5

See Carter (1992).

Panel 6

Given that it is well established that testosterone causes aggression in males and affects sexual behaviour it was hypothesised that male sexual offenders might have abnormal amounts of testosterone in their body. However, research suggests that the levels of testosterone in these individuals are not abnormal. The majority of studies have found that sexual offenders have an average amount of testosterone (e.g. Lang, FLor-Henry & Frenzel, 1990). However, a few studies have found lower levels and some studies have found higher levels (see Rösler & Witztum, 1998).

▶ **PAGE 164**

Panel 1

The menstrual cycle is categorised as a cyclical release of a number of different hormones that affect the level of fertility in women.

Panel 4

See Adams, Gold and Burt (1978) and Udry and Morris (1968).

Panel 5

See Slob *et al.*, (1996).

Panel 6

Penton-Voak *et al.* (1999) found that during their peri-ovulatory period, women participants preferred more 'masculine' looking men's faces in photos as possible sexual partners. Outside of their peri-ovulatory period, these women preferred more 'feminine' looking men's faces.

▶ **PAGE 165**

Panel 1

As Garrett (2003) has pointed out, if we find out why some people prefer the same gender, this might allow us some insight into heterosexuality as well.

A particularly tricky aspect of this type of research is that it is difficult to find out exactly how many people are homosexual. Michael *et al.* (1994) conducted a survey in the United States that suggested that 9 per cent of men and 4 per cent of women are homosexual. Other, similar surveys, have suggested slightly lower percentages however.

Panel 2

There are two general hypotheses that have been suggested to explain the 'causes' of homosexuality. The first is the *social influence* hypothesis that argues that homosexuality is a result of parental influences as a child. The research has tended to focus on early sexual experiences.

However, Bell, Weinberg and Hammersmith (1982) conducted a large survey of both homosexual and heterosexual men and found no significant difference in their early sexual experiences. In fact most of the research conducted in this area (see, for example, Van Wyk & Geist, 1984) has only found evidence of sexual experiences that could be interpreted as reflecting an early demonstration of homosexuality rather than a cause of homosexuality.

The alternative hypothesis is known as the *biological* hypothesis. This posits that homosexuality has a biological cause. There have therefore been attempts to demonstrate a genetic, hormonal or neural explanation for homosexuality.

▶ **PAGE 166**

Panels 2 and 3

In fact the figures are:

Related to a homosexual man

Monozygotic twin:	Homosexual	52%
	Heterosexual	48%
Dizygotic twin:	Homosexual	22%
	Heterosexual	78%
Adopted brother:	Homosexual	11%
	Heterosexual	89%

Related to a homosexual woman

Monozygotic twin:	Homosexual	48%
	Heterosexual	52%
Dizygotic twin:	Homosexual	16%
	Heterosexual	84%
Adopted sister:	Homosexual	6%
	Heterosexual	94%

The above figures come from Kalat (2004) based on Bailey and Pillard (1991) and Bailey, Pillard, Nale and Agyei (1993).

CHAPTER 8
SLEEP AND BIOLOGICAL RHYTHMS

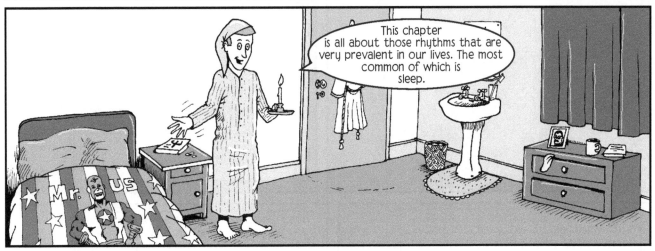

This chapter is all about those rhythms that are very prevalent in our lives. The most common of which is sleep.

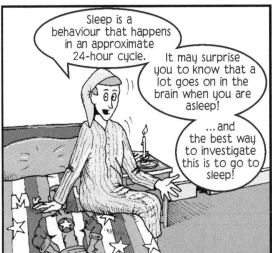

Sleep is a behaviour that happens in an approximate 24-hour cycle.

It may surprise you to know that a lot goes on in the brain when you are asleep!

...and the best way to investigate this is to go to sleep!

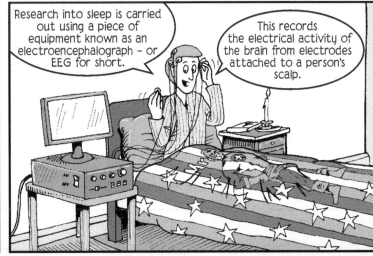

Research into sleep is carried out using a piece of equipment known as an electroencephalograph – or EEG for short.

This records the electrical activity of the brain from electrodes attached to a person's scalp.

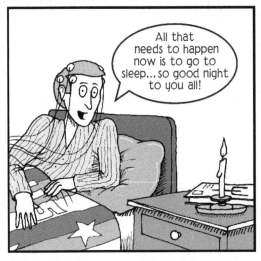

All that needs to happen now is to go to sleep... so good night to you all!

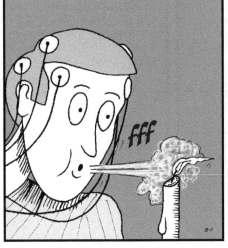

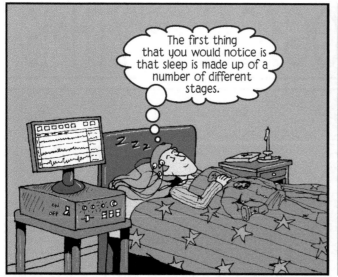

The first thing that you would notice is that sleep is made up of a number of different stages.

These stages are characterised by different patterns of EEG activity.

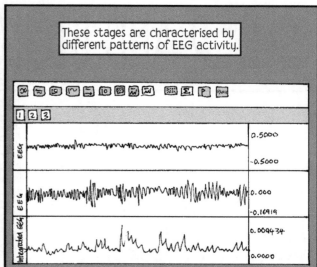

Before sleep, the EEG pattern is mostly BETA WAVES when you are awake and ALPHA WAVES during times of quiet relaxation.

Stage 1 of sleep is a general state of drowsiness that is defined by the presence of Theta Waves in the EEG pattern.

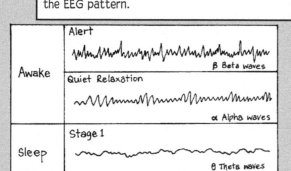

	Alert	
Awake	Alert waveform — β Beta waves	
	Quiet Relaxation — α Alpha waves	
Sleep	Stage 1 — θ Theta waves	

Theta Waves are quite fast and erratic waves that are just a little slower than the waves shown during times of relaxation.

George, WAKE up!

Aah... What? I wasn't sleeping!

People that are woken during Stage 1 of sleep often will claim that they were not actually asleep!

Stage 2 of sleep is characterised by slower and longer waves accompanied by sleep spindles – short bursts of fast activity.

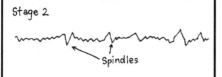

Stage 2

Spindles

The third stage of sleep has waves that are even slower and larger – known as DELTA WAVES.

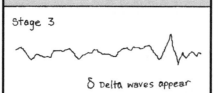

Stage 3

δ Delta waves appear

During the fourth stage of sleep, the body's metabolism is at its slowest and the EEG pattern is almost exclusively made up of DELTA waves.

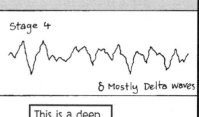

Stage 4

δ Mostly Delta waves

This is a deep stage of sleep.

8-2

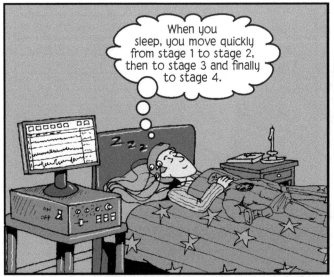

When you sleep, you move quickly from stage 1 to stage 2, then to stage 3 and finally to stage 4.

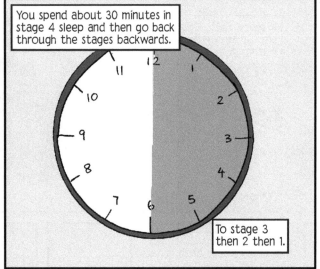

You spend about 30 minutes in stage 4 sleep and then go back through the stages backwards.

To stage 3 then 2 then 1.

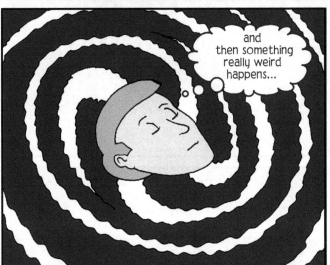

and then something really weird happens...

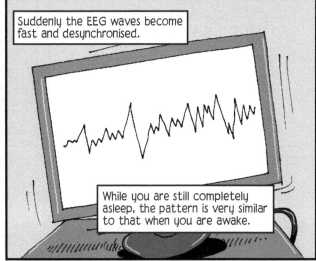

Suddenly the EEG waves become fast and desynchronised.

While you are still completely asleep, the pattern is very similar to that when you are awake.

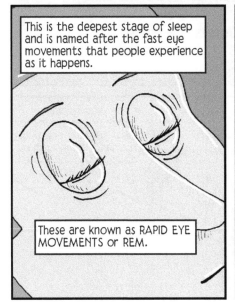

This is the deepest stage of sleep and is named after the fast eye movements that people experience as it happens.

These are known as RAPID EYE MOVEMENTS or REM.

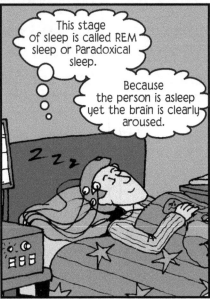

This stage of sleep is called REM sleep or Paradoxical sleep.

Because the person is asleep yet the brain is clearly aroused.

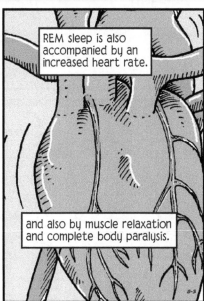

REM sleep is also accompanied by an increased heart rate.

and also by muscle relaxation and complete body paralysis.

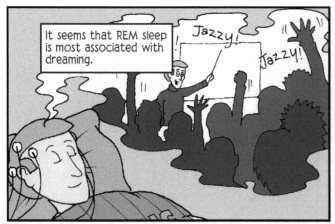

It seems that REM sleep is most associated with dreaming.

Jazzy!

Jazzy!

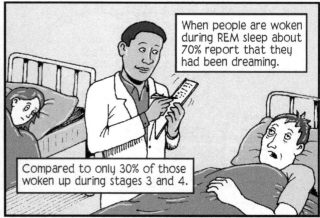

When people are woken during REM sleep about 70% report that they had been dreaming.

Compared to only 30% of those woken up during stages 3 and 4.

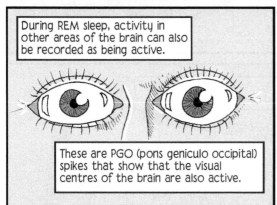

During REM sleep, activity in other areas of the brain can also be recorded as being active.

These are PGO (pons geniculo occipital) spikes that show that the visual centres of the brain are also active.

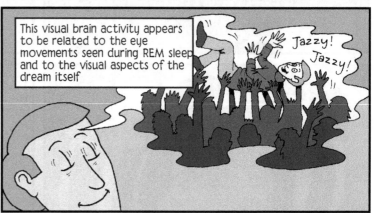

This visual brain activity appears to be related to the eye movements seen during REM sleep and to the visual aspects of the dream itself

Jazzy!

Jazzy!

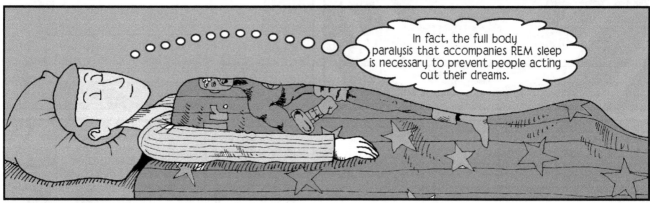

In fact, the full body paralysis that accompanies REM sleep is necessary to prevent people acting out their dreams.

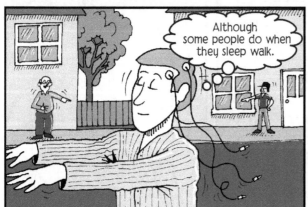

Although some people do when they sleep walk.

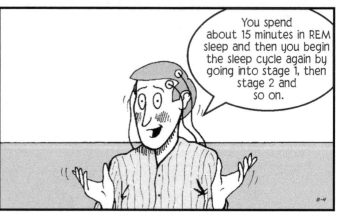

You spend about 15 minutes in REM sleep and then you begin the sleep cycle again by going into stage 1, then stage 2 and so on.

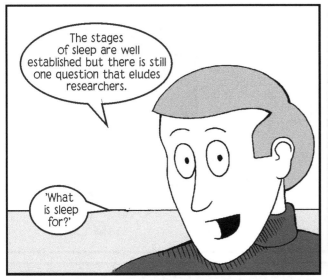

The stages of sleep are well established but there is still one question that eludes researchers.

'What is sleep for?'

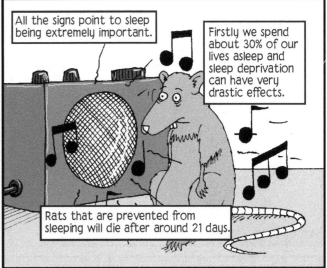

All the signs point to sleep being extremely important.

Firstly we spend about 30% of our lives asleep and sleep deprivation can have very drastic effects.

Rats that are prevented from sleeping will die after around 21 days.

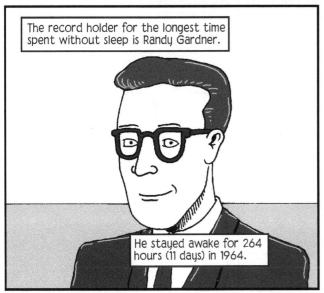

The record holder for the longest time spent without sleep is Randy Gardner.

He stayed awake for 264 hours (11 days) in 1964.

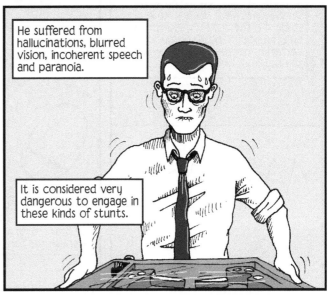

He suffered from hallucinations, blurred vision, incoherent speech and paranoia.

It is considered very dangerous to engage in these kinds of stunts.

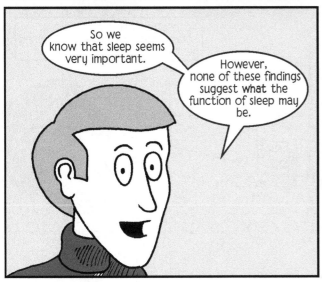

So we know that sleep seems very important.

However, none of these findings suggest what the function of sleep may be.

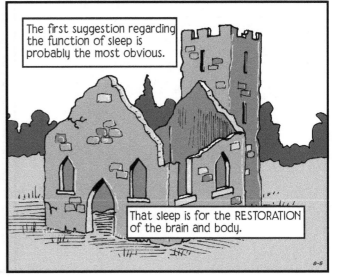

The first suggestion regarding the function of sleep is probably the most obvious.

That sleep is for the RESTORATION of the brain and body.

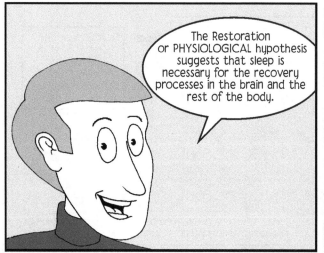

The Restoration or PHYSIOLOGICAL hypothesis suggests that sleep is necessary for the recovery processes in the brain and the rest of the body.

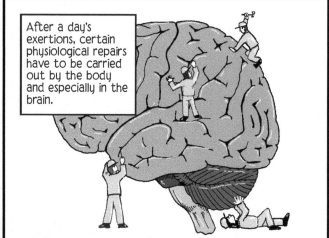

After a day's exertions, certain physiological repairs have to be carried out by the body and especially in the brain.

During slow wave sleep – like in stage 4 – the brain is peaceful but the body is busily producing certain hormones that help with the repair of body tissues.

Stage 4

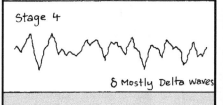

δ Mostly Delta waves

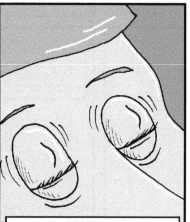

It was Oswald (1980) who suggested that REM sleep is used for brain repair while slow wave sleep is used for bodily repair.

Support for this hypothesis comes from the finding that newborn babies have proportionately more REM sleep.

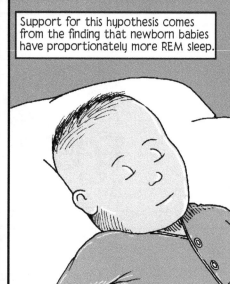

Horne (1988) however, suggested that in humans, both slow wave and REM sleep is used for brain repair.

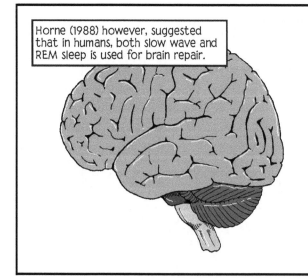

According to Horne, in humans, body repairs are carried out during periods of relaxed wakefulness.

NICE SMELLS

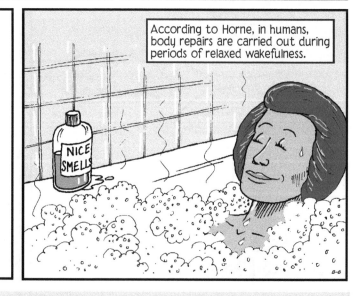

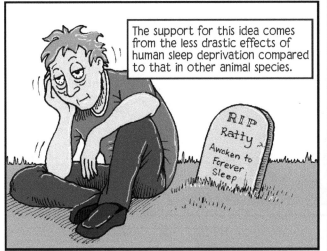

The support for this idea comes from the less drastic effects of human sleep deprivation compared to that in other animal species.

RIP
Ratty
Awoken to
Forever
Sleep

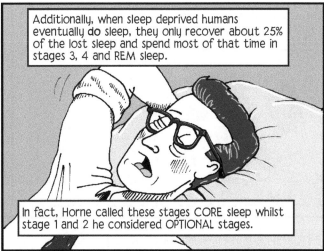

Additionally, when sleep deprived humans eventually **do** sleep, they only recover about 25% of the lost sleep and spend most of that time in stages 3, 4 and REM sleep.

In fact, Horne called these stages CORE sleep whilst stage 1 and 2 he considered OPTIONAL stages.

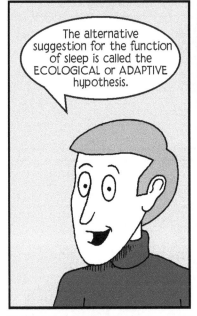

The alternative suggestion for the function of sleep is called the ECOLOGICAL or ADAPTIVE hypothesis.

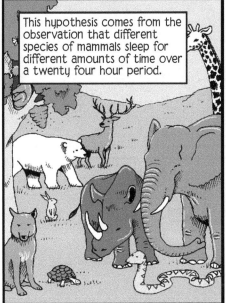

This hypothesis comes from the observation that different species of mammals sleep for different amounts of time over a twenty four hour period.

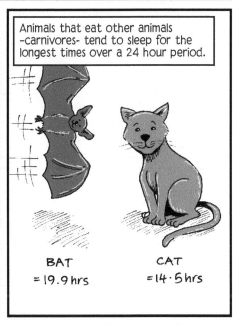

Animals that eat other animals -carnivores- tend to sleep for the longest times over a 24 hour period.

BAT
= 19.9 hrs

CAT
= 14.5 hrs

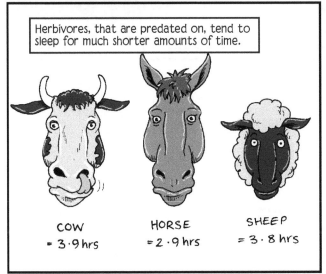

Herbivores, that are predated on, tend to sleep for much shorter amounts of time.

COW
= 3.9 hrs

HORSE
= 2.9 hrs

SHEEP
= 3.8 hrs

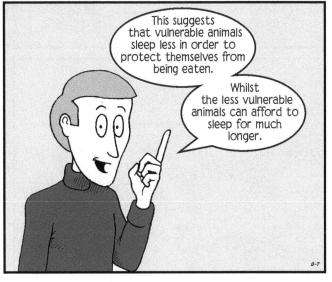

This suggests that vulnerable animals sleep less in order to protect themselves from being eaten.

Whilst the less vulnerable animals can afford to sleep for much longer.

183

However, whilst the adaptive hypothesis seems appropriate to explain these differences, there is an alternative explanation.

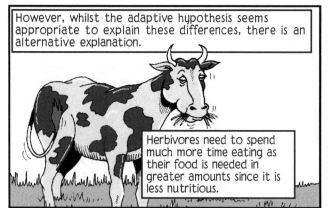

Herbivores need to spend much more time eating as their food is needed in greater amounts since it is less nutritious.

So while sleep may be unsafe for a herbivore, that may not be the only reason different species sleep for different amounts of time.

In reality, herbivores cannot sleep as long as carnivores simply because they need to spend much more time awake eating!

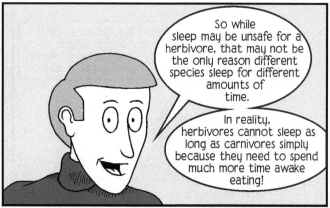

It may be that different animal species will have different functions for sleep.

The bottlenose dolphin, for example, sleeps one brain hemisphere at a time to prevent it drowning whilst asleep!

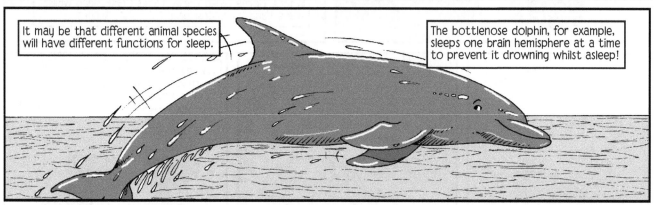

It may simply be that the function of sleep is to conserve energy.

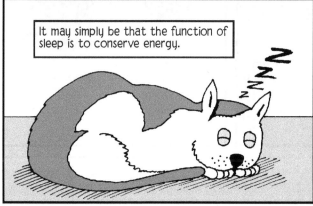

The real answer to the function of sleep is clearly a long way away.

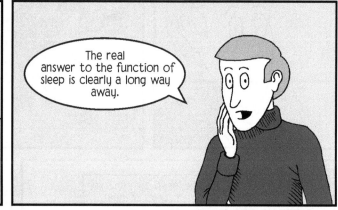

However, the restorative and the adaptive hypotheses are not incompatible.

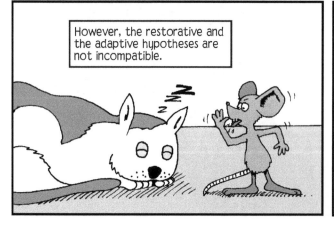

If sleep is indeed restorative, it would also make adaptive sense to vary sleep depending on issues of food consumption, safety from predation and energy conservation.

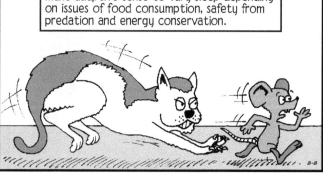

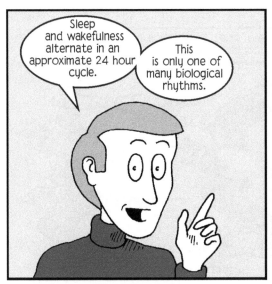

Sleep and wakefulness alternate in an approximate 24 hour cycle.

This is only one of many biological rhythms.

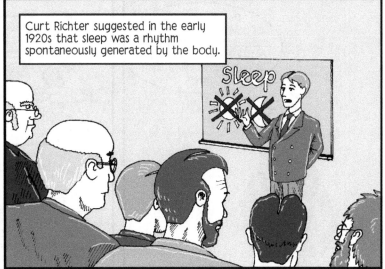

Curt Richter suggested in the early 1920s that sleep was a rhythm spontaneously generated by the body.

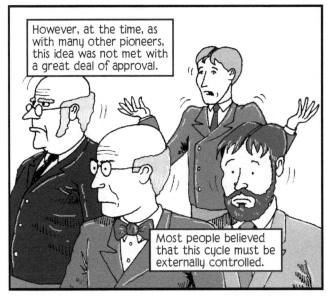

However, at the time, as with many other pioneers, this idea was not met with a great deal of approval.

Most people believed that this cycle must be externally controlled.

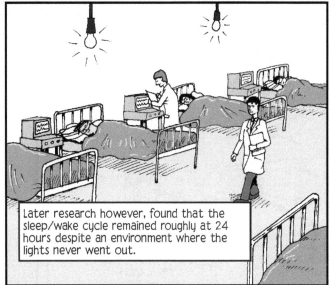

Later research however, found that the sleep/wake cycle remained roughly at 24 hours despite an environment where the lights never went out.

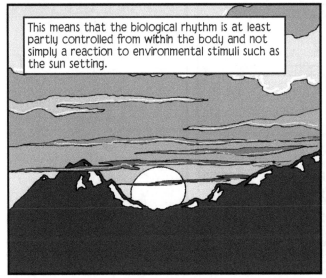

This means that the biological rhythm is at least partly controlled from within the body and not simply a reaction to environmental stimuli such as the sun setting.

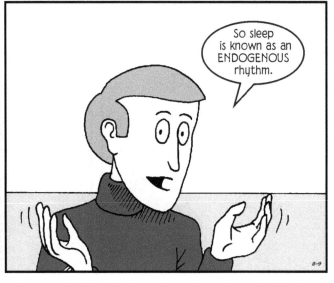

So sleep is known as an ENDOGENOUS rhythm.

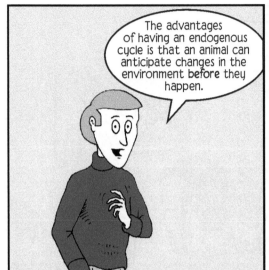

The advantages of having an endogenous cycle is that an animal can anticipate changes in the environment **before** they happen.

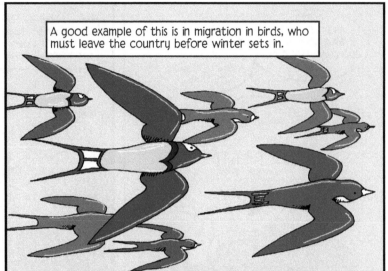

A good example of this is in migration in birds, who must leave the country before winter sets in.

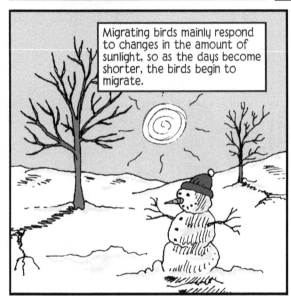

Migrating birds mainly respond to changes in the amount of sunlight, so as the days become shorter, the birds begin to migrate.

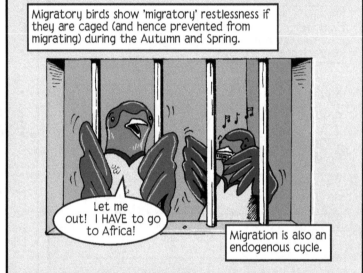

Migratory birds show 'migratory' restlessness if they are caged (and hence prevented from migrating) during the Autumn and Spring.

Let me out! I HAVE to go to Africa!

Migration is also an endogenous cycle.

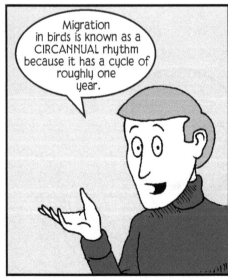

Migration in birds is known as a CIRCANNUAL rhythm because it has a cycle of roughly one year.

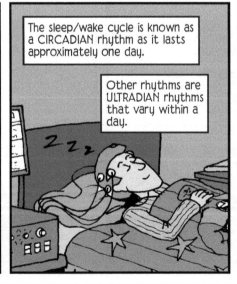

The sleep/wake cycle is known as a CIRCADIAN rhythm as it lasts approximately one day.

Other rhythms are ULTRADIAN rhythms that vary within a day.

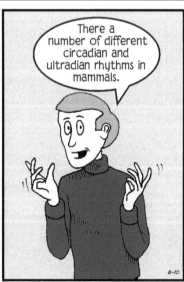

There a number of different circadian and ultradian rhythms in mammals.

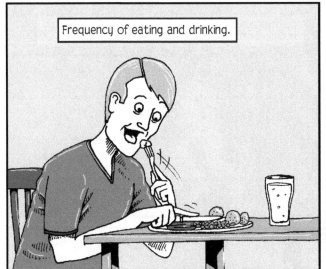

Frequency of eating and drinking.

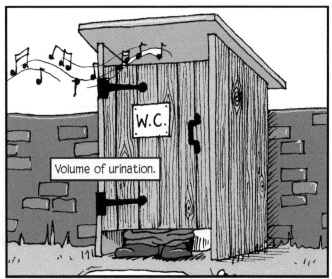

Volume of urination.

W.C.

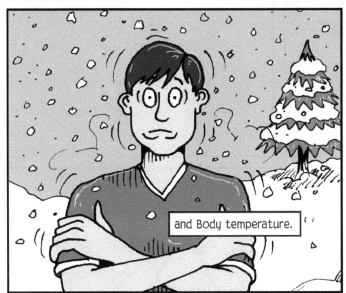

and Body temperature.

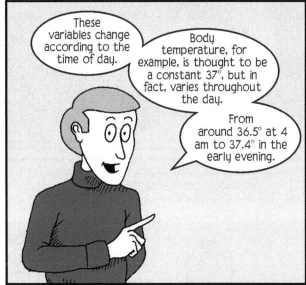

These variables change according to the time of day.

Body temperature, for example, is thought to be a constant 37°, but in fact, varies throughout the day.

From around 36.5° at 4 am to 37.4° in the early evening.

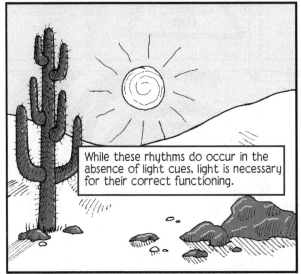

While these rhythms do occur in the absence of light cues, light is necessary for their correct functioning.

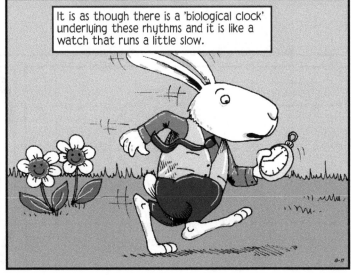

It is as though there is a 'biological clock' underlying these rhythms and it is like a watch that runs a little slow.

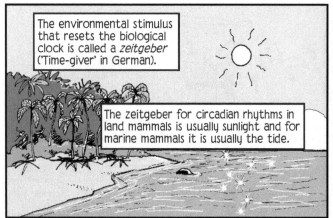

The environmental stimulus that resets the biological clock is called a *zeitgeber* ('Time-giver' in German).

The zeitgeber for circadian rhythms in land mammals is usually sunlight and for marine mammals it is usually the tide.

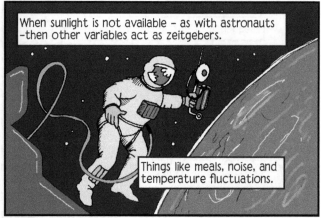

When sunlight is not available – as with astronauts –then other variables act as zeitgebers.

Things like meals, noise, and temperature fluctuations.

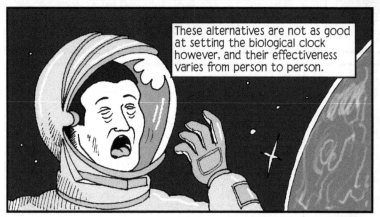

These alternatives are not as good at setting the biological clock however, and their effectiveness varies from person to person.

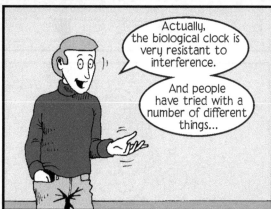

Actually, the biological clock is very resistant to interference.

And people have tried with a number of different things...

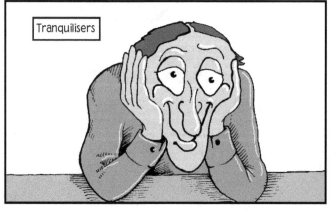

Food and water deprivation.

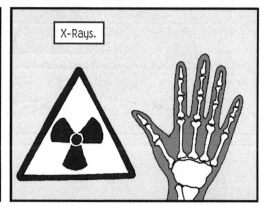

X-Rays.

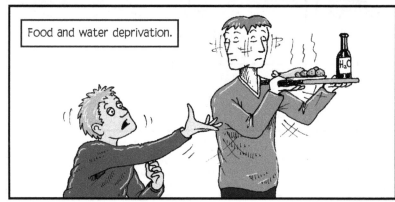

Tranquilisers

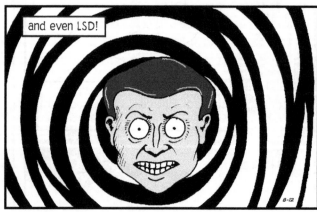

and even LSD!

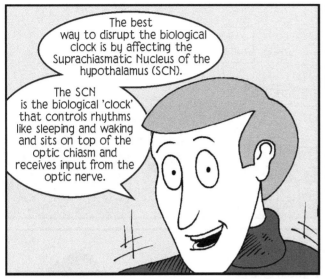

The best way to disrupt the biological clock is by affecting the Suprachiasmatic Nucleus of the hypothalamus (SCN).

The SCN is the biological 'clock' that controls rhythms like sleeping and waking and sits on top of the optic chiasm and receives input from the optic nerve.

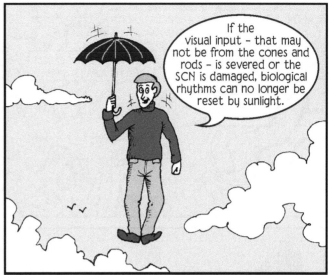

If the visual input - that may not be from the cones and rods - is severed or the SCN is damaged, biological rhythms can no longer be reset by sunlight.

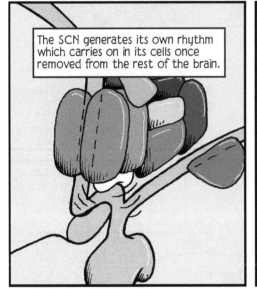

The SCN generates its own rhythm which carries on in its cells once removed from the rest of the brain.

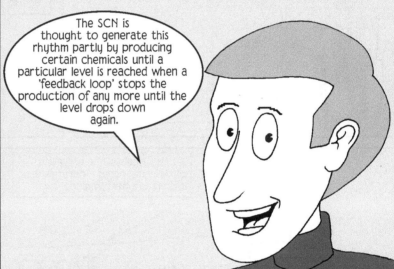

The SCN is thought to generate this rhythm partly by producing certain chemicals until a particular level is reached when a 'feedback loop' stops the production of any more until the level drops down again.

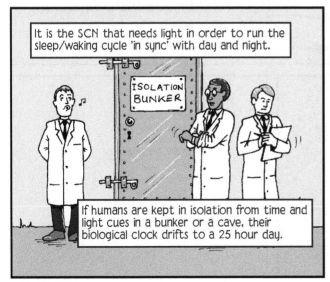

It is the SCN that needs light in order to run the sleep/waking cycle 'in sync' with day and night.

ISOLATION BUNKER

If humans are kept in isolation from time and light cues in a bunker or a cave, their biological clock drifts to a 25 hour day.

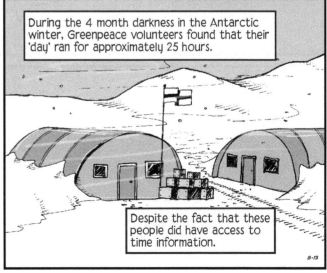

During the 4 month darkness in the Antarctic winter, Greenpeace volunteers found that their 'day' ran for approximately 25 hours.

Despite the fact that these people did have access to time information.

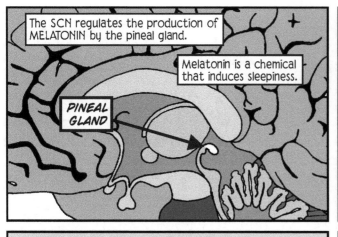

The SCN regulates the production of MELATONIN by the pineal gland.

Melatonin is a chemical that induces sleepiness.

PINEAL GLAND

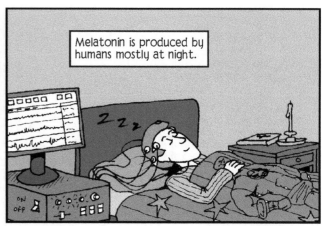

Melatonin is produced by humans mostly at night.

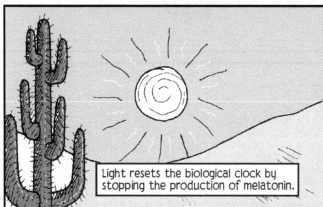

Light resets the biological clock by stopping the production of melatonin.

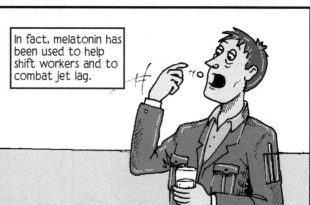

In fact, melatonin has been used to help shift workers and to combat jet lag.

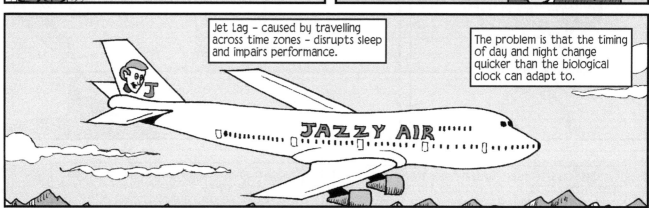

Jet Lag – caused by travelling across time zones – disrupts sleep and impairs performance.

The problem is that the timing of day and night change quicker than the biological clock can adapt to.

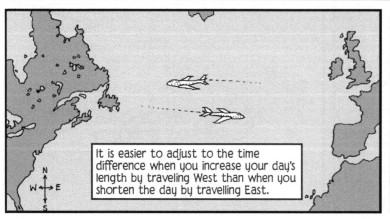

It is easier to adjust to the time difference when you increase your day's length by traveling West than when you shorten the day by travelling East.

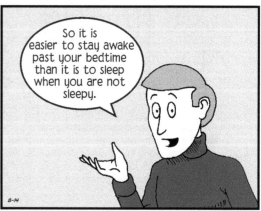

So it is easier to stay awake past your bedtime than it is to sleep when you are not sleepy.

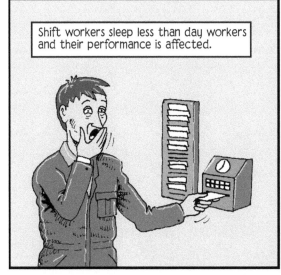

Shift workers sleep less than day workers and their performance is affected.

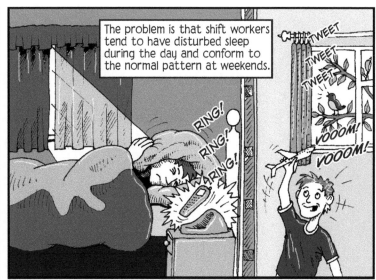

The problem is that shift workers tend to have disturbed sleep during the day and conform to the normal pattern at weekends.

CHIRP TWEET TWEET TWEET VOOOM! VOOOM!

RING! RING! RING!

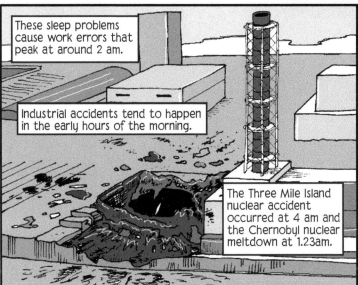

These sleep problems cause work errors that peak at around 2 am.

Industrial accidents tend to happen in the early hours of the morning.

The Three Mile Island nuclear accident occurred at 4 am and the Chernobyl nuclear meltdown at 1.23am.

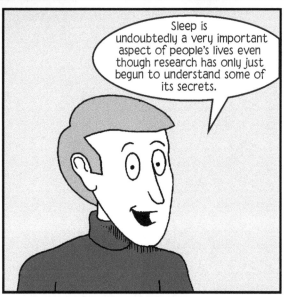

Sleep is undoubtedly a very important aspect of people's lives even though research has only just begun to understand some of its secrets.

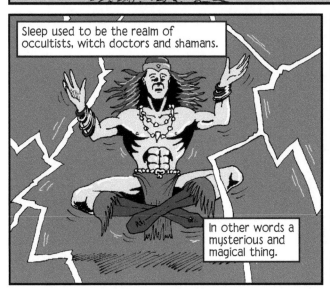

Sleep used to be the realm of occultists, witch doctors and shamans.

In other words a mysterious and magical thing.

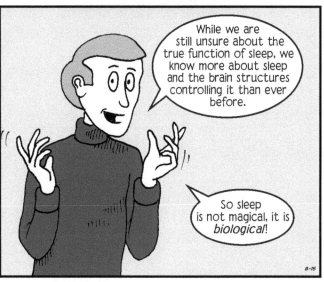

While we are still unsure about the true function of sleep, we know more about sleep and the brain structures controlling it than ever before.

So sleep is not magical, it is *biological*!

Sleep and biological rhythms

▶ **PAGE 177**

Panel 4

The *electroencephalograph* or EEG, is a way of measuring the electrical activity of the brain. Small electrodes (usually up to around eight) are attached to the scalp at various points using some kind of adhesive. Each electrode measures the average amount of electricity created by the collection of neurons just below it. This measure is then amplified and recorded.

The advantage of using the EEG to record brain activity is that you don't have to cut into the brain to take measurements. One of the problems is that since the EEG measures such a huge number of neurons at a time it is difficult to do much with the results except in general terms. Despite this, however, from the output of the EEG trained individuals can tell if someone is asleep, awake, or excited for example. Some abnormalities in the EEG can also suggest problems with the brain, like the presence of a tumour.

▶ **PAGE 178**

Panel 2

In the past, EEG results were recorded on paper although most of it is now carried out using computers.

Panel 3

Slow wave EEG activity shows that all the neurons are synchronised; in other words, all firing at the same time.

▶ **PAGE 179**

Panel 5

REM sleep was accidentally discovered in the 1950s by two separate sets of researchers: Jouvet in France and Arenski and Kleitman in the United States.

Panel 7

REM sleep is also accompanied by penile erections in men and vaginal moistening in women.

▶ **PAGE 180**

Panel 2

The finding that REM sleep is accompanied by dreaming was reported by Dement and Kleitman (1957), although other research later found that when people were woken during non-REM sleep they also reported dreaming. It does appear, however, that REM sleep dreaming is accompanied by more visual imagery.

▶ **PAGE 182**

Panel 2

During sleep, the brain makes proteins and replaces lost energy. However, the brain doesn't recover in the same way that, say runners recover their breath after running. In general, people do not sleep significantly more after a particularly mentally or physically taxing day (Horne & Minard, 1985; Shapiro *et al.*, 1981). So the length of sleep is not dependent on the amount of activity we have carried out.

In addition, people vary a great deal in the amount of sleep they need. Jones and Oswald (1968) found two men who regularly only slept for about 3 hours a night and seemed to suffer no problems as a result. Meddis, Peason and Langford (1973) reported the case of a 70-year-old woman who only slept for 1 hour per night and sometimes did not sleep at all.

The former Prime Minister of the United Kingdom, Margaret Thatcher, famously boasted that she only needed 5 hours sleep per night during her time in office. However, she was in her 60s at the time and it is not uncommon for people of this age to need less sleep.

▶ **PAGE 183**

Panel 3

See Kleitman (1963) and Webb (1974).

The adaptive hypothesis is a little like the idea of hibernation. By sleeping, animals can conserve energy at a time when food is less available. The approximate 1°C drop in body temperature that accompanies sleep helps to conserve energy. The adaptive hypothesis is supported by the finding that animals sleep longer at times of food shortage (Berger & Phillips, 1995).

▶ **PAGE 184**

Panel 5

We spend a lot of our time asleep and a lot of that time in REM sleep. This has led to the suggestion that REM sleep has an important function. In addition, the fact that many birds and mammals have been shown to have REM sleep leads to the suggestion that it is part of our evolutionary past and therefore has an important survival role.

When animal species are compared, there is a lot of variation in the amount of REM sleep that occurs. Generally those animals that sleep the most also spend the most time in REM sleep (Siegel, 1995). As we age, we spend less time asleep and this is accompanied by less time spent in REM sleep. Babies spend more time asleep generally and thus spend more time in REM sleep than adults.

Dement (1960) found that deprivation of REM sleep for 4 to 7 nights has a number of effects. He found these by waking subjects as soon as they entered REM sleep thus preventing them from engaging in any REM sleep at all. The effects were firstly that the sleeper increases the amount of REM sleep they engage in on subsequent nights. Participants in this study also reported mild personality changes, increased anxiety, impaired concentration, increased appetite and increased weight.

When these participants were allowed to sleep normally after the study was over, they spent more time than usual in REM sleep as if they needed to catch up.

There are a number of hypotheses that attempt to explain the need for REM sleep:

Memory Storage

One of the major ideas is that REM sleep is needed for memory consolidation and storage. However, the findings in this area are not very conclusive. Some studies show that learning is better if followed by sleep (Stickgold, James & Hobson, 2000; Stickgold *et al.*, 2000), although it is not determined if the crucial aspect in these cases is REM sleep rather than sleep in general. However, there is also evidence that people who take drugs that inhibit REM sleep do not report any memory problems (Parent, Habib & Baker, 1999).

Oxygen Supply to the Corneas

A more recent suggestion is that REM sleep is necessary to shake the eyeballs so that enough oxygen can reach the cornea (Maurice, 1998). When the eyes are open, the corneas receive most of their oxygen supply from the air and some from the fluid behind the eyes. When the eyes are still, the fluid loses much of its oxygen. According to this suggestion, REM sleep is necessary to arouse the sleeper enough to cause the movement of the eyeballs. This idea still lacks substantive support but is an interesting alternative.

There are two hypotheses that attempt to explain the function of dreaming:

Activation-synthesis Hypothesis

This hypothesis suggests that dreaming is the brain's way of making sense of the information it receives whilst you are asleep. During the early part of sleep, the pons activates various areas of the brain, but other areas are not activated. This hypothesis posits that during dreams, the brain is just trying to tie up these sources of information and make some sort of sense of it (Hobson & McCarley, 1977; Hobson, Pace-Schott & Stickgold, 2000, McCarley & Hobson, 1981).

Dreams of falling or being unable to move are dreams that support this hypothesis. During sleep you are lying down and without all the other sensory information, the brain may interpret this as falling. Furthermore, the muscle paralysis that accompanies REM sleep may account for the reports of people dreaming about not being able to move.

One criticism of this theory (which involves a detailed knowledge of the areas of the brain that are active during sleep) is that the predictions from it are quite vague. So, for example, if we dream of falling because we are lying down whilst asleep, why don't we always dream of falling? Another criticism is that patients with damage to the pons still report dreams (Solms, 1997).

Clinico-anatomical Hypothesis

This is very similar to the activation-synthesis hypothesis except that it does not ascribe special importance to the function of the pons. Here, dreams are still seen as the brain's attempt to make sense of information from the senses, recent memories and brain area activity. It is useful to think of this hypothesis as saying that when we dream we are simply thinking without all the usual set of information.

During sleep the brain is deprived of much of the information from the senses and therefore can generate images without interference from, for example, the visual system.

▶ **PAGE 185**

Panel 2

See Richter (1922).

▶ **PAGE 186**

Panel 2

Actually, the influence of an endogenous cycle on the northern return of migratory birds is quite remarkable. In southern climates, where these birds spend the winter months, there is very little difference in the length of day/night throughout the year since these countries are nearer to the earth's equator. This means that the birds must be almost entirely reliant on their endogenous cycle to trigger their return to the north.

▶ **PAGE 187**

Panel 6

Richter (1967) introduced the concept of the brain generating its own internal rhythm and therefore introduced the idea of a 'biological clock'.

▶ **PAGE 188**

Panels 5 to 8

See Richter (1967).

▶ **PAGE 189**

Panel 1

See Refinetti and Menaker (1992).

Panel 3

See Earnest *et al.* (1999), Inouye and Kawamura (1979) and Herzog, Kakahashi and Block (1998).

Panel 4

See Gillette and McArthur (1996).

▶ **PAGE 190**

Panel 1

The pineal gland is an endocrine gland that secretes hormones. It is found just behind the thalamus in the brain.

Panel 5

What we call 'jet lag' is a disruption in the normal circadian rhythms that occurs after you cross time zones. Basically, your zeitgebers of daylight and your internal clock become 'out-of-sync'. The effects are sleepiness during the day and sleeplessness during the night. Other effects are depression and loss of concentration.

▶ **PAGE 191**

Panel 1

The best way for shift workers to adjust to night work is to work in very bright lights and sleep in a very dark room (Czeisler *et al.*, 1990).

CHAPTER 9
MEMORY AND LEARNING

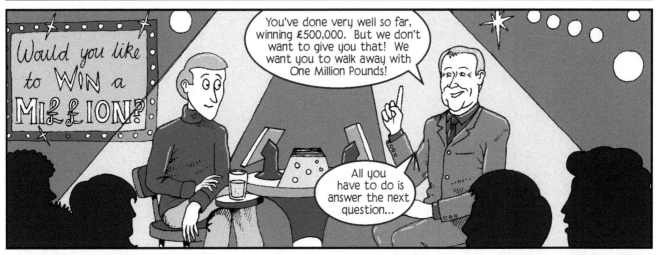

You've done very well so far, winning £500,000. But we don't want to give you that! We want you to walk away with One Million Pounds!

All you have to do is answer the next question...

Would you like to WIN a MILLION?

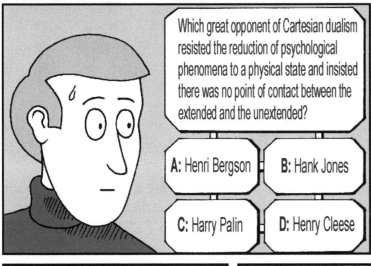

Which great opponent of Cartesian dualism resisted the reduction of psychological phenomena to a physical state and insisted there was no point of contact between the extended and the unextended?

A: Henri Bergson **B:** Hank Jones

C: Harry Palin **D:** Henry Cleese

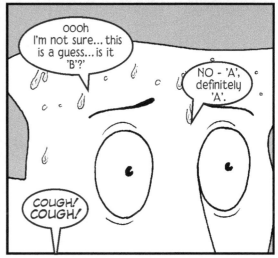

oooh I'm not sure... this is a guess... is it 'B'?

NO - 'A', definitely 'A'.

COUGH! COUGH!

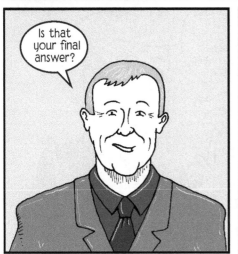

Is that your final answer?

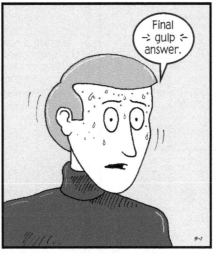

Final → gulp ← answer.

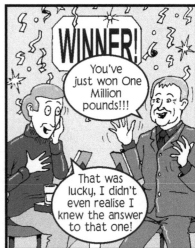

WINNER!

You've just won One Million pounds!!!

That was lucky, I didn't even realise I knew the answer to that one!

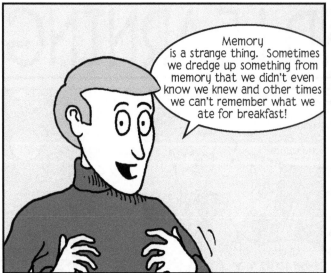

Memory is a strange thing. Sometimes we dredge up something from memory that we didn't even know we knew and other times we can't remember what we ate for breakfast!

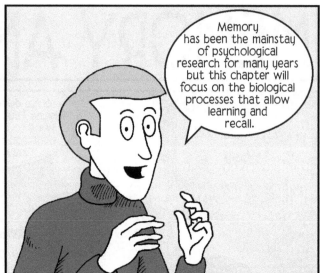

Memory has been the mainstay of psychological research for many years but this chapter will focus on the biological processes that allow learning and recall.

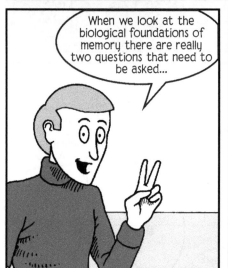

When we look at the biological foundations of memory there are really two questions that need to be asked...

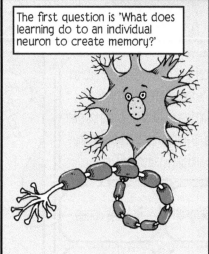

The first question is 'What does learning do to an individual neuron to create memory?'

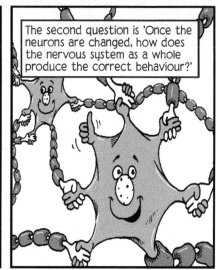

The second question is 'Once the neurons are changed, how does the nervous system as a whole produce the correct behaviour?'

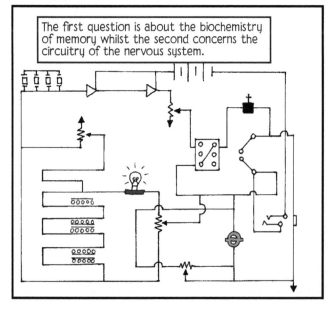

The first question is about the biochemistry of memory whilst the second concerns the circuitry of the nervous system.

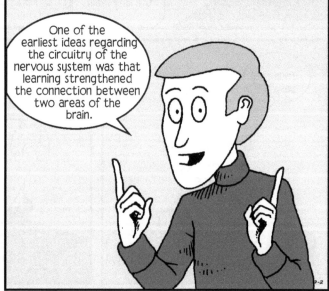

One of the earliest ideas regarding the circuitry of the nervous system was that learning strengthened the connection between two areas of the brain.

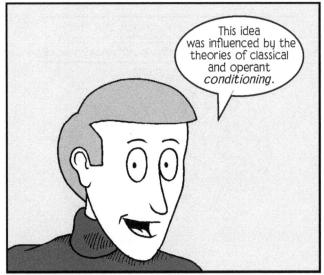

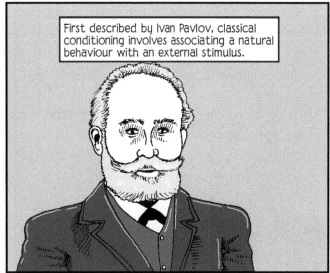

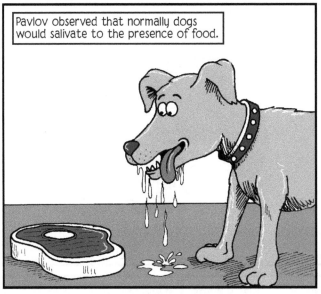

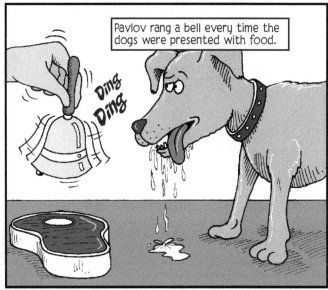

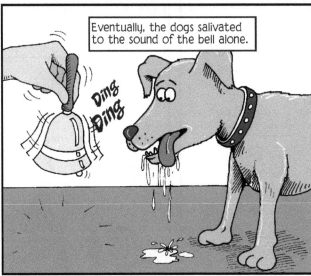

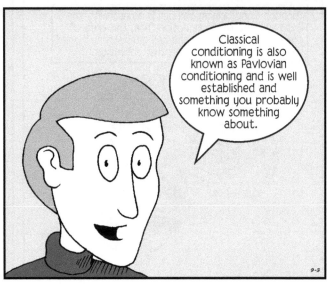

Pavlov thought that conditioning represented the strengthening of a physical connection between two areas of the brain.

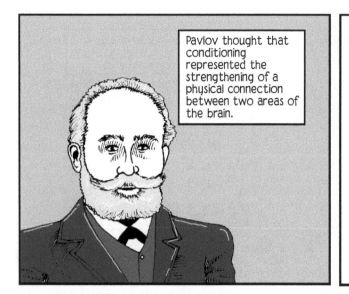

This idea begins with the concept that there is a particular area of the brain that represents the detection of the presence of food.

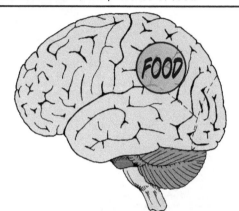

Normally, this section of the brain is physically connected to another area of the brain representing salivation, so that when food is detected by the brain nerve impulses are sent to the area representing salivation.

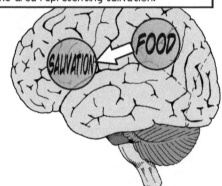

The area of the brain representing the bell is not at all connected to the area representing either food or salivation.

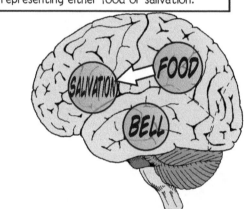

Through conditioning the bell is paired with the food so that the connection from the area of the brain representing the bell gets strengthened so that the bell alone will cause salivation.

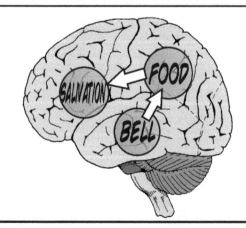

Bear in mind that this idea was largely theoretical and that the areas shown on the brain are just arbitrary and are not where these types of information are actually processed in the brain.

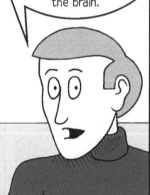

Karl Lashley set out to test Pavlov's idea by searching for the physical representation of conditioning – what he called the **Engram**.

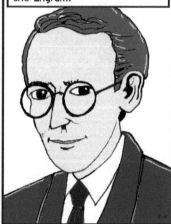

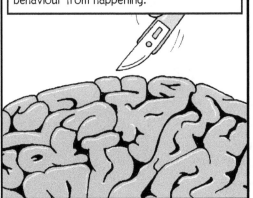

Lashley argued that a cut somewhere in the brain would break the connection between the two areas of the brain connected by the conditioning and so prevent the learned behaviour from happening.

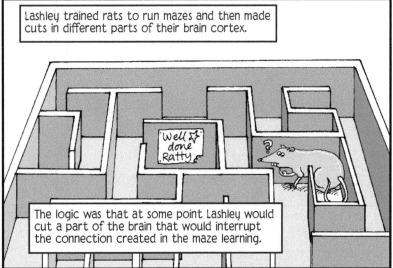

Lashley trained rats to run mazes and then made cuts in different parts of their brain cortex.

Well done Ratty

The logic was that at some point Lashley would cut a part of the brain that would interrupt the connection created in the maze learning.

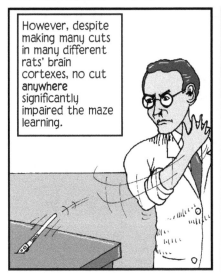

However, despite making many cuts in many different rats' brain cortexes, no cut **anywhere** significantly impaired the maze learning.

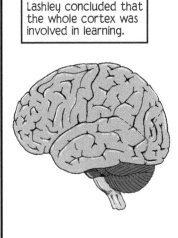

Lashley concluded that the whole cortex was involved in learning.

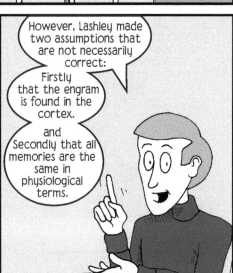

However, Lashley made two assumptions that are not necessarily correct:

Firstly that the engram is found in the cortex.

and Secondly that all memories are the same in physiological terms.

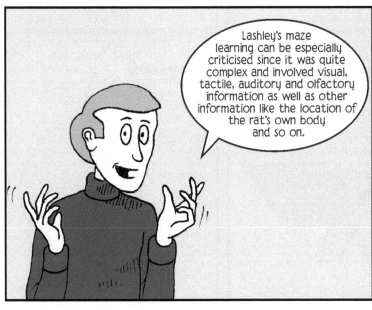

Lashley's maze learning can be especially criticised since it was quite complex and involved visual, tactile, auditory and olfactory information as well as other information like the location of the rat's own body and so on.

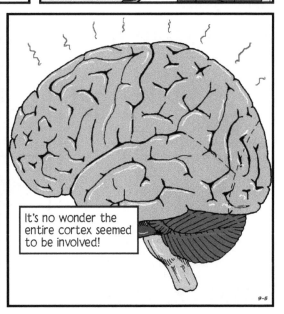

It's no wonder the entire cortex seemed to be involved!

9-5

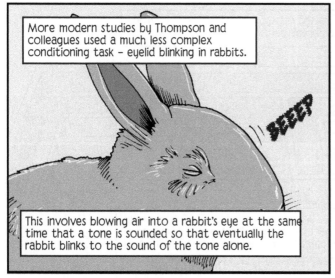

More modern studies by Thompson and colleagues used a much less complex conditioning task – eyelid blinking in rabbits.

This involves blowing air into a rabbit's eye at the same time that a tone is sounded so that eventually the rabbit blinks to the sound of the tone alone.

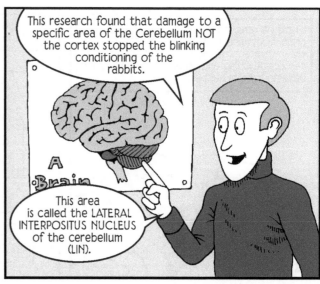

This research found that damage to a specific area of the Cerebellum NOT the cortex stopped the blinking conditioning of the rabbits.

This area is called the LATERAL INTERPOSITUS NUCLEUS of the cerebellum (LIN).

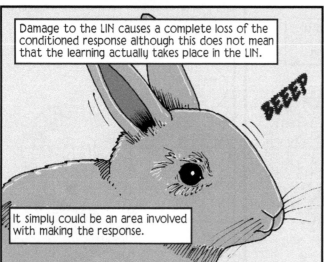

Damage to the LIN causes a complete loss of the conditioned response although this does not mean that the learning actually takes place in the LIN.

It simply could be an area involved with making the response.

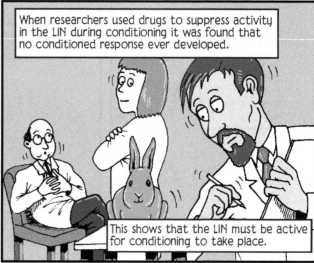

When researchers used drugs to suppress activity in the LIN during conditioning it was found that no conditioned response ever developed.

This shows that the LIN must be active for conditioning to take place.

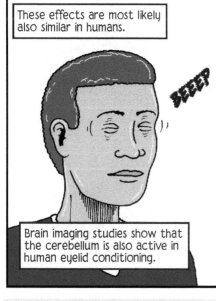

These effects are most likely also similar in humans.

Brain imaging studies show that the cerebellum is also active in human eyelid conditioning.

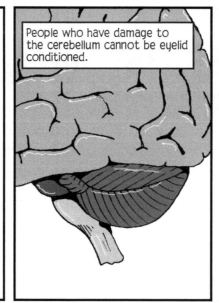

People who have damage to the cerebellum cannot be eyelid conditioned.

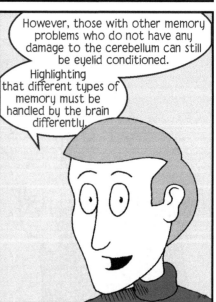

However, those with other memory problems who do not have any damage to the cerebellum can still be eyelid conditioned.

Highlighting that different types of memory must be handled by the brain differently.

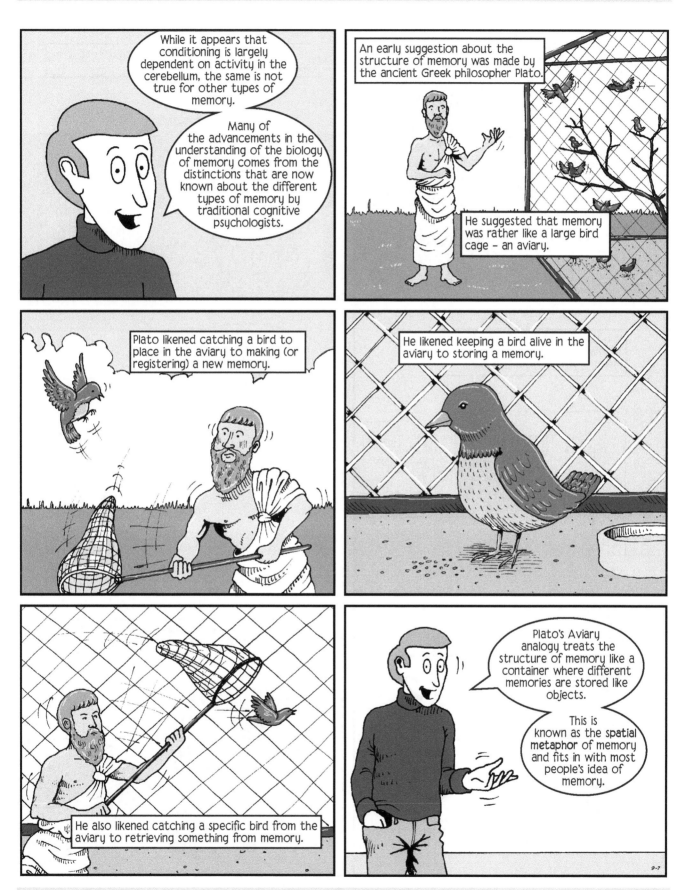

While it appears that conditioning is largely dependent on activity in the cerebellum, the same is not true for other types of memory.

Many of the advancements in the understanding of the biology of memory comes from the distinctions that are now known about the different types of memory by traditional cognitive psychologists.

An early suggestion about the structure of memory was made by the ancient Greek philosopher Plato.

He suggested that memory was rather like a large bird cage – an aviary.

Plato likened catching a bird to place in the aviary to making (or registering) a new memory.

He likened keeping a bird alive in the aviary to storing a memory.

He also likened catching a specific bird from the aviary to retrieving something from memory.

Plato's Aviary analogy treats the structure of memory like a container where different memories are stored like objects.

This is known as the spatial metaphor of memory and fits in with most people's idea of memory.

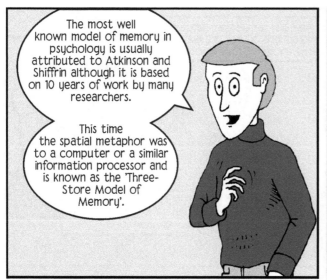

The most well known model of memory in psychology is usually attributed to Atkinson and Shiffrin although it is based on 10 years of work by many researchers.

This time the spatial metaphor was to a computer or a similar information processor and is known as the 'Three-Store Model of Memory'.

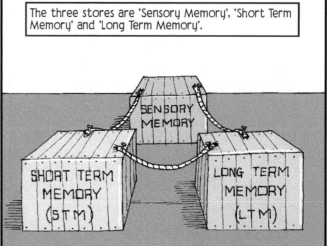

The three stores are 'Sensory Memory', 'Short Term Memory' and 'Long Term Memory'.

SENSORY MEMORY

SHORT TERM MEMORY (STM)

LONG TERM MEMORY (LTM)

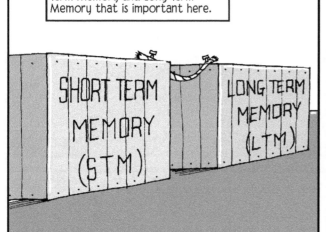

It is the distinction between Short Term Memory and Long Term Memory that is important here.

SHORT TERM MEMORY (STM)

LONG TERM MEMORY (LTM)

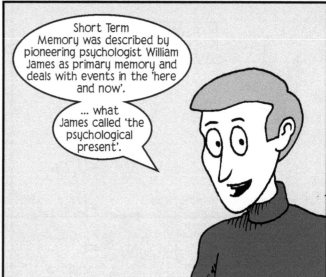

Short Term Memory was described by pioneering psychologist William James as primary memory and deals with events in the 'here and now'.

... what James called 'the psychological present'.

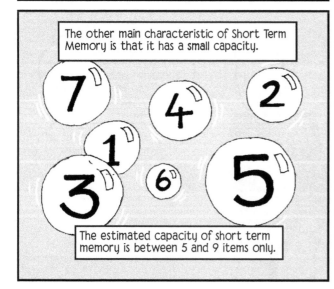

The other main characteristic of Short Term Memory is that it has a small capacity.

7   4   2
3 1   6   5

The estimated capacity of short term memory is between 5 and 9 items only.

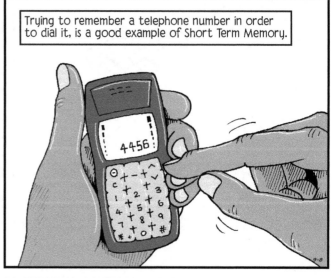

Trying to remember a telephone number in order to dial it, is a good example of Short Term Memory.

4456

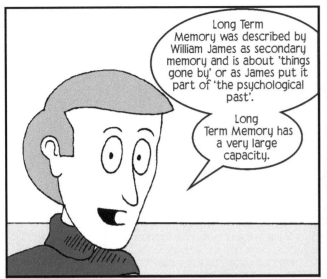

Long Term Memory was described by William James as secondary memory and is about 'things gone by' or as James put it part of 'the psychological past'.

Long Term Memory has a very large capacity.

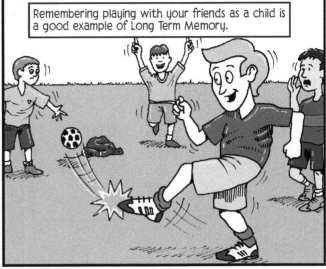

Remembering playing with your friends as a child is a good example of Long Term Memory.

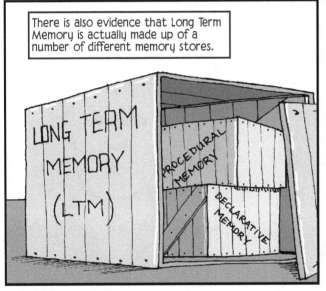

There is also evidence that Long Term Memory is actually made up of a number of different memory stores.

LONG TERM MEMORY (LTM)

PROCEDURAL MEMORY

DECLARATIVE MEMORY

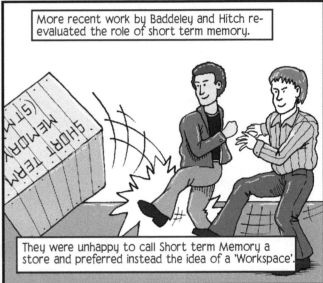

More recent work by Baddeley and Hitch re-evaluated the role of short term memory.

SHORT TERM MEMORY (STM)

They were unhappy to call Short term Memory a store and preferred instead the idea of a 'Workspace'.

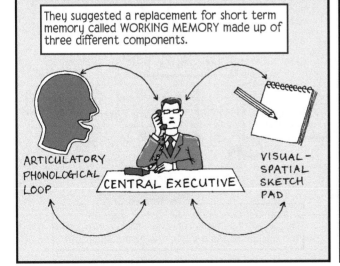

They suggested a replacement for short term memory called WORKING MEMORY made up of three different components.

ARTICULATORY PHONOLOGICAL LOOP

CENTRAL EXECUTIVE

VISUAL - SPATIAL SKETCH PAD

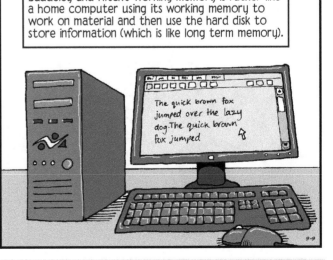

Baddeley and Hitch's working memory is rather like a home computer using its working memory to work on material and then use the hard disk to store information (which is like long term memory).

The quick brown fox jumped over the lazy dog. The quick brown fox jumped

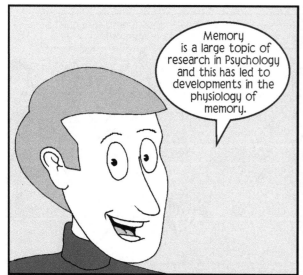

Memory is a large topic of research in Psychology and this has led to developments in the physiology of memory.

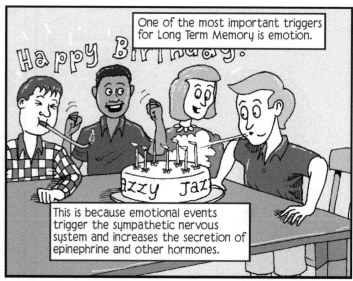

One of the most important triggers for Long Term Memory is emotion.

This is because emotional events trigger the sympathetic nervous system and increases the secretion of epinephrine and other hormones.

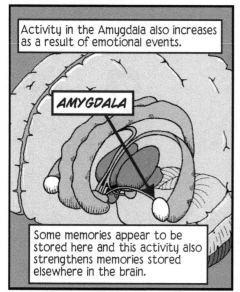

Activity in the Amygdala also increases as a result of emotional events.

AMYGDALA

Some memories appear to be stored here and this activity also strengthens memories stored elsewhere in the brain.

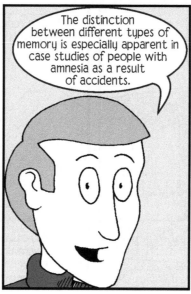

The distinction between different types of memory is especially apparent in case studies of people with amnesia as a result of accidents.

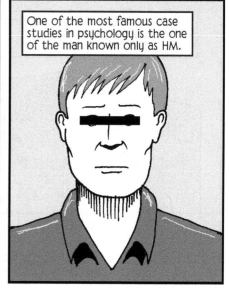

One of the most famous case studies in psychology is the one of the man known only as HM.

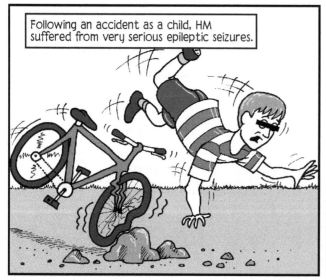

Following an accident as a child, HM suffered from very serious epileptic seizures.

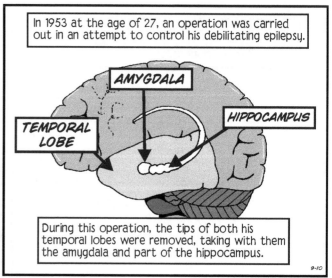

In 1953 at the age of 27, an operation was carried out in an attempt to control his debilitating epilepsy.

AMYGDALA

TEMPORAL LOBE

HIPPOCAMPUS

During this operation, the tips of both his temporal lobes were removed, taking with them the amygdala and part of the hippocampus.

9-10

Following his operation, HM seemed remarkably unaffected.

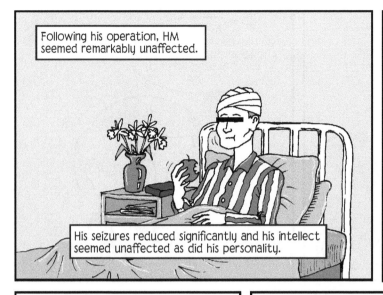

His seizures reduced significantly and his intellect seemed unaffected as did his personality.

In terms of his memory, HM could remember almost everything up to the moment of his operation.

Although his recall of events between 1 and 3 years before the operation was a bit patchy.

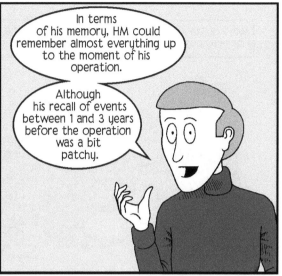

His most severe problem came from the memories he had for the time after his operation.

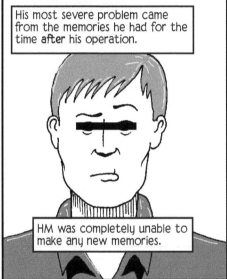

HM was completely unable to make any new memories.

HM was able to read the same magazine over and over again as new, he wouldn't recognise his doctor from one visit to the next and he had difficulty working out where his parents' new home was.

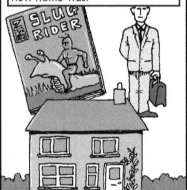

However, HM was able to learn some new skills like a small finger maze.

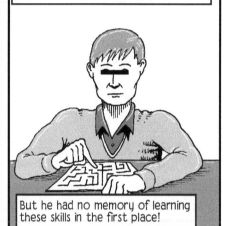

But he had no memory of learning these skills in the first place!

Case studies of amnesics like HM show that not all aspects of memory are lost equally.

This implies that there are several distinct types of memory that are independent of each other and are likely to have different biological bases.

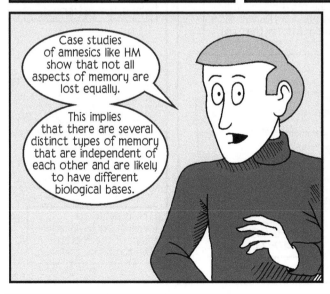

The damage to HM's brain was mainly to the amygdala – whose role in emotion and memory has already been described – and the hippocampus.

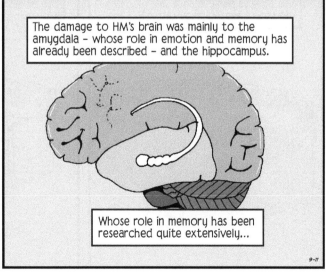

Whose role in memory has been researched quite extensively...

9-11

209

Most of the research concerning the role of the hippocampus in memory has been carried out using rats.

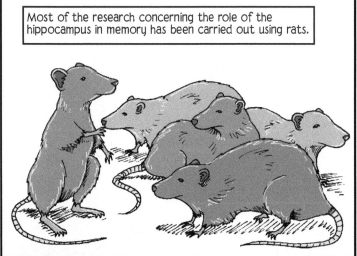

As with HM, damage to a rat's hippocampus affects some memory tasks and not others.

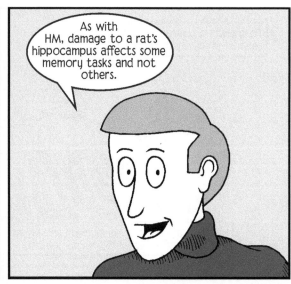

Radial maze experiments have trained rats to find food in specific arms of these mazes.

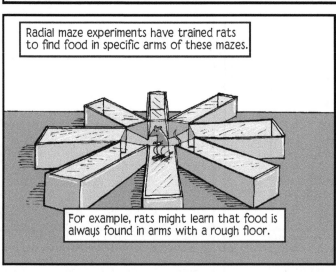

For example, rats might learn that food is always found in arms with a rough floor.

Rats without damage to the hippocampus learn quickly the rule about the radial arms and seldom re-visit arms they have already collected food from.

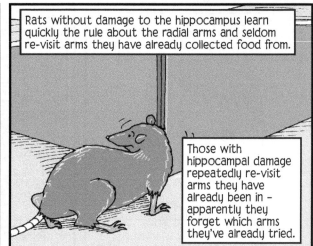

Those with hippocampal damage repeatedly re-visit arms they have already been in – apparently they forget which arms they've already tried.

Hippocampus damage in rats also affects performance on the Morris Water maze task.

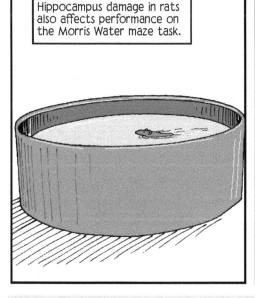

In this task, the rat is placed in a vat of milky liquid. In the vat there is a submerged platform that the rat needs to find to stop swimming.

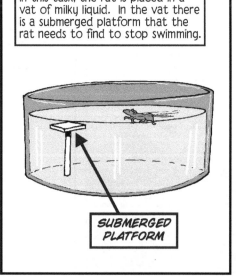

SUBMERGED PLATFORM

Normal rats quickly learn where the platform is.

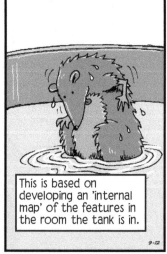

This is based on developing an 'internal map' of the features in the room the tank is in.

A rat with damage to the hippocampus however, repeatedly swims around trying to find the platform by chance.

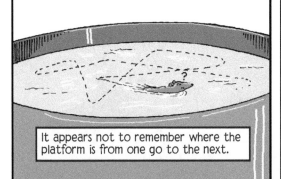

It appears not to remember where the platform is from one go to the next.

The hippocampus therefore seems to be involved in developing a spatial map.

For this reason one of the suggestions for the function of the hippocampus has been as the storage for a Cognitive Map.

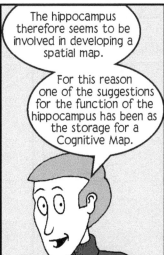

Here the hippocampus stores information about the relative position in space of various things in the environment.

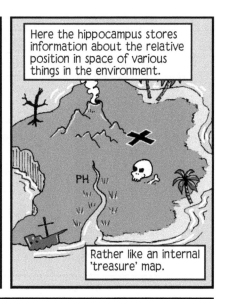

Rather like an internal 'treasure' map.

Compelling evidence for the idea of the hippocampus as a cognitive map comes from comparing the hippocampus of different species of birds.

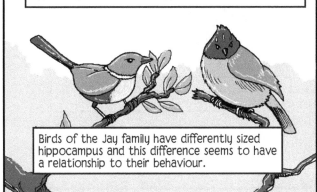

Birds of the Jay family have differently sized hippocampus and this difference seems to have a relationship to their behaviour.

Clarke's Nutcracker is a Jay that during the winter relies on finding food it has buried during the spring and summer.

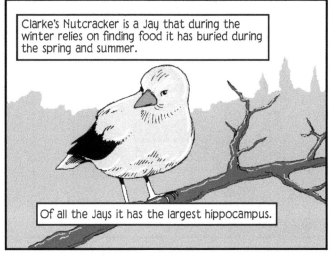

Of all the Jays it has the largest hippocampus.

Pinyon Jays are much less dependent on buried food during the winter and their hippocampus is smaller than Clarke's Nutcracker.

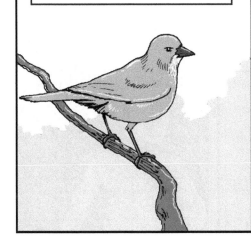

Scrub and Mexican Jays don't bury their food at all so don't have to find any of it during the winter and have the smallest hippocampus.

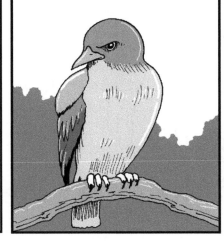

It would seem that if for survival a Jay **needs** to be able to remember accurately where it has buried its food, then it has developed a large hippocampus in which to 'store' the 'maps to the food'.

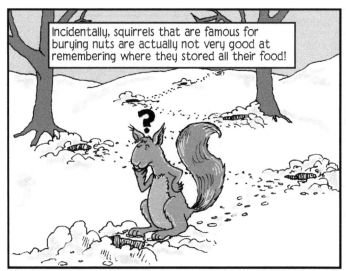

Incidentally, squirrels that are famous for burying nuts are actually not very good at remembering where they stored all their food!

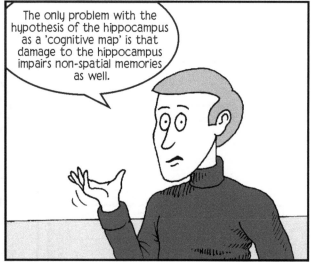

The only problem with the hypothesis of the hippocampus as a 'cognitive map' is that damage to the hippocampus impairs non-spatial memories as well.

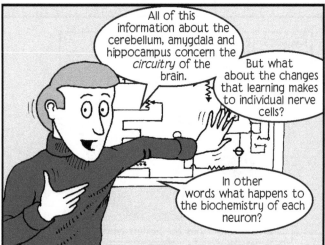

All of this information about the cerebellum, amygdala and hippocampus concern the *circuitry* of the brain.

But what about the changes that learning makes to individual nerve cells?

In other words what happens to the biochemistry of each neuron?

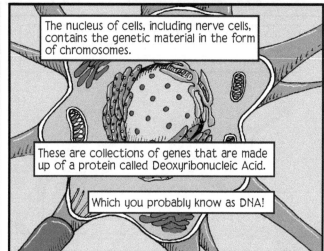

The nucleus of cells, including nerve cells, contains the genetic material in the form of chromosomes.

These are collections of genes that are made up of a protein called Deoxyribonucleic Acid.

Which you probably know as DNA!

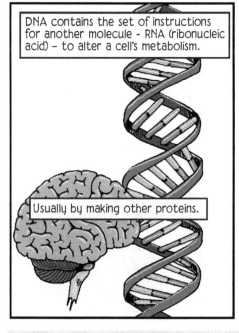

DNA contains the set of instructions for another molecule - RNA (ribonucleic acid) - to alter a cell's metabolism.

Usually by making other proteins.

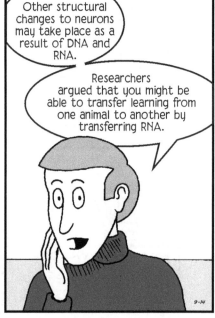

Other structural changes to neurons may take place as a result of DNA and RNA.

Researchers argued that you might be able to transfer learning from one animal to another by transferring RNA.

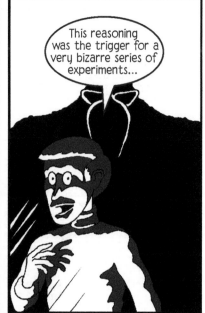

This reasoning was the trigger for a very bizarre series of experiments...

McConnell was one of the first to attempt one of these experiments.

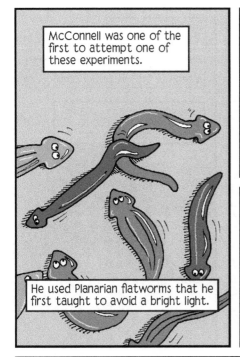

He used Planarian flatworms that he first taught to avoid a bright light.

He then chopped up and fed the trained worms to some untrained ones!

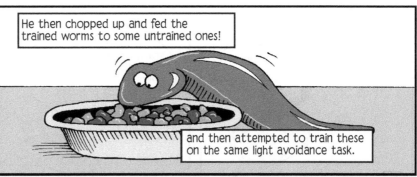

and then attempted to train these on the same light avoidance task.

McConnell found that the untrained worms became conditioned to avoid the light much quicker than those that had not fed on trained worms.

McConnell reasoned that the RNA in the trained worms had transferred the learning to the untrained worms through their 'food stuffs'.

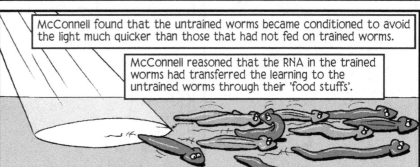

While McConnell's studies seemed promising, they have been criticised...

The main criticism being that it is very difficult to work out if planarian worms have actually learnt anything at all!

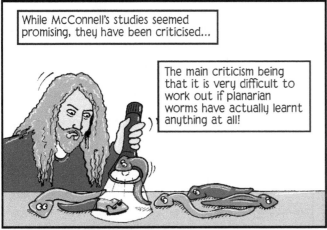

In the 1970s these transfer studies were carried out using animals that are usually easy to condition...

...Rats!

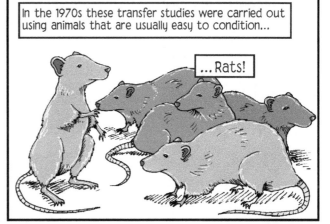

This work involved training a rat, extracting the RNA from its brain and then injecting this into an untrained rat.

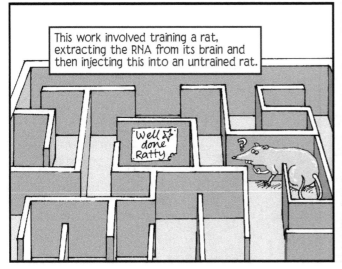

Well done Ratty

Overall, these studies only produced inconsistent results.

Furthermore, the most effective results involved tranferring peptide molecules not RNA or DNA.

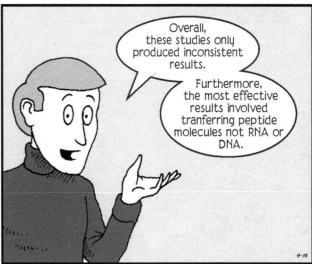

9-15

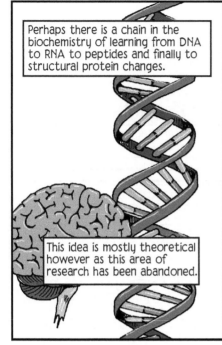

Perhaps there is a chain in the biochemistry of learning from DNA to RNA to peptides and finally to structural protein changes.

This idea is mostly theoretical however as this area of research has been abandoned.

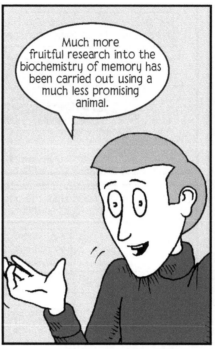

Much more fruitful research into the biochemistry of memory has been carried out using a much less promising animal.

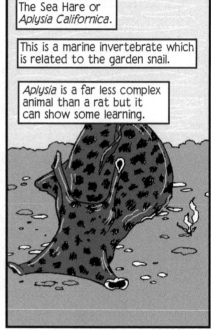

The Sea Hare or *Aplysia Californica*.

This is a marine invertebrate which is related to the garden snail.

Aplysia is a far less complex animal than a rat but it can show some learning.

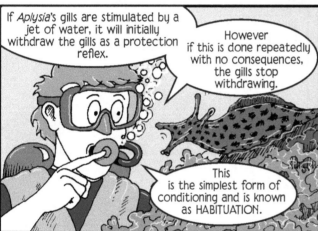

If *Aplysia*'s gills are stimulated by a jet of water, it will initially withdraw the gills as a protection reflex.

However if this is done repeatedly with no consequences, the gills stop withdrawing.

This is the simplest form of conditioning and is known as HABITUATION.

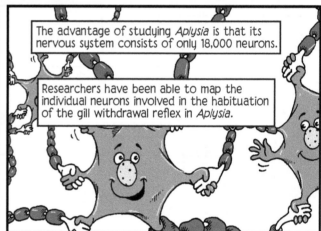

The advantage of studying *Aplysia* is that its nervous system consists of only 18,000 neurons.

Researchers have been able to map the individual neurons involved in the habituation of the gill withdrawal reflex in *Aplysia*.

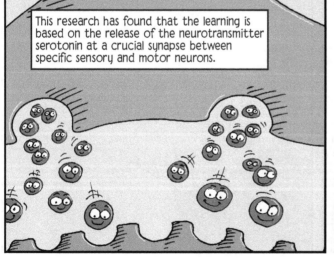

This research has found that the learning is based on the release of the neurotransmitter serotonin at a crucial synapse between specific sensory and motor neurons.

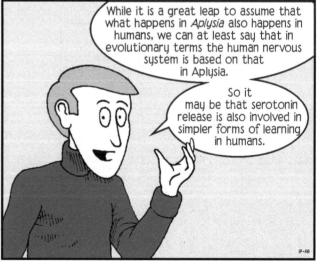

While it is a great leap to assume that what happens in *Aplysia* also happens in humans, we can at least say that in evolutionary terms the human nervous system is based on that in Aplysia.

So it may be that serotonin release is also involved in simpler forms of learning in humans.

9-16

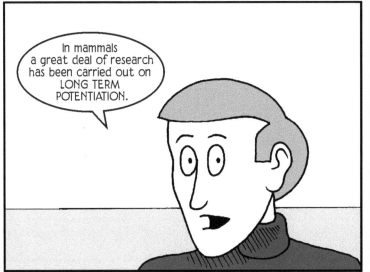

In mammals a great deal of research has been carried out on LONG TERM POTENTIATION.

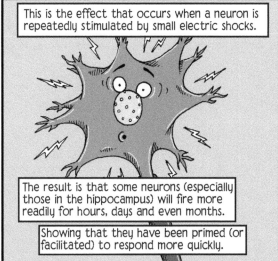

This is the effect that occurs when a neuron is repeatedly stimulated by small electric shocks.

The result is that some neurons (especially those in the hippocampus) will fire more readily for hours, days and even months.

Showing that they have been primed (or facilitated) to respond more quickly.

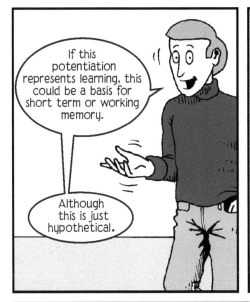

If this potentiation represents learning, this could be a basis for short term or working memory.

Although this is just hypothetical.

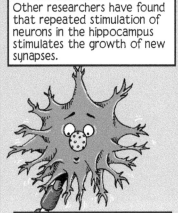

Other researchers have found that repeated stimulation of neurons in the hippocampus stimulates the growth of new synapses.

This could represent the basis for long term changes in circuitry and so a basis for long term memory.

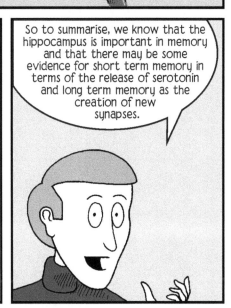

So to summarise, we know that the hippocampus is important in memory and that there may be some evidence for short term memory in terms of the release of serotonin and long term memory as the creation of new synapses.

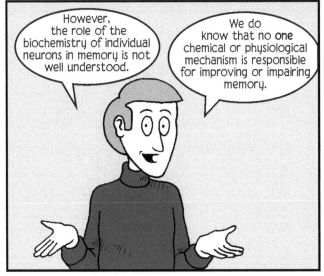

However, the role of the biochemistry of individual neurons in memory is not well understood.

We do know that no **one** chemical or physiological mechanism is responsible for improving or impairing memory.

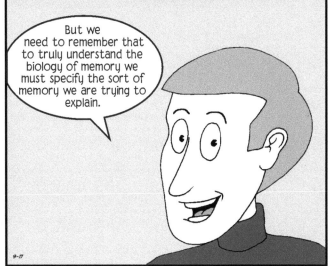

But we need to remember that to truly understand the biology of memory we must specify the sort of memory we are trying to explain.

9-17

215

Memory and learning

▶ **PAGE 200**

Panel 2

The connection between learning and memory is not straightforward. Learning is demonstrated by many different animals. Even single-celled organisms can be shown to have 'learnt' something. These learnt behaviours tend to be quite simple though. Things like avoiding swimming towards a light. A problem arises with the retention of this information. These simple animals don't remember the learning after a short period of time. In other words, they do not create any memories for the learning. So while learning is necessary for memory, memories are not always a consequence of learning.

▶ **PAGE 201**

Panel 2

See Pavlov (1927).

Panel 6

There are three types of conditioning according to Learning Theory:

Classical Conditioning ('Learning by Association')

This is also called Pavlovian conditioning and involves learning by association. A 'natural' behaviour, that is normally triggered by one event, is associated with an external stimulus so that eventually the stimulus alone causes the behaviour. It tends to occur in behaviours that you don't have much control over like salivating or blinking. Emotional responses are also said to be classically conditioned.

Operant Conditioning ('Learning by Consequences')

This type of conditioning involves learning by consequences. Behaviour that an animal has conscious control over (i.e. voluntary) is repeated if the consequences of that behaviour have positive benefits for the animal. Conversely behaviours that have negative consequences will not be repeated. This type of conditioning is associated with B. F. Skinner who developed 'skinner' boxes where animals (usually rats) had to learn to press levers to obtain a food reward.

Social Learning Theory ('Learning by Imitation')

This type of learning is associated with Albert Bandura who suggested that in addition to learning by association and consequences, we also learn by copying others. We will copy behaviours that we see others obtaining rewards for and stop those behaviours we see others being punished for.

▶ **PAGE 202**

Panel 7

See Lashley (1929, 1950).

▶ **PAGE 203**

Panel 4

Lashley's conclusions were a little more complex than is suggested here. Because he found that no cut in a rat's cortex could interfere with learning, he suggested two principles about the biology of memory.

Firstly, he said that there was a principle of *Equipotentiality* whereby all parts of the cortex are involved in the control of complex behaviour and that any damaged part can be replaced by any other.

Secondly, he suggested the principle of *Mass Action*. Here he was suggesting that the cortex works as a whole rather than different tasks being carried out by different parts of the cortex.

While these seemed reasonable conclusions at the time, Lashley did not account for the complexity of the learning tasks that he had taught to the rats. The tasks involved the whole cortex because many aspects of the rats' behaviour were needed to carry out them out.

▶ **PAGE 204**

Panel 2

See Thompson (1986).

Panel 5

A PET scan or Positron Emission Tomography is a brain imaging technique that involves injecting a radioactive chemical into the blood that is taken up by parts of the brain. Active parts of the brain will take up more of this chemical than non-active parts. The PET scanner can then detect which areas of the brain are most active during a particular behaviour. In this way we can determine what parts of the brain are activated when we do something.

Using PET scans Logan and Grafton (1995) found that the classical conditioning of eyelid blinking in young adults showed increased activity in the cerebellum and other areas.

Other imaging methods are CAT scans (Computerised Axial Tomography) and MRI scans (Magnetic Resonance Imaging).

Panel 6

See Woodruff-Pak, Papka and Ivry (1996).

▶ **PAGE 206**

Panel 1

See Atkinson and Shiffrin (1968).

Panel 4

See James (1890).

Panel 5

Miller (1956), in a classic paper in Cognitive Psychology, reviewed several different studies on short-term memory and found that its capacity was limited to about seven items of information plus or minus two. In other words the capacity was between 5 and 9 items. What constitutes an 'item' varies. It can mean a single number or letter or a meaningful combination of a few numbers or letters.

▶ **PAGE 207**

Panel 4

See Baddeley and Hitch (1974).

▶ **PAGE 208**

Panel 5

The case of HM, sometimes known as Henry M., was described by Scoville and Milner (1957). At the age of 7, HM was involved in a bicycle accident that was thought to have been the cause of his minor epileptic seizures that started three years later. At the age of 16, HM had his first major seizure. Eventually these became more frequent and he was forced to give up his job in a local factory. Given that anti-convulsant drugs were no longer helping him, it was decided that experimental surgery had to be performed. As a result, in 1953, at the age of 27, HM underwent surgery that removed most of both of his temporal lobes where the seizures originated.

The results upon his epilepsy were quite successful. With the aid of drugs, his seizures became much milder and the major ones were reduced to one a year.

In terms of side-effects of the procedure, HM seemed amazingly unaffected. His personality and intelligence were not affected and in fact his IQ score increased.

However, in terms of memory, HM was severely impaired by any definition. Technically speaking he had severe *anterograde anmesia*. This refers the fact that his memories for events that occurred after the surgery were almost non-existent. He also suffered from mild *retrograde amnesia* for events that occurred about one year before the surgery. This refers to the fact that his memories for events prior to the surgery remained intact (apart for some events that happened a little time before the operation). This basically means that whilst his old memories remained intact, HM was unable to create any new memories.

This had a profound effect on HM's life. He was said to be a man who perpetually 'lived in the past' and always spoke as if he was still living in the 1950s. One of the best descriptions of his condition is by HM himself:

'Every day is alone in itself, whatever enjoyment I've had, and whatever sorrow I've had…Right now, I'm wondering: Have I done or said something amiss? You see, at this moment everything looks clear to me, but what happened just before? That's what worries me. It's like waking from a dream; I just don't remember' (Milner, 1970, p. 37).

▶ PAGE 210

Panel 1

There are three hypotheses that suggest how the hippocampus is involved in memory:

The Hippocampus and Declarative Memory

Squire (1992) has suggested that the hippocampus is essential for what is described as declarative memory. This is memory for events in your life that you declare about. One example of declarative memory is to recall what occurred during your holidays.

This idea fits in well with HM and other cases of amnesia. Most amnesiacs lose the ability to recount events but are able to learn new skills. However, it is difficult to obtain much animal study support for this hypothesis since animals cannot declare anything.

Despite this problem, there is some evidence for this idea in rats and chimpanzees, but it is a little mixed and open to other criticisms (for example see Fortin, Agster & Eichenbaum, 2002; Kesner, Gilbert & Barua, 2002; and Zola *et al.*, 2000)

The Hippocampus and Spatial Memory

This suggestion is that the hippocampus is especially important for the development of memory for spatial locations. This is the work that involves the radial search maze, the Morris Search task and the comparative work on Jays described in this chapter.

Human evidence for this study comes from work on brain imaging studies in London Taxi drivers. Maguire, Frackowiak and Frith (1997) found that the hippocampus was activated when the taxi drivers were asked questions about how to go from one London landmark to another. Bohbot, Allen and Nadel (2000) found that people with damage to the hippocampus had difficulty on tests of spatial memory.

Overall, whilst the hippocampus is indeed involved in spatial memories, this is not its only memory function. Damage to the hippocampus also causes a number of non-spatial impairments.

The Hippocampus and Configural Learning

The last suggestion is that the hippocampus is involved in memory for tasks that require a response to a number of different stimuli and the combinations between them. So, for example, an animal might need to learn that the colour red means food, the colour green also means food but red **and** green means no food.

There are studies which show that damage to the hippocampus causes impairment in configural learning tasks (Rickard & Grafman, 1998). However, this finding is not exclusive and the idea that the hippocampus is **essential** for configural learning has been changed.

A more recent suggestion is that the hippocampus stores a kind of 'map' for working out where all the different memories for a single event are stored in the brain so that the cortex can bring them all together.

The last suggestion concerning the function of the hippocampus is that damage to it causes an interruption in the production of certain hormones from the adrenal glands. Hippocampal damage in rats results in increased levels of adrenal hormones (e.g. cortisol) AND a disruption of spatial memories. Roozendaal *et al.* (2001) found that if these rats are given drugs that block the effects of the cortisol then their spatial memories return.

▶ **PAGE 213**

Panel 1

See McConnell (1962).

Panel 5

See Babich *et al.* (1965), Dyal (1971) and Fjerdingstad (1973).

Babich *et al.* (1965) trained rats to follow a clicking sound in order to find food. Once they established that the rats had adequately learnt this skill, they removed their brains and extracted the RNA within. After this, they injected the extracted RNA into untrained rats. These rats learned to follow the clicking sound in fewer trials than before.

This research led to a rush of similar studies that unfortunately found it difficult to replicate Babich *et al.*'s (1965) findings. Eventually this line of research was completely abandoned.

▶ **PAGE 214**

Panels 3 and 4

See, for example, Kupferman *et al.* (1970).

▶ **PAGE 215**

Panel 1

See, for example, Bliss & Lømo (1973) and Weinberger, Javid & Lepan (1995).

CHAPTER 10
EVOLUTIONARY PSYCHOLOGY

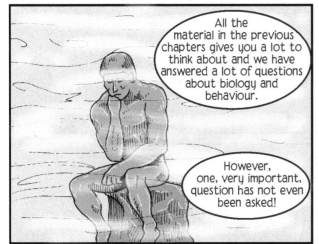

All the material in the previous chapters gives you a lot to think about and we have answered a lot of questions about biology and behaviour.

However, one, very important, question has not even been asked!

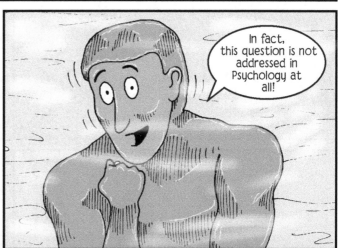

In fact, this question is not addressed in Psychology at all!

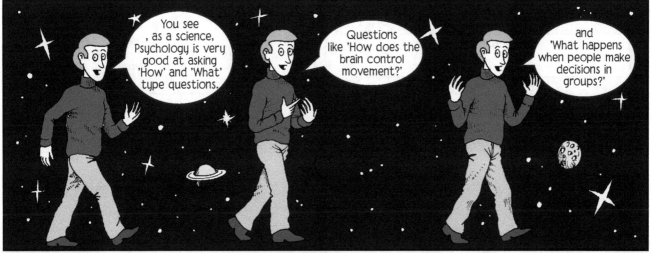

You see, as a science, Psychology is very good at asking 'How' and 'What' type questions.

Questions like 'How does the brain control movement?'

and 'What happens when people make decisions in groups?'

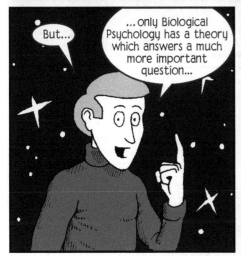

But...

...only Biological Psychology has a theory which answers a much more important question...

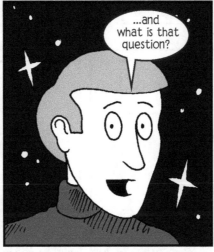

...and what is that question?

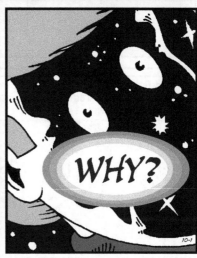

WHY?

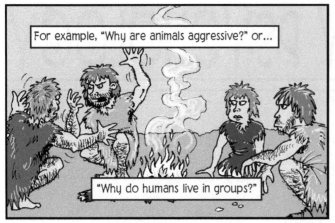

For example, "Why are animals aggressive?" or...

"Why do humans live in groups?"

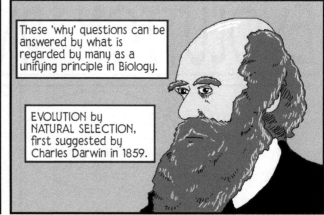

These 'why' questions can be answered by what is regarded by many as a unifying principle in Biology.

EVOLUTION by NATURAL SELECTION, first suggested by Charles Darwin in 1859.

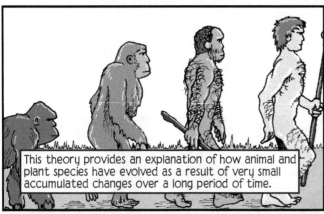

This theory provides an explanation of how animal and plant species have evolved as a result of very small accumulated changes over a long period of time.

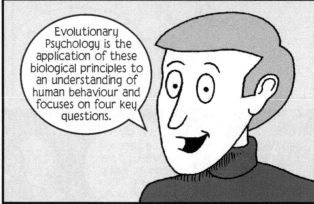

Evolutionary Psychology is the application of these biological principles to an understanding of human behaviour and focuses on four key questions.

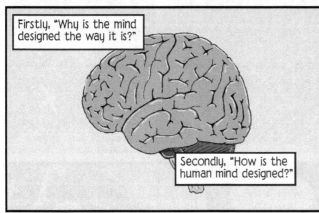

Firstly, "Why is the mind designed the way it is?"

Secondly, "How is the human mind designed?"

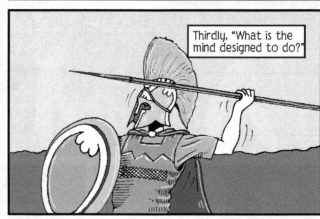

Thirdly, "What is the mind designed to do?"

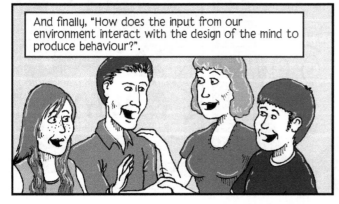

And finally, "How does the input from our environment interact with the design of the mind to produce behaviour?".

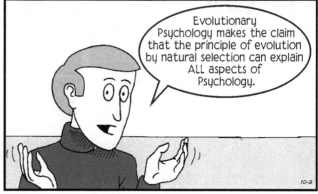

Evolutionary Psychology makes the claim that the principle of evolution by natural selection can explain ALL aspects of Psychology.

10-2

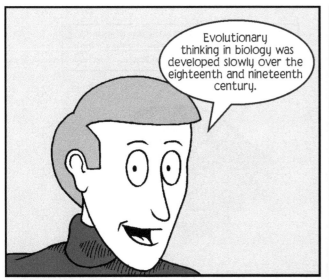

Evolutionary thinking in biology was developed slowly over the eighteenth and nineteenth century.

Before 1859 and Charles Darwin, it was well known that animal species had changed over time.

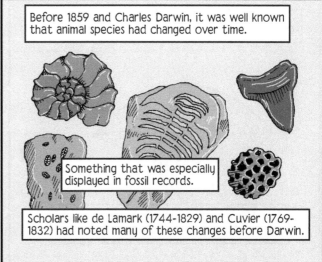

Something that was especially displayed in fossil records.

Scholars like de Lamark (1744-1829) and Cuvier (1769-1832) had noted many of these changes before Darwin.

However, it was Darwin's contribution of a method by which these changes take place that really revolutionised thinking in this area.

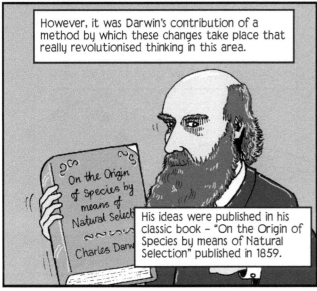

On the Origin of Species by means of Natural Selection

Charles Darwin

His ideas were published in his classic book – "On the Origin of Species by means of Natural Selection" published in 1859.

Darwin's ideas can be traced back to a five year trip he took around the world as a naturalist on board the ship the H.M.S. Beagle between 1831 and 1836.

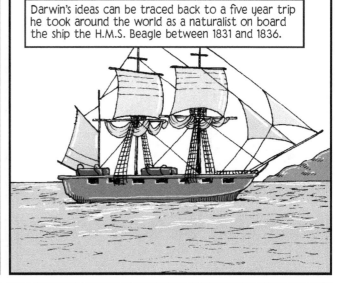

His important observations are often linked to the time Darwin spent on the Galapagos Islands off the coast of Ecuador.

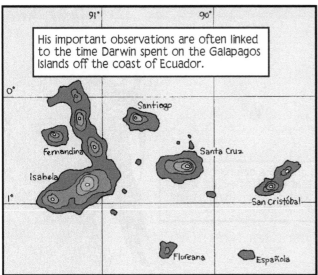

Darwin observed that Finches – a species of bird – on the different islands obviously came from a common ancestor but each had a different beak.

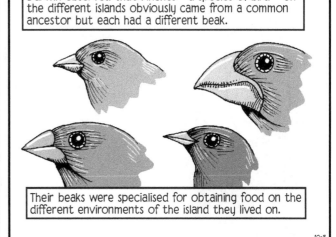

Their beaks were specialised for obtaining food on the different environments of the island they lived on.

10-3

225

Darwin observed that all of these finches appeared to be modified versions of a seed eating finch.

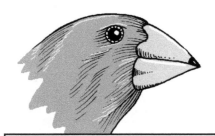

The different islands offered different types of food for the finches to adapt to.

On one island, where insects were abundant, the finch species had pointed beaks which enabled them to catch insects.

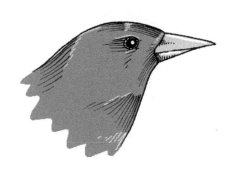

On another island, where fruit was plentiful, the finches had developed a larger beak that was suited to eating fruit and buds from plants.

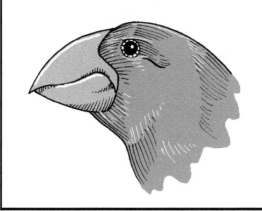

This appeared to be the case for several other species of finch. The type of food each island provided seemed to have influenced the development of the finch's beaks from that common seed eating ancestor. As Darwin wrote:

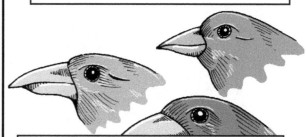

"One might really fancy that, from an original paucity of birds in this archipelago, one species had been taken and modified for different ends."

Whilst Darwin observed these species' changes, his goal was to devise a theory that explained HOW living things changed...

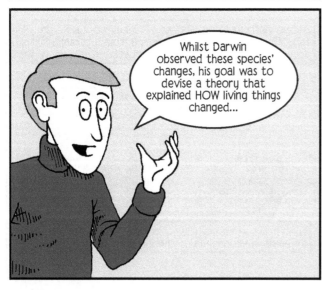

...from the different ways that plants distribute their seeds to the different ways animals find their food.

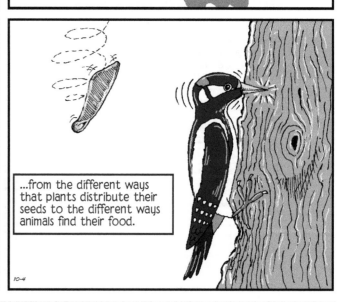

10-4

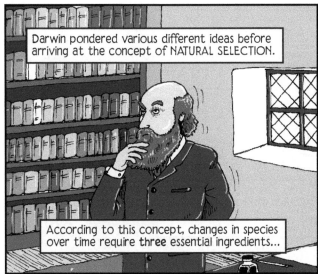

Darwin pondered various different ideas before arriving at the concept of NATURAL SELECTION.

According to this concept, changes in species over time require **three** essential ingredients...

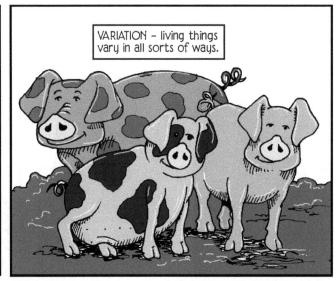

VARIATION – living things vary in all sorts of ways.

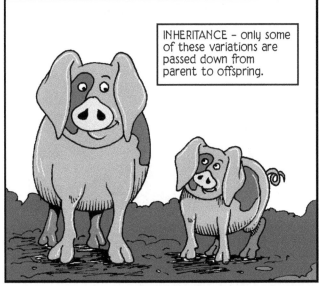

INHERITANCE – only some of these variations are passed down from parent to offspring.

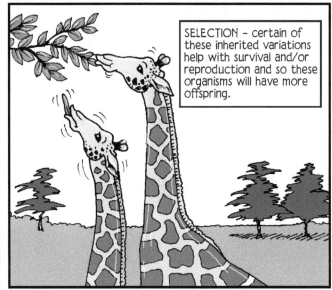

SELECTION – certain of these inherited variations help with survival and/or reproduction and so these organisms will have more offspring.

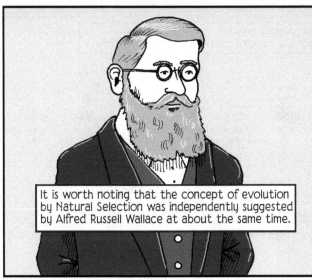

It is worth noting that the concept of evolution by Natural Selection was independently suggested by Alfred Russell Wallace at about the same time.

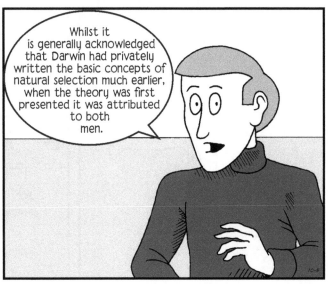

Whilst it is generally acknowledged that Darwin had privately written the basic concepts of natural selection much earlier, when the theory was first presented it was attributed to both men.

The most important concept in Natural Selection is that the possession of certain inherited factors increases or decreases a living thing's chances of survival and hence the chances of reproduction.

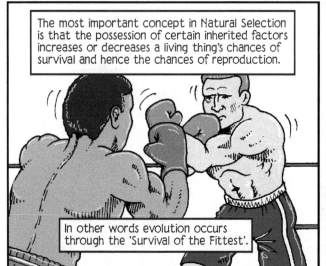

In other words evolution occurs through the 'Survival of the Fittest'.

Darwin used the concept of *differential reproductive success* to explain the comparative reproductive success of different individuals in a species.

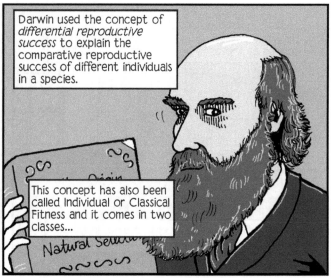

This concept has also been called Individual or Classical Fitness and it comes in two classes...

A role in Survival like taste allows an animal to choose the correct food to eat.

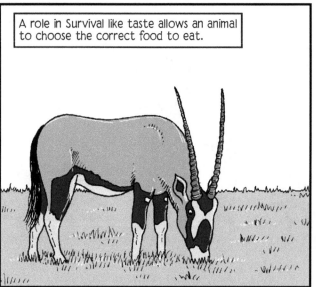

And a role in Reproduction like the song of a male songbird that attracts a mate.

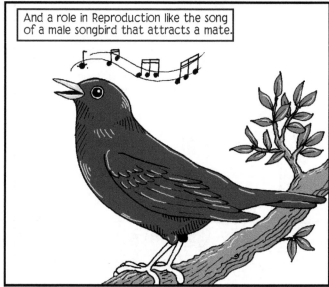

However, evolution is NOT intentional and does not work towards a goal. Natural selection acts upon all heritable variations that exist, favouring those that allow survival in the current environment.

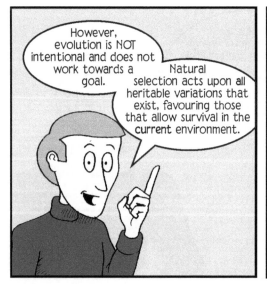

The changes brought about by natural selection happen over a very long time period.

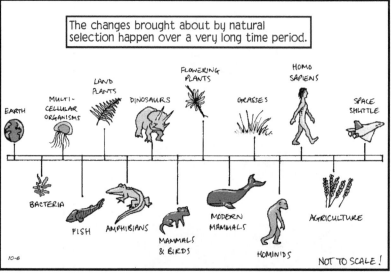

Evolution connects ALL living things into a large 'tree of descent' so that all species are connected to one another through common ancestors.

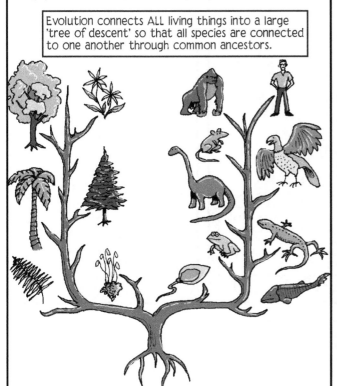

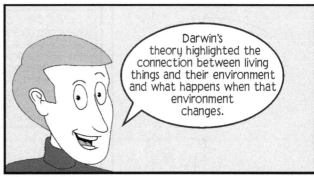

Darwin's theory highlighted the connection between living things and their environment and what happens when that environment changes.

Imagine a time when Giraffes had short necks...

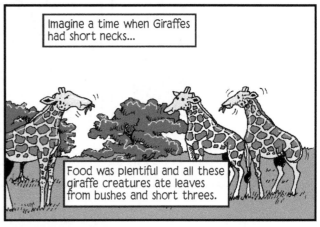

Food was plentiful and all these giraffe creatures ate leaves from bushes and short threes.

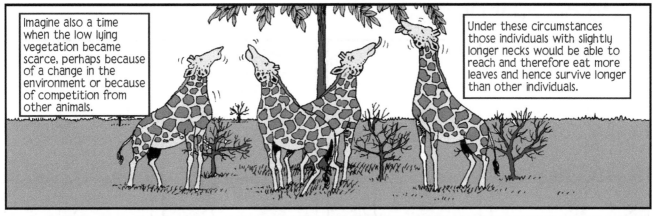

Imagine also a time when the low lying vegetation became scarce, perhaps because of a change in the environment or because of competition from other animals.

Under these circumstances those individuals with slightly longer necks would be able to reach and therefore eat more leaves and hence survive longer than other individuals.

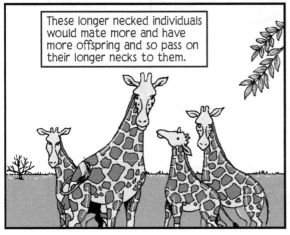

These longer necked individuals would mate more and have more offspring and so pass on their longer necks to them.

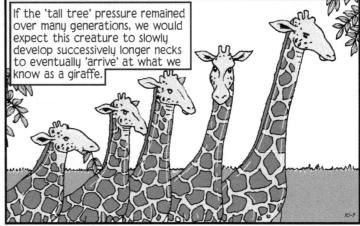

If the 'tall tree' pressure remained over many generations, we would expect this creature to slowly develop successively longer necks to eventually 'arrive' at what we know as a giraffe.

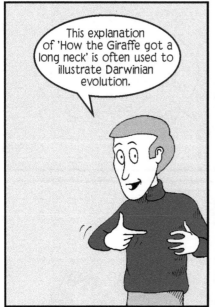

This explanation of 'How the Giraffe got a long neck' is often used to illustrate Darwinian evolution.

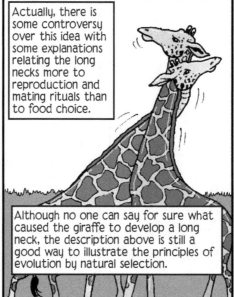

Actually, there is some controversy over this idea with some explanations relating the long necks more to reproduction and mating rituals than to food choice.

Although no one can say for sure what caused the giraffe to develop a long neck, the description above is still a good way to illustrate the principles of evolution by natural selection.

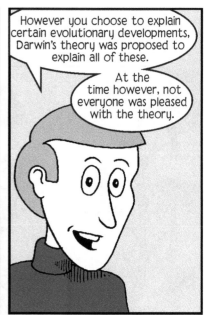

However you choose to explain certain evolutionary developments, Darwin's theory was proposed to explain all of these.

At the time however, not everyone was pleased with the theory.

The first criticism of Darwin's theory concerned the usefulness of early stages of evolutionary changes. For example, how could a partial wing be an advantage?

GOOD OL' CHARLIE D BY EWAN MEE

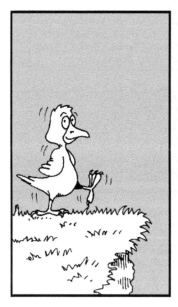

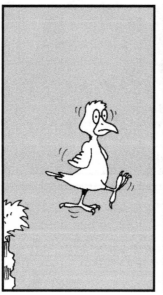

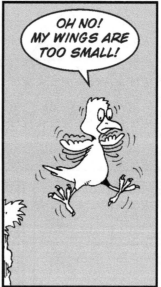

OH NO! MY WINGS ARE TOO SMALL!

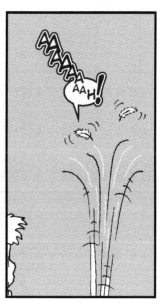

AAH!

Darwin's point was that partial physical changes MUST convey a reproductive or survival advantage regardless of whether we can imagine how.

10-8

Darwin's greatest critics were those who believed in religious creation.

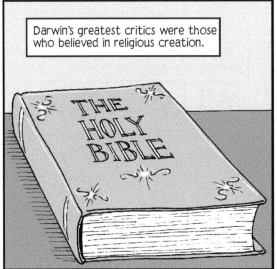

At the time Darwin published his theory, most people believed that all living things were created by a deity and were therefore unchanging.

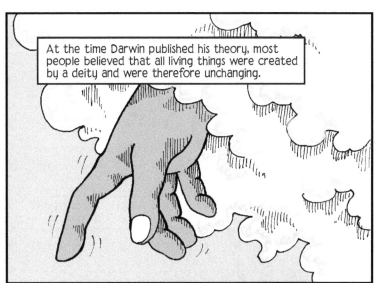

The additional problem for Creationists was that Darwin suggested that humans had developed as a result of random natural selection rather than as a part of 'God's Great Plan'.

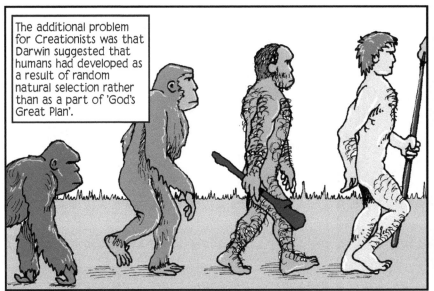

Darwin realised the religious issues that his theory would raise and agonised about publishing his book.

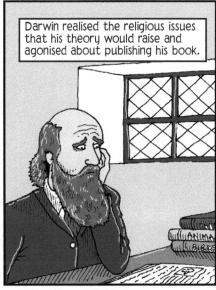

The last objection to Darwin's theory was the lack of a developed theory of inheritance.

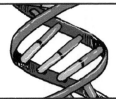

Darwin was unaware of genetics and favoured a theory whereby parents' inherited factors were blended in offspring. So that a tall man and a short woman would have average height children for example.

Through work on genes after Darwin, we now know that the blending theory is incorrect.

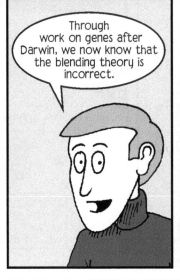

The true nature of inheritance was discovered by a contemporary of Darwin's.

He was an Austrian Monk called Gregor Mendel.

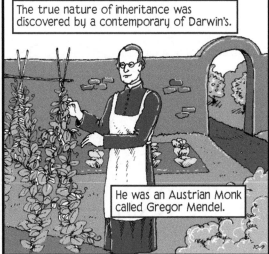

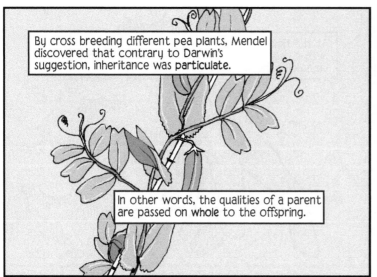

By cross breeding different pea plants, Mendel discovered that contrary to Darwin's suggestion, inheritance was **particulate**.

In other words, the qualities of a parent are passed on **whole** to the offspring.

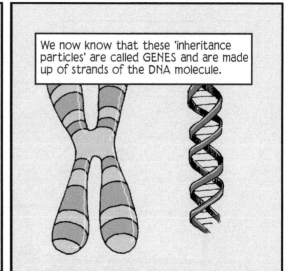

We now know that these 'inheritance particles' are called GENES and are made up of strands of the DNA molecule.

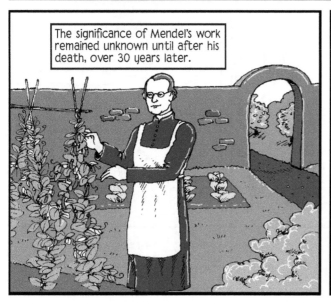

The significance of Mendel's work remained unknown until after his death, over 30 years later.

It is possible that Darwin could have been vaguely aware of Mendel's work since his library contained books by W. O. Focke and H. Hoffmann, both of whom referred to Mendel.

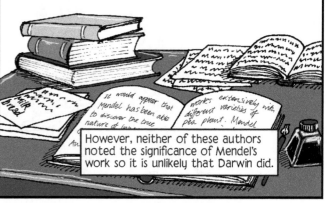

However, neither of these authors noted the significance of Mendel's work so it is unlikely that Darwin did.

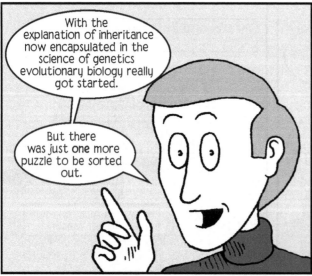

With the explanation of inheritance now encapsulated in the science of genetics evolutionary biology really got started.

But there was just **one** more puzzle to be sorted out.

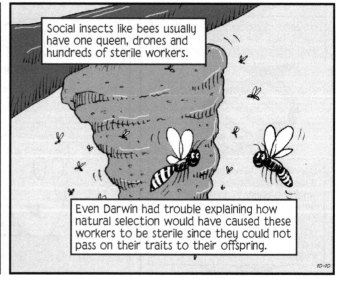

Social insects like bees usually have one queen, drones and hundreds of sterile workers.

Even Darwin had trouble explaining how natural selection would have caused these workers to be sterile since they could not pass on their traits to their offspring.

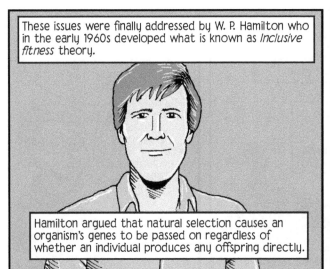

These issues were finally addressed by W. P. Hamilton who in the early 1960s developed what is known as *Inclusive fitness* theory.

Hamilton argued that natural selection causes an organism's genes to be passed on regardless of whether an individual produces any offspring directly.

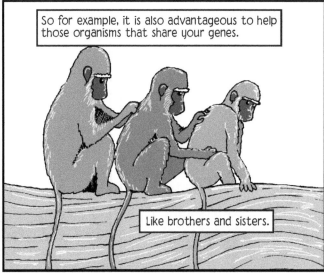

So for example, it is also advantageous to help those organisms that share your genes.

Like brothers and sisters.

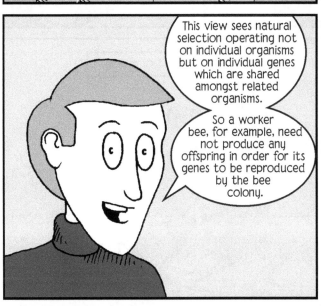

This view sees natural selection operating not on individual organisms but on individual genes which are shared amongst related organisms.

So a worker bee, for example, need not produce any offspring in order for its genes to be reproduced by the bee colony.

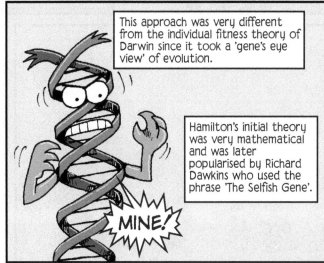

This approach was very different from the individual fitness theory of Darwin since it took a 'gene's eye view' of evolution.

Hamilton's initial theory was very mathematical and was later popularised by Richard Dawkins who used the phrase 'The Selfish Gene'.

MINE!

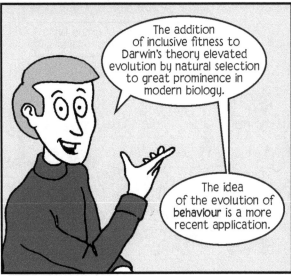

The addition of inclusive fitness to Darwin's theory elevated evolution by natural selection to great prominence in modern biology.

The idea of the evolution of **behaviour** is a more recent application.

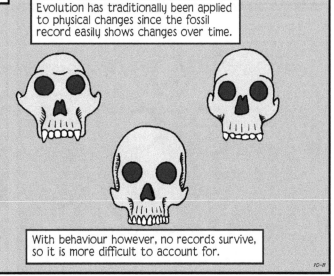

Evolution has traditionally been applied to physical changes since the fossil record easily shows changes over time.

With behaviour however, no records survive, so it is more difficult to account for.

10-11

233

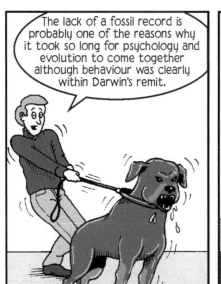

The lack of a fossil record is probably one of the reasons why it took so long for psychology and evolution to come together although behaviour was clearly within Darwin's remit.

Darwin argued that natural selection must play a part in, for example, aggression in dogs since aggressive dog breeds have been developed by cross breeding.

Early attempts to use evolutionary theory to explain behaviour concentrated on animals and was called ETHOLOGY.

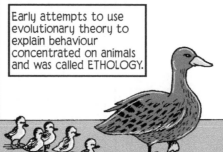

This looked at concepts like imprinting that describes how a new born duck follows the first thing it sees when it hatches.

Modern evolutionary psychology attempts to explain ALL human psychological phenomena using the concepts of natural selection.

There are four areas that are covered in explaining behaviour from an evolutionary perspective...

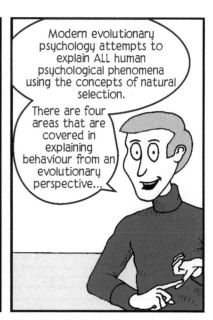

Problems of survival and growth...

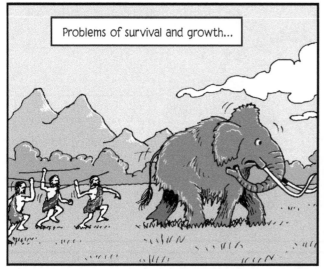

Problems of mating...

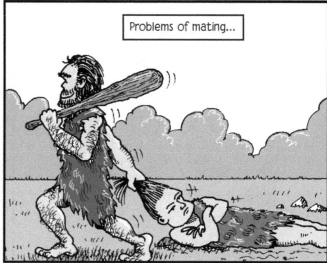

Problems of parenting...

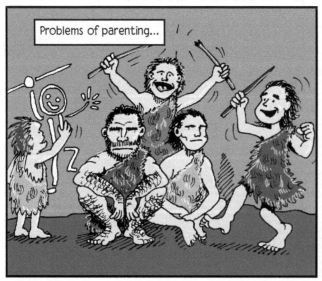

and problems of group living and aiding genetic relatives.

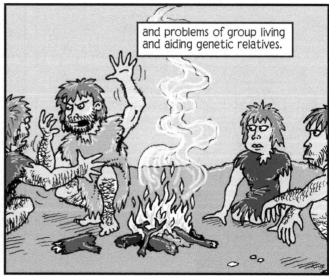

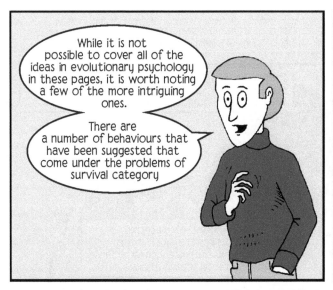

While it is not possible to cover all of the ideas in evolutionary psychology in these pages, it is worth noting a few of the more intriguing ones.

There are a number of behaviours that have been suggested that come under the problems of survival category

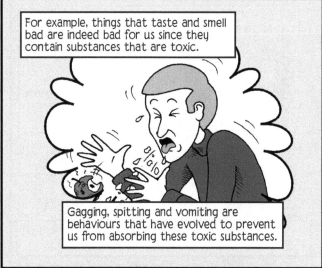

For example, things that taste and smell bad are indeed bad for us since they contain substances that are toxic.

Gagging, spitting and vomiting are behaviours that have evolved to prevent us from absorbing these toxic substances.

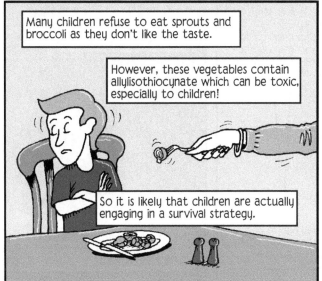

Many children refuse to eat sprouts and broccoli as they don't like the taste.

However, these vegetables contain allylisothiocynate which can be toxic, especially to children!

So it is likely that children are actually engaging in a survival strategy.

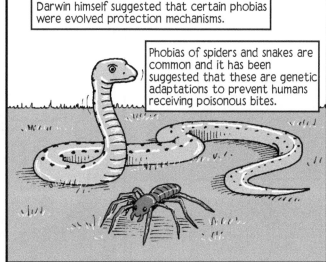

Darwin himself suggested that certain phobias were evolved protection mechanisms.

Phobias of spiders and snakes are common and it has been suggested that these are genetic adaptations to prevent humans receiving poisonous bites.

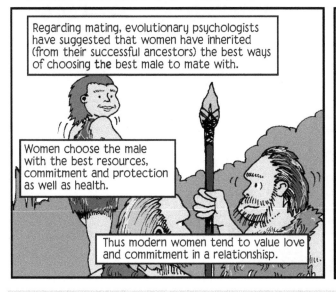

Regarding mating, evolutionary psychologists have suggested that women have inherited (from their successful ancestors) the best ways of choosing **the** best male to mate with.

Women choose the male with the best resources, commitment and protection as well as health.

Thus modern women tend to value love and commitment in a relationshisp.

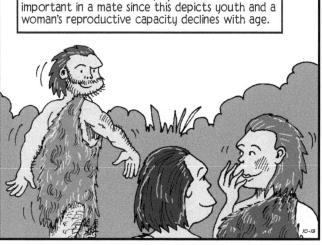

Men have evolved to find physical attraction important in a mate since this depicts youth and a woman's reproductive capacity declines with age.

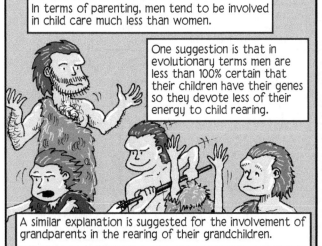

In terms of parenting, men tend to be involved in child care much less than women.

One suggestion is that in evolutionary terms men are less than 100% certain that their children have their genes so they devote less of their energy to child rearing.

A similar explanation is suggested for the involvement of grandparents in the rearing of their grandchildren.

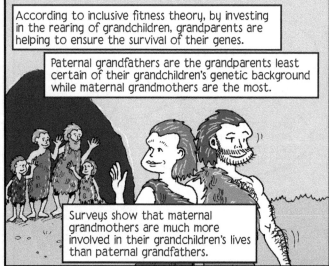

According to inclusive fitness theory, by investing in the rearing of grandchildren, grandparents are helping to ensure the survival of their genes.

Paternal grandfathers are the grandparents least certain of their grandchildren's genetic background while maternal grandmothers are the most.

Surveys show that maternal grandmothers are much more involved in their grandchildren's lives than paternal grandfathers.

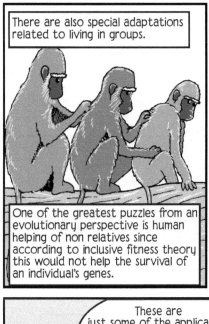

There are also special adaptations related to living in groups.

One of the greatest puzzles from an evolutionary perspective is human helping of non relatives since according to inclusive fitness theory this would not help the survival of an individual's genes.

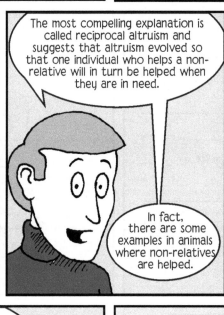

The most compelling explanation is called reciprocal altruism and suggests that altruism evolved so that one individual who helps a non-relative will in turn be helped when they are in need.

In fact, there are some examples in animals where non-relatives are helped.

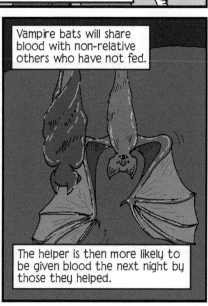

Vampire bats will share blood with non-relative others who have not fed.

The helper is then more likely to be given blood the next night by those they helped.

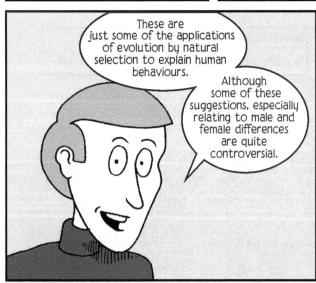

These are just some of the applications of evolution by natural selection to explain human behaviours.

Although some of these suggestions, especially relating to male and female differences are quite controversial.

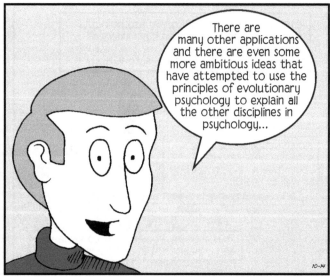

There are many other applications and there are even some more ambitious ideas that have attempted to use the principles of evolutionary psychology to explain all the other disciplines in psychology...

10-14

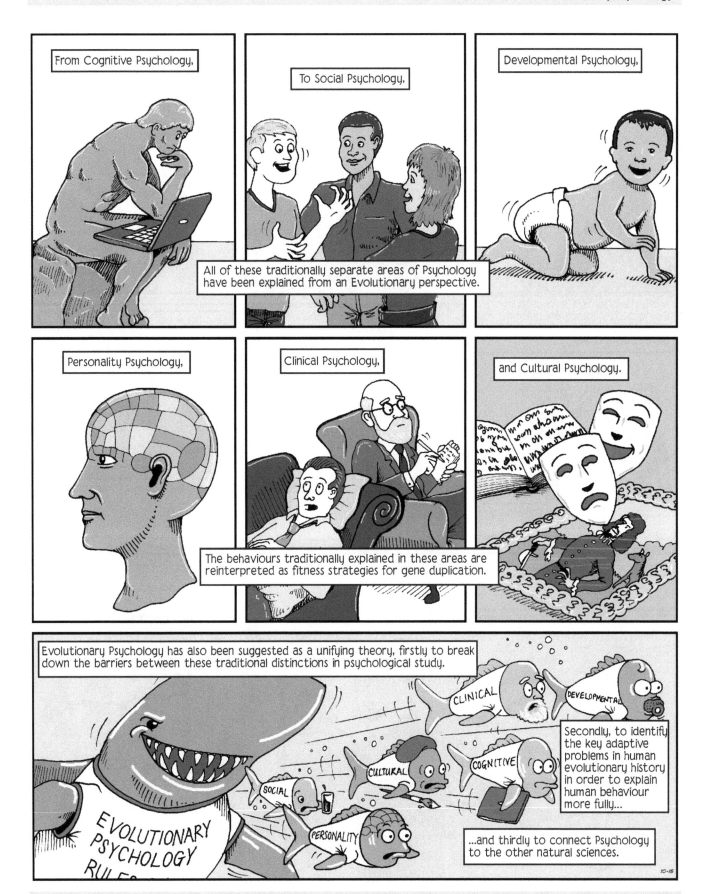

From Cognitive Psychology,

To Social Psychology,

Developmental Psychology,

All of these traditionally separate areas of Psychology have been explained from an Evolutionary perspective.

Personality Psychology,

Clinical Psychology,

and Cultural Psychology.

The behaviours traditionally explained in these areas are reinterpreted as fitness strategies for gene duplication.

Evolutionary Psychology has also been suggested as a unifying theory, firstly to break down the barriers between these traditional distinctions in psychological study.

CLINICAL

DEVELOPMENTAL

CULTURAL

COGNITIVE

SOCIAL

PERSONALITY

EVOLUTIONARY PSYCHOLOGY RULES

Secondly, to identify the key adaptive problems in human evolutionary history in order to explain human behaviour more fully...

...and thirdly to connect Psychology to the other natural sciences.

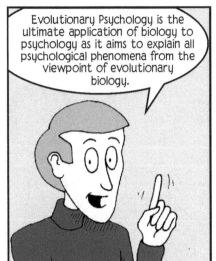

Evolutionary Psychology is the ultimate application of biology to psychology as it aims to explain all psychological phenomena from the viewpoint of evolutionary biology.

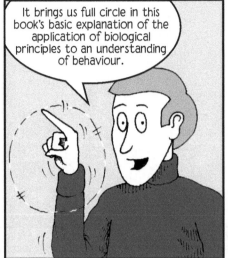

It brings us full circle in this book's basic explanation of the application of biological principles to an understanding of behaviour.

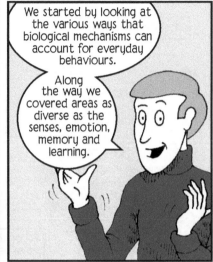

We started by looking at the various ways that biological mechanisms can account for everyday behaviours.

Along the way we covered areas as diverse as the senses, emotion, memory and learning.

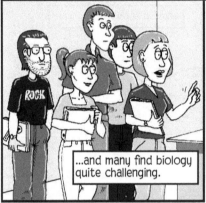

Many students first encountering Biological Psychology are quite nervous, especially if they haven't studied any biology beforehand...

...and many find biology quite challenging.

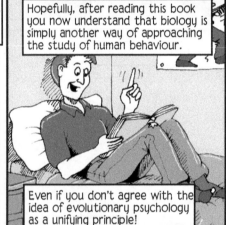

Hopefully, after reading this book you now understand that biology is simply another way of approaching the study of human behaviour.

Even if you don't agree with the idea of evolutionary psychology as a unifying principle!

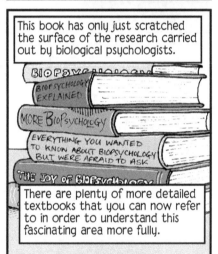

This book has only just scratched the surface of the research carried out by biological psychologists.

BIOPSYCHOLOGY
BIOPSYCHOLOGY EXPLAINED
MORE BIOPSYCHOLOGY
EVERYTHING YOU WANTED TO KNOW ABOUT BIOPSYCHOLOGY BUT WERE AFRAID TO ASK
THE JOY OF BIOPSYCHOLOGY

There are plenty of more detailed textbooks that you can now refer to in order to understand this fascinating area more fully.

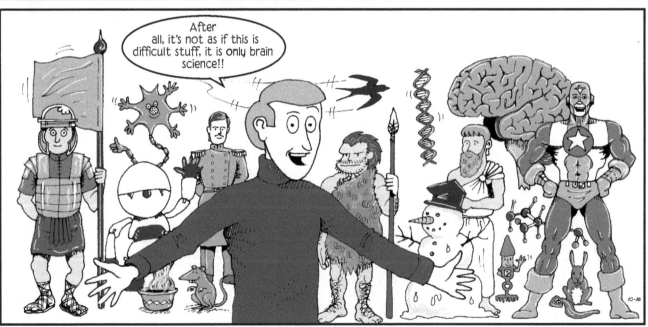

After all, it's not as if this is difficult stuff, it is only brain science!!

Evolutionary psychology

Most introductory books on Biological Psychology do not have a separate chapter on evolution and evolutionary psychology. It is true that all of these mention evolution and natural selection at some point but choose not to highlight this on its own. It is included here because it follows from the aim of this book to apply biological principles to an understanding of psychology. This chapter is an acknowledgement that Darwinian evolution is another biological theory that needs to be considered when attempting to understand human behaviour. Additionally, it is hoped that the basic principles introduced here will allow a better understanding of those texts that do refer to evolution in the course of their, more detailed, explanations of other areas.

▶ PAGE 224

Panel 3

This image (and many other common variations) is based on a painting by Rudy Zallinger usually referred to as 'The March of Progress'. It was used as the cover to a book called *Early Man* published in the 1970s. See the notes on the implications of this image below (Page 229 Panel 1).

▶ PAGE 225

Panel 2

The idea that living things change over time was originally known as *transmutation* (see Hosler, 2003). Darwin's ideas, observations and experiments on what he eventually termed *natural selection* were written over decades in journals that Darwin called 'The Transmutation Notebooks'. Transmutation is what we now know as *evolution*.

Panel 3

Common misunderstandings of Darwin's ideas often attribute to him the idea of evolution. He did not 'invent' the idea of evolution. Darwin's real breakthrough was the contribution of a method by which species evolve: Natural Selection.

Panel 4

Darwin was not originally brought on to the Beagle as a naturalist. He was accepted on the Beagle's five-year voyage (the ship's mission was to map and survey the coast of South America) as a dinner companion for the Captain, Robert Fitzroy. Apparently, Fitzroy wanted someone of a similar social standing to keep him company. When the ship's surgeon-come-naturalist Robert McCormick left, Darwin became the ship's full time naturalist even though he was not really qualified (he had failed to study Medicine at

Cambridge University and had then scraped through a Bachelor of Arts course – something his father hoped would qualify Darwin as a clergyman!).

As the ship's naturalist, Darwin excelled at carefully documenting the variety in the geology, the plants, animals and fossils in the places he visited. He collected an enormous number of fossils, many of animals unknown to science at the time. Some of these fossils fuelled his ideas on natural selection as they showed extinct versions of modern animals such as giant sloths. Before Darwin came to prominence as a result of his ideas on natural selection, he had become quite well known amongst the scientific community for the fossils that he had shipped back to England while he was still on the voyage. Darwin spent more time on land than on the ship over the five years which was probably a good thing since he suffered terribly from seasickness!

Panel 5

The Beagle visited the Galapagos Islands in 1835. The islands lie in the Pacific Ocean approximately 1000 km from the South American coast, either side of the Equator. There are a total of 13 large islands, 6 smaller ones and 107 islets and rocks. The islands have a total area of around 8000 km2. They are volcanic in origin and there are still several active volcanoes upon them. Currently, some of the islands are inhabited as was the case when Darwin visited.

Panel 6

Darwin's ideas on the finches were not developed until after he had returned to England. The birds he had thought were merely different varieties of 'mockingbirds' turned out, when examined by an expert, to be different species related to the finch. This led Darwin to wonder whether the different islands of the Galapagos – with their different environments – were the reason these finches were different. Unfortunately, Darwin had not labelled his stuffed specimens of these birds by island! Luckily other members of the Beagle's crew, including Robert Fitzroy, had been more meticulous in labelling their specimens.

▶ **PAGE 227**

Panels 5 and 6

Darwin had secretly pondered and worked on his theory since around 1838. He had only confided his ideas with two friends: Charles Lyell and Joseph Hooker. In 1858, however, he received a letter (dated 18 June) from a young naturalist called Alfred Russell Wallace, with whom he had previously corresponded. In it Wallace described a very similar evolutionary mechanism and asked Darwin to pass it on for publication. This prompted Darwin to finally want to present his ideas in public and it was decided that both Darwin and Wallace should present the theory jointly to the Linnaean Society on 1 July 1858 (although Darwin did not attend as his son had recently died of scarlet fever). However, there is absolutely no question that Darwin's ideas came first. Darwin's book *On the Origin of Species* was published the following year.

The full title of Darwin's book was 'On the Origin of Species by means of Natural Selection or The Preservation of the favoured races in the struggle for life' (it is normally just referred to as 'On the Origin of Species').

▶ **PAGE 228**

Panel 6

Evolution by natural selection is **very** gradual. It has taken dozens, hundreds, thousands and sometimes millions of generations to arrive at the animal and plant species that are alive today. Some changes are relatively quick while some are extremely slow; it all depends on the specific conditions. There are even situations where a great deal of time goes by without any evolutionary changes at all, followed by a relatively swift change called 'punctuated equilibrium' (Gould & Eldredge, 1977). Bear in mind that even a sudden change results in only very small adaptations.

▶ **PAGE 229**

Panel 1

The idea of visualising evolution as a tree rather than on a line, as was the convention at the time, was another contribution made by Charles Darwin.

The problem with the 'tree of life' image is that it suggests that those species on the lower branches are somehow 'less evolved' than those at the top and that there is a sort of 'march of progress' (see Page 224 Panel 3) whereby single celled organisms are 'waiting' to change into the more complex species above. However, there is nothing in natural selection that suggests that a move towards complexity is its 'goal'. It is wrong to think of evolution as having any 'goal'. As Hosler (2003) puts it '…evolution isn't necessarily a process of increasing complexity. It is a process of surviving the prevailing environmental conditions' (p.148). From this viewpoint, the most successful living things on this planet are also the least complex: bacteria. These livings things thrive in the harshest environments and attest to the success of their simple design. For an excellent discussion of these issues see chapter 3 in Pinker (1997).

Panels 3 to 6

The visualisations of these early 'giraffes' are invented and bear no resemblance to any actual scientific ideas.

▶ **PAGE 230**

Panel 2

Darwin himself suggested the long neck of the giraffe as a feeding strategy in the sixth edition of *On the Origin of the Species* in 1872. However, there a few problems with the idea:

1) The longer necked giraffes would be able to reach taller branches but would also be much heavier and therefore require more food.
2) Pincher (1949) pointed out that male giraffes are about one metre taller than females and so if the long neck was for feeding, the males would have been able to reach taller branches and the females would have died, killing off the entire species!
3) Ginnett and Demment (1997) found that female giraffes tend to feed from branches at their belly height which seems contrary to the idea of long necks as a feeding strategy. Other giraffe feeding studies including Leuthold and Leuthold (1972); Pellew (1984); Woolnough and du Toit (2001);

and Young and Isbell (1991) cast further doubt on the feeding strategy hypothesis. These show that giraffes actually do most of their feeding at shoulder height and during dry spells (when the theory suggests they should eat from higher branches) they seek out food from bushes below shoulder height.

4) There are other ways to eat from taller trees. Goats, for example, have been known to climb trees in order to eat from their top branches (Butzer, 2000) and elephants sometimes rear on their back legs to reach food.

Several other ideas have been suggested to account for the evolution of the giraffe's long neck. Pincher (1949) suggested that it was the giraffe's long legs that gave it the advantage of being faster and more able to escape predators while Brownlee (1967) suggested that the long neck and larger bulk of the giraffe would create a larger surface area to help with cooling down. It was Simons and Scheepers (1996) who suggested that it was sexual selection that caused the lengthening of the male giraffe's neck. However, none of these (and other) explanations are without their criticisms.

Panels 4 to 7

The issue of 'intermediary' advantages is something which caused Darwin a great deal of criticism. For example, how could a partial eye help an animal if it is insufficient for seeing things? Darwin's theory of natural selection requires each intermediary stage to offer some kind of advantage to the organism. So a partial eye must be an adaptive change. As Dawkins (1982) has pointed out, simply because someone cannot imagine the usefulness of a particular intermediate structure is not a good way to discredit the theory.

▶ PAGE 231

Panels 1 to 3

The controversy of religious creation continues to this day. It is the application of the theory to humans that creates the greatest resistance.

Darwin himself worried a great deal about the religious implications of his theory and is one of the reasons he took so long to publish his ideas. His wife, Emma, was devotedly religious and was openly worried about Darwin's theory, going so far as to be concerned for his soul.

▶ PAGE 231 (Panels 6 to 7) and PAGE 232 (Panels 1 to 2)

The significance of the work of Gregor Mendel remained unknown to the scientific community for 30 years. It was not until the 1900s that his work was rediscovered and its importance noted.

The combination of Darwin's theory of natural selection with Mendel's work on genetics occurred in the 1930s and 1940s and was called the *Modern Synthesis* (see Dobzhansky, 1937; Huxley, 1942; Mayr, 1942; Simpson, 1944).

Panel 4

Many writers have claimed that Mendel had sent Darwin copies of his papers and that these remained unopened or their significance un-noted by Darwin. However, none of these papers have been found amongst Darwin's collection which still survives (Sclater, 2003). Furthermore, even if Darwin had read these papers, he (like everyone else at the time) is unlikely to have fully understood their significance.

▶ **PAGE 233**

Panel 1

Hamilton's theory was developed as part of his doctoral dissertation. It was eventually published in 1964 (Hamilton, 1964). Buss (1999) suggests that this publication caused a 'revolution' that completely changed the field of biology.

Panel 4

Richard Dawkins popularised Hamilton's inclusive fitness theory in *The Selfish Gene* (Dawkins, 1989).

▶ **PAGE 234**

Panel 2

The application of evolutionary principles to behaviour is quite obvious. This is because firstly, all behaviour requires physical structures to operate. For instance, people need legs to be able to walk somewhere! Secondly, it is known that certain animals can be bred to exhibit certain behaviours. Dogs, for example, have been selectively bred by people over the years to produce breeds that are known to be aggressive. Breeds such as the Pit-bull, the Rottweiler, the Doberman and so on are well known to be aggressive.

Ethology

Ethology is in essence the study of animal behaviour. The principles developed were not meant to be applied to human behaviour (that application came later). The origins of ethology can be traced to the naturalists of the 1800s. Von Pernau and Spalding both investigated the behaviour of birds and concentrated on what was termed their 'innate' behaviour (see Plotkin, 1997).

The real start of the ethology movement was begun by Konrad Lorenz in the 1930s. One of the first phenomena to be investigated by Lorenz was *imprinting*. Lorenz found that baby ducks will follow the first moving object they see the moment they hatch. This is called imprinting. Normally this will be the ducks' mother and the young ducks will then follow the mother around. Lorenz found that if he exposed newly hatched ducks to his leg, they then followed **him** rather than their mother (see Lorenz, 1965). This behaviour, it was argued, was an evolved behavioural adaptation that followed Darwinian principles. It was upon this basis that ethology was founded as a branch of biology.

The other notable researcher in this area was Niko Tinbergen who is known for defining the subject matter of ethology (Tinbergen, 1951). These were:

1) The *immediate* causes of behaviour.
   In the case of imprinting in baby ducks, this is the mother's movement.
2) The *developmental* causes of behaviour.
   – such as the events in the baby duck's life.

3) The *function* of behaviour or its *adaptive purpose.*
   – keeping a baby duck close to its mother helps it to survive.
4) The *evolutionary* causes of behaviour.
   – the events, in evolutionary terms, that have led to the development of imprinting in ducks.

Ethology developed a number of other important concepts including *fixed action patterns*. These are sequences of behaviour that animals make that are started by a well defined stimulus. An example of a fixed action pattern is the courtship ritual of a male duck when exposed to a female duck.

Buss (1999) suggested that ethology 'died' out because it ran into three problems: firstly, concepts like imprinting acted more like labels than explanations; secondly, ethologists tended to ignore anything 'internal' that was not observable and hence did not try to understand the internal mechanisms that controlled animals' behaviour; thirdly, as a discipline, ethology did not develop adequate criteria for investigating behavioural adaptations.

However, Buss also stated that in ethology were the 'glimmers' of modern evolutionary psychology because it focused attention on the adaptive nature of behaviour and pointed psychologists in the direction of evolution as an explanation for human behaviour.

Sociobiology

The next major advancement in the application of Darwinian principles to human behaviour was outlined in a book by Wilson (1975) called *Sociobiology: The New Synthesis*. This was an in-depth examination of a large variety of biological and psychological principles and it argued that both animals and humans were unified by the principles of evolution. This was a controversial publication, especially the chapter dealing with humans. Many were appalled that Wilson suggested that a number of uniquely human phenomena, such as culture, ethics, religion, consciousness, rationalisation and so on, could be explained by evolution rather than the established psychological and sociological theories.

Buss (1999) suggested that the extreme reaction to Wilson's ideas (which did not include a great deal of 'new' theory or supporting evidence for human behaviour) was due to four common misunderstandings of evolutionary theory. It is worth detailing these here as they shed some light on the ideas themselves.

Common Misunderstandings of Darwin's Theory

There are five common misunderstandings that are sometimes made by both lay and more scholarly individuals:

1) The first misunderstanding is that to accept evolutionary theory is to accept that human behaviour is therefore genetically determined.
   – it is often said that evolution is about genetic determinism. This is the theory that behaviour is wholly determined by genes rather than environment since it is the genes that are passed on from generation to generation. However, evolutionary theory does not suggest this. In fact, for natural selection to occur there needs to be a true interaction between genes and the environment. Genetic changes through natural selection are a result of adaptations to changes to the environment.
2) The second is that if behaviour is determined by evolution it means that the behaviour cannot be changed.
   – this misunderstanding is related to the one above concerning genetic determinism. However, this is both a misunderstanding of evolution and genetics. Human beings constantly change their

environment so that evolutionary adaptations are no longer applicable. Often used examples are calluses. The skin on our feet has been developed, through evolutionary forces, to harden when friction is applied. This would have helped to protect feet over harsh terrain. However, in modern times people wear shoes that prevent the application of friction, so the skin adaptation is no longer necessary. Therefore discovering that feet are adapted to develop callused skin does not mean that we should suddenly stop wearing shoes! Behavioural adaptations that may be evolutionary adaptations also do not have to be slavishly adhered to. In fact, knowing about behavioural adaptations gives us the power to change that behaviour for the better.

3) The third misunderstanding is that evolutionary theory requires complicated mathematical abilities in animals.

   – some critics of natural selection have focused on Hamilton's inclusive fitness theory. As mentioned before, this theory is very mathematical and it suggests that the likelihood people would, for example, help a relative's child depends on their genetic relationship which is expressed in a complex mathematical formula. Critics have argued that it is improbable to suggest that people would make decisions (about whether to help a relative for example) based on the complicated mathematical formulas developed by Hamilton. In other words, people cannot have the mathematical ability to behave in such ways, so inclusive fitness cannot be correct.

   However, again this is incorrect. No one expects a spider to use a calculator to make a web that can clearly be described in mathematical terms like angles and formulae (Dawkins, 1979). Nevertheless, a spider's web is clearly seen as a behavioural adaptation. The web is constructed using 'rules of thumb', that are complex but do not require the spider to be a maths 'whizz'. Similar mechanisms are thought to exist in humans and their adapted behaviour towards relatives.

   The point is that while we may need mathematics to describe adaptations (either helping relatives or spiders' webs!) this does not mean that the animal or person needs to have knowledge of this mathematics.

4) The fourth misunderstanding is that current behaviours are the best that they can be.

   – again, this misunderstanding is related to the two above regarding both the genetic and the unchangeable nature of adaptations. There is often the additional assumption that any current adaptations that are identified must be 'optimally designed'. This is often phrased in terms of if something is an adaptation it is therefore 'natural' and hence it is the best way to behave. In fact, there are many reasons that current adaptations will not be perfect. Two of them are especially important to mention here.

   Firstly, there is a time lag for the adaptations. Since it takes at least hundreds of generations for a species to adapt to an environmental change it follows that our current adaptations are necessarily out of date for our current needs. As Buss (1999) has stated 'we carry around a stone-aged brain in a modern environment' (p. 20).

   Secondly, all adaptations have an associated cost. Therefore there is often a trade-off between an ideal adaptation and the cost to the organism of doing that. For example, if everyone was given such an extreme fear of spiders that they never ventured outside, then the chances of people ever being killed by venomous spider bites would be reduced to nothing. However, this 'ideal adaptation' would have associated the costs of people not being able to go out and find food or to meet others to reproduce. A preferable alternative would be to give people a moderate fear of spiders to reduce the likelihood that someone would be bitten and to allow other behaviours to occur. Therefore any adaptation is balanced against the associated cost it may have for the organism. Natural selection favours adaptations where the benefits outweigh any costs, not the best adaptations that are possible.

5) The last misunderstanding is that evolutionary theory implies that human motivation is to maximise gene reproduction.

– we all have goals in our lives. Some are small, such as saving for a summer holiday, while others are larger, such as getting a degree or raising children successfully to adulthood. However, in all likelihood you do not see 'maximising gene reproduction' as a goal in your life. Natural selection does not suggest that the ultimate human motivation is to reproduce our genes. The expression of this is made through other mechanisms like the drive to survive by avoiding predators, obtaining food, finding a mate, helping relatives and so on.

From a theoretical point of view, since gene reproduction (in evolutionary terms) cannot be seen in one lifetime this cannot constitute a human motivation since one individual can never see the results of their actions. Furthermore, the factors that affect gene reproduction are different for males and females and also for children in different situations. Hence, maximising gene reproduction cannot be the overt motivation in an organism.

Panels 4 to 7

These four areas were highlighted by Buss (1999).

▶ PAGE 235

Panel 3

See Nesse and Williams (1994).

Panel 4

That common human fears have an evolutionary background is discussed by Darwin (1877) and Nesse (1990) amongst others.

Panel 5

Women's preference for mates with good resources was reported by a number of researchers including Buss (1989) and Kendrick, Sadalla, Groth and Trost (1990). Women's preference for commitment was investigated by Buss *et al*. (1990). Women's preference for men with symmetrical faces has been suggested as an indicator of health in men (e.g see Gangestad & Thornhill, 1997).

Please note that women's long-term mating strategies have received detailed investigation in a number of other, more specific, areas.

Panel 6

See Buss (1989) and Kendrick and Keefe (1992).

The research in this area is much more detailed than is suggested in the body of the chapter.

▶ **PAGE 236**

Panel 1

The idea that fathers are less than 100 per cent sure that their children have their genes is called the *paternity uncertainty hypothesis*. This is only one of three suggestions concerning the question of why men tend to be less involved in the parenting of their children (see Alcock, 1993 and Pedersen, 1991).

Panel 2

This idea has become known as the *grandmother hypothesis* (Hill & Hurtado, 1991).

There are also similar studies concerning other relatives like aunts and uncles that show similar patterns with maternal aunts, on average, investing more time in their relationships with their nieces and nephews (Gaulin, McBurney & Brademan-Wartell, 1997).

Panels 3 to 4

See, for example, Cosmides and Tooby (1992).

Panel 5

Vampire bat blood sharing was reported by Wilkinson (1984).

▶ **PAGE 237**

Panel 6

Pinker (1997) provides a good discussion of the application of evolutionary principles to an understanding of culture. In the final chapter of this book, he discusses the possible adaptive value of art, music, films and humour.

▶ **PAGE 238**

Panel 6

There are many books on the market that have detailed information on most of the issues discussed in the present text. The best advice we can offer is that you examine as many of these as you can before deciding on any one.

References

Adams, D. B., Gold, A. R. & Burt, A. D. (1978). Rise in female-initiated sexual activity at ovulation and its suppression by oral contraceptives. *New England Journal of Medicine, 299*, 1145–1150.

Adler, E., Hoon, M. A., Mueller, K. L., Chandrashekaer, J., Ryba, N. J. P., & Zuker, C. S. (2000). A novel family of mammalian taste receptors. *Cell, 100*, 693–702.

Allcock, J. (1993). *Animal Behaviour: An Evolutionary Approach* (5th ed.). Sunderland, MA: Sinauer.

Amoore, J. E. (1977). Specific asnomia and the concept of primary odors. *Chemical Senses and Flavor, 2*, 267–281.

Andersen, J. L., Klitgaard, H., & Slatin, B. (1994). Myosin heavy chain isoforms in single fibres from m. vastus lateralis of sprinters: Influence of training. *Acta Physiologica Scandinavica, 151*, 135–142.

Appley, M. H. (1991). Motivation, equilibrium, and stress. In R. Dienstbier (ed.), *Nebraska Symposium on Motivation 1990.* Lincoln: University of Nebraska Press.

Archer, J. & Lloyd, B., (1985). *Sex and Gender* (2nd ed.). New York: Cambridge University Press.

Atkinson, R. C. & Shiffrin R. M. (1968). Human memory: A proposed system and its control processes. In K. W. Spence and J. T. Spence (eds.), *The Psychology of Learning and Motivation: Advances in Research and Theory.* New York: Academic Press.

Avenet, P. & Lindeman, B. (1989). Perspectives of taste reception. *Journal of Membrane Biology, 112*, 1–8.

Babich, F. R., Jacobson, A. L., Bubash, S., & Jacobson, A. (1965). Transfer of a response to naïve rats by injection of ribonucleic acid extracted from trained rats. *Science, 149*, 656–657.

Baddeley, A. D. & Hitch, G. (1974). Working memory. In G. H. Bower (ed.), *The Psychology of Learning and Motivation Vol. 8.* New York: Academic Press.

Bailey, J. M. & Pillard, R. C. (1991). A genetic study of male sexual orientation. *Archives of General Psychiatry, 48*, 1089–1096.

Bailey, J. M., Pillard, R. C., Neale, M. C., & Agyei, Y. (1993). Heritable factors influence sexual orientation in women. *Archives of General Psychiatry, 50*, 217–223.

Basbaum, A. I. & Fields, H. L. (1984). Endogenous pain control systems: Brainstem spinal pathways and endorphin circuitry. *Annual Review of Neuroscience, 7*, 309–338.

Bard, P. (1929). The central representation of the sympathetic system. *Archives of Neurology and Psychiatry, 22*, 230–246.

Bard, P. (1934). On emotional expression after decortication with some remarks on certain theoretical views. *Psychological Review, 41*, 309–329.

Bartoshuk, L. M. & Beauchamp, G. K. (1994). Chemical senses. In L. W. Porter and M. R. Rosenzweig, *Annual Review of Psychology*, Vol. 45. Palo Alto: Annual Reviews Inc.

Baum, M. J. & Vreeburg, J. T. M. (1973). Copulation in castrated male rats following combined treatment with estradiol and dihydrotestosterone. *Science, 182*, 283–285.

Bell, A. P., Weinberg, M. S., & Hammersmith, S. K. (1981). *Sexual Preference.* Bloomington: Indiana University Press.

Berenbaum, S. A. (1999). Effects of early androgens on sex-typed activities and interests in adolescents with congenital hyperplasia. *Hormones and Behaviour, 35*, 102–110.

Berger, R. J. & Phillips, N. H. (1995). Energy conservation and sleep. *Behavioural Brain Research, 69*, 65–73.

Bigelow, H. J. (1850). Dr. Harlow's case of recovery from the passage of an iron bar through the head. *American Journal of the Medical Sciences, 19*, 13–22.

Bliss, T. V. P. & Lømo, T. (1973). Long lasting potentiation of synaptic transmission in the dentate area of the anaesthetized rabbit following stimulation of the perforant path. *Journal of Physiology* (London), *232*, 331–356.

Bohbot, V. D., Allen, J. J. B., & Nedel, L. (2000). Memory deficits characterized by patterns of lesions to the hippocampus and parahippocampal cortex. *Annals of the New York Academy of Sciences, 911*, 355–368.

Bolles, R. C. (1975). *Theory of Motivation.* New York: Harper & Row.

Brownlee, A. (1963). Evolution of the giraffe. *Nature, 200*, 1022.

Buss, D. M. (1989). Sex differences in human mate preferences: Evolutionary hypotheses testing in 37 cultures. *Behavioral Brain Sciences, 12*, 1–49.

Buss, D. M. (1999). *Evolutionary Psychology.* Needham Heights, MA: Allyn & Bacon.

Buss, D. M., Abbott, M., Angleitner, A, Asherian, A., Biaggio, A, & 45 other co-authors. (1990). International preferences in selecting mates: A study of 37 cultures. *Journal of Cross-Cultural Psychology, 21*, 5–47.

Butzer, K. (2000). The human role in environmental history. *Nature. 287*, 2427–2428.

Campfield, L. A., Smith, F. J., & Burn, P. (1998). Strategies and potential molecular targets for obesity treatment. *Science, 280*, 1383–1387.

Carlson, N. R. (2001). *Physiology of Behaviour* (7th ed.). Needham Heights, AZ: Pearson.

Carter, C. S. (1992). Hormonal influences on human sexual behaviour. In J. B. Becker, S. M. Breedlove, and D. Crews, *Behavioral Endocrinology.* Cambridge, MA: MIT Press.

Chaudari, N., Landin, A. M., & Roper, S. D. (2000). A metabotropic glutamate receptor variant functions as a taste receptor. *Nature Neuroscience, 3*, 113–119.

Cosmides, L. & Tooby, J. (1992). Cognitive adaptations for social exchange. In J. Barkow, L. Cosmides, & J. Tooby (eds.), *The Adapted Mind.* New York: Oxford University Press.

Critchley, H. D. & Rolls, E. T. (1996). Hunger and satiety modify the responses of olfactory and visual neurons in the primate orbitofrontal cortex. *Journal of Neurophysiology, 75*, 1673–1686.

Czeisler, C. A., Johnson, M. P., Dufy, J. F., Brown, E. N, Ronda, J. M., & Kronauer, R. E. (1990). Exposure to bright light and darkness to treat physiologic maladaptation to night work. *New England Journal of Medicine, 322*, 1253–1259.

Damasio, A. (1994). *Descartes' Error: Emotion, Reason and the Human Brain.* New York: Gossett/Putman.

Damasio, A. (1999). *The Felling of What Happens.* New York: Putnam's Sons.

Damasio, H., Grabowski, T., Frank, R., Galaburda, A. M., & Damasio, A. R. (1994). The return of Phineas Gage: Clues about the brain from the skull of a famous patient. *Science, 264*, 1102–1105.

Darwin, C. (1859). *On the Origin of Species.* London: Murray.

Darwin, C. (1872). *The Expression of Emotions in Man and Animals.* Oxford: Oxford University Press.

Darwin, C. (1877). A biographical sketch of an infant. *Mind, 2*, 285–294.

Daum, I., Ackerman, H., Schugens, M. M., Reimold, C., Dichgans, J., & Birbaumer, N. (1993). The cerebellum and cognitive functions in humans. *Behavioral Neuroscience, 107*, 411–419.

Dawkins, R. (1979). Twelve misunderstandings of kin selection. *Zeitschrift fur Tierpsychologie, 51*, 184–200.

Dawkins, R. (1982). *The Extended Phenotype.* Oxford; W. H. Freeman & Co.

Dawkins, R. (1989). *The Selfish Gene.* New York: Oxford University Press.

de Castro, J. M. & Plunkett, S. (2002). A general model of intake regulation. *Neuroscience and Behavioral Reviews, 26*, 581–595.

Dement, W. (1960). The effect of dream deprivation. *Science, 131*, 1705–1707.

Dement, W. & Kleitman, N. (1957). The relation of eye movements during sleep to dream activity: An objective method for the study of dreaming. *Journal of Experimental Psychology, 53*, 339–346.

Deutsch, J. A., Young, W. G., & Kalogeris, T. J. (1978). The stomach signals satiety. *Science, 201*, 165–167.

Dobzhansky, T. (1937). *Genetics and the Origin of Species.* New York: Columbia University Press.

Drasdo, N. (1977). The neural representation of visual space. *Nature, 266*, 554–556.

Dyal, J. A. (1971). Transfer of behavioural bias: Reality and specificity. In E. J. Fjerdingstad (ed.), *Chemical Transfer of Learned Information*. New York: American Elsevier.

Earnest, D. J., Liang, F.-Q., Ratcliff, M., & Cassone, V. M. (1999). Immortal time: Circadian clock properties of rat suprachiasmatic cell lines. *Science, 283*, 693–695.

Eberhart, J. A., Keverne, E. B., & Miller, R. E. (1980). Social influence on plasma testosterone in male talapoin monkeys. *Hormones and Behaviour, 14*, 247–266.

Ekman, P. (1977). Biological and cultural contributions to body and facial movement. In J. Blacking (ed.) *The Anthropology of the Body*. A.S.A. Monograph 15. London: Academic Press.

Ekman, P. (1992). Facial expressions of emotion: New findings, new questions. *Psychological Sciences, 3*, 34–38.

Ekman, P. & Friesen, W. V. (1975). *Unmasking the Face: A Guide to Recognising Emotions and Facial Cues*. Englewood Cliff, NJ: Prentice- Hall.

Ekman, P., Friesen, W. V., & Ellsworth, P. (1982). What are the similarities and differences in facial behaviour across cultures? In P. Ekman (ed.). *Emotion in the Human Face* (2nd ed.). New York: Cambridge University Press.

Ekman, P. & Oster, H. (1979). Facial expressions of emotion. *Annual Review of Psychology, 30*, 527–554.

Erickson, R. P., DiLorenzo, P. M., & Woodbury, M. A. (1994). Classification of taste responses in brain stem: Membership in fuzzy sets. *Journal of Neurophysiology, 71*, 2139–2150.

Etgen, A. M., Chu, H.-P., Fiber, J. M., Karkanias, G. B., & Morales, J. M. (1999). Hormonal integration of neurochemical and sensory signals governing female reproductive behaviour. *Behavioural Brain Research, 105*, 93–103.

Finger, S. & Roe, D. (1996). Gustave Dax and the early history of cerebral dominance. *Archives of Neurology, 53*, 806–813.

Fiske, D. W. & Maddi, S. R. (1961). *A Conceptual Framework*. In D. W. Fiske & S. R. Maddi (eds.), *Functions of Varied Experience*. Homewood, IL: Dorsey Press.

Fjerdingstad, E. J. (1973). Transfer of learning in rodents and fish. In W. B. Essman and S. Nakajima (eds.), *Current Biochemical Approaches to Learning and Memory*. New York: Spectrum.

Forman, R. F., & McCauley, C. (1986). Validity of the positive control polygraph test using the field practice model. *Journal of Applied Psychology, 71*, 691–698.

Fortin, N. J., Agster, K. L., & Eichenbaum, H. B. (2002). Critical role of the hippocampus in memory for sequences of events. *Nature Neuroscience, 5*, 458–462.

Fritsch, G., & Hitzig, E. (1870). Uber die elektrische Errebbarkeit des Grosshirns [Concerning the electrical stimulability of the cerebrum]. *Archive fur Anatomie Physiologie und Wissenshcaftliche Medicin*. 300–332.

Fukuwatari, T., Kawada, T., Tsuruta, M., Hiraoka, T., Iwanaga, T., Sugimoto, E., & Fushiki, T. (1997). Expression of the putative membrane fatty acid transporter (FAT) in taste buds of the circumvallate papillaein rats. *FEBS Letters, 414*, 461–464.

Galef, B. G. Jr. (1992). Weaning from mother's milk to solid foods: The developmental psychobiology of self-selection of foods by rats. *Annals of the New York Academy of Sciences, 662*, 37–52.

Gangestad, S. W. & Thornhill, R. (1997). Human sexual selection and developmental stability. In J. A. Simpson and D. T. Kendrick (eds.), *Evolutionary Social Psychology*. Mahwah, NJ: Erlbaum.

Garrett, B. (2003). *Brain and Behaviour*. Toronto: Thompson.

Gaulin, S. J. C., McBurney, D. H., & Brakeman-Wartell, S. L. (1997). Matrilateral biases in the investment of aunts and uncles. *Human Nature, 8*, 139–151.

Gazzaniga, M. S. (1967). The split brain in man. *Scientific American, 217*, 24–29.

Gilbertson, T. A., Fontenot, D. T., Liu, L., Zhang, H., & Monroe, W.T. (1997). Fatty acid modulation of K+ channels in taste receptor cells: Gustatory cues for dietary fat. *American Journal of Physiology, 272*, C1203–C1210.

Ginnett, T, & Demment, M. (1997). Sex differences in giraffe foraging behavior at two spatial scales. *Oecologia, 110*, 291–300.

Gillette, M. U. & McArthur, A. J. (1996). Circadian actions of melatonin at the suprachiasmatic nucleus. *Behavioural Brain Research, 73*, 135–139.

Goldstein, A. (1980). Thrills in response to music and other stimuli. *Physiological Psychology, 8*, 126–129.

Gould, S. & Eldridge, N. (1977). Punctuated equilibria: The tempo and mode of evolution reconsidered. *Paleobiology, 3*, 115–151.

Green, S. (1994). *Principles of Biopsychology.* Hove: Psychology Press.

Hamilton, W. D. (1964). The genetic evolution of social behaviour. I and II. *Journal of Theoretical Biology, 7*, 1–52.

Harris, C. R. (1999). The mystery of ticklish laughter. *American Scientist, 87(4)*, 344–351.

Hennig, R. & Lømo, T., (1985). Firing patterns of motor units in normal rats. *Nature, 314*, 164–166.

Herzog, E. D., Takahashi, J. S., & Block, G. D. (1998). Clock controls circadian period in isolated suprachiasmatic nucleus neurons. *Nature Neuroscience, 1*, 708–713.

Hettinger, T. P. & Frank, M. E. (1992). Information processing in the mammalian gustatory system. *Current opinion in Neurobiology, 2*, 469–478.

Hill, K. & Hurtado, A. M. (1991). The evolution of premature reproductive senescence and menopause in human females. *Human Nature, 2*, 313–50.

Hobson, J. A. & McCarley, R. W. (1977). The brain as a dream state generator: an activation-synthesis hypothesis of the dream process. *American Journal of Psychiatry, 134*, 1335–1348.

Hobson, J. A., Pace-Schott, E. F., & Stickgold, R. (2000). Dreaming and the brain: Toward a cognitive neuroscience of conscious states. *Behavioural and Brain Sciences, 23*, 793–1121.

Horne, J. A. & Minard, A. (1985). Sleep and sleepiness following a behaviourally active "active" day. *Ergonomics, 28*, 567–575.

Hosler, J. (2003). *The Sandwalk Adventures.* Columbus OH: Active Synapse.

Huang, W., Sved, A. F., & Stricker, E. M. (2000). Water ingestion provides an early signal inhibiting osmotically stimulated vasopressin secretion in rats. *American Journal of Physiology, 279*, R756–R760.

Hubel, D. H. & Wiesel, T. N. (1959). Receptive fields of single neurons in the cat's striate cortex. *Journal of Physiology, 148*, 574–591.

Hubel, D. H. & Wiesel, T. N. (1979). Brain mechanisms of vision. *Scientific American, 241*, 150–162.

Hull, C. L. (1951). *Essentials of Behaviour.* New Haven, CT: Yale University Press.

Hunt, S. P. & Mantyh, P. W. (2001). The molecular dynamics of pain control. *Nature Reviews Neuroscience, 2*, 83–91.

Huxley, J. S. (1942). *Evolution: The Modern Synthesis.* London: Allen & Unwin.

Hurvich, L. M. & Jameson, D. (1957). An opponent-process theory of colour vision. *Psychological Review, 64*, 384–404.

Inouye, S. T. & Kawamura, H. (1979). Persistence of circadian rhythmicity in mammalian hypothalamic "island" containing the suprachiasmatic nucleus. *Proceedings of the National Academy of Sciences USA, 76*, 5962–5966.

Izard, C. E. (1971). *The Face of Emotion.* New York: Appleton.

Izard, C. E. (1977). *Human Emotions.* New York: Plenum Press.

James. W. (1890). *The Principles of Psychology.* New York: Holt, Rinehart & Winston.

Johnson, W. G. & Wildman, H. E. (1983). Influence of external and covert food stimuli on insulin secretion in obese and normal subjects. *Behavioral Neuroscience, 97*, 1025–1028.

Jones, H. S. & Oswald, I. (1968). Two cases of healthy insomnia. *Electroencephalography and Clinical Neurophysiology, 24*, 378–380.

Jordan, H. A. (1969). Voluntary intragastric feeding. *Journal of Comparative and Physiological Psychology, 68*, 498–506.

Kalat, J. W. (2004). *Biological Psychology* (8th ed.). Toronto: Wadsworth.

Kendrick, D. T., Sadalla, E. K., Groth, G., & Trost, M. R. (1990). Evolution, traits, and stages of human courtship; Qualifying the parental investment model. *Journal of Personality, 58*, 97–116.

Kendrick, D. T. & Keefe, R.C. (1992). Age preferences in mates reflect sex differences in reproductive strategies. *Behavioral and Brain Sciences, 15*, 75–133.

Kesner, R. P., Gilbert, P. E., & Barua, L. A. (2002). The role of the hippocampus in meaning for the temporal order of a sequence of odors. *Behavioral Neuroscience, 116*, 286–290.

Keverne, E. B., (1999). The vomeronasal organ. *Science, 286*, 716–720.

Kinnamon, S. C. & Cummings, T. A. (1992). Chemosensory transduction mechanisms in taste. *Annual Review of Physiology, 54*, 715–731.

Kinnamon, S. C., Dionne, V. E., & Beam, K. G. (1988). Apical localization of k$^+$ channels in taste cells provides the basis for sour taste transduction. *Proceedings of the National Academy of Sciences, 85*, 7023–7027.

Kirk-Smith, M., Both, D. A., Carroll, D., & Davies, P. (1978). Human social attitudes affected by androstenol. *Research Communications in Psychology Psychiatry and Behavior, 3*, 379–384.

Kleitman, N. (1963). *Sleep and Wakefulness*. Chicago: University of Chicago Press.

Kluger, M. J. (1991). Fever: Role of pyrogens and cryogens. *Physiological Reviews, 71*, 93–127.

Komisaruk, B. R., Adler, N. T., & Hutchinson, J. (1972). Genital sensory field: Enlargement by estrogen treatment in female rats. *Science, 178*, 1295–1298.

Kupferman I., Castelucci, V., Pinsker, H., & Kandel, E. (1970). Neuronal correlates of habituation and dishabituation of the gill withdrawal reflex in *Aplysia. Science, 167*, 1743–1745.

Kurahashi, T., Lowe, G., & Gold, G. H. (1994). Suppression of odorant responses by odorants in olfactory receptor cells. *Science, 265*, 118–120.

Kurihara, K. (1987). Recent progress in taster receptor mechanisms. In Y. Kawamura and M. R. Kare (eds.) *Umami: A Basic Taste*. New York: Dekker.

Lang, R. A., Flor-Henry, P., & Frenzel, R. R. (1990). Sex hormone profiles in pedophilic and incestuous men. *Annals of Sex Research, 3*, 59–74.

Lashley, K. S. (1927). *Brain Mechanisms and Intelligence*. Chicago: University of Chicago Press.

Lashley, K. S. (1950). In search of the engram. *Symposia of the Society for Experimental Psychology, 4*, 454–482.

Leibowitz, S. F., Hammer, N. J., & Chang, K. (1981). Hypothalamic paraventricular nucleus lesions produce overeating and obesity in the rat. *Physiology and Behaviour, 27*, 1031–1040.

Leibowitz, S. F., & Hoebel, B. G. (1998). Behavioral neuroscience of obesity. In G. A. Bray, C. Bouchard, & P. T. James (eds.), *Handbook of Obesity*. New York: Dekker.

Leshem, M. (1999). The ontogeny of salt hunger in the rat. *Neuroscience and Biobehavioral Reviews, 23*, 649–659.

Lester, L. S. & Fanselow, M. S. (1985). Exposure to a cat produces opioid analgesia in rats. *Behavioral Neuroscience, 99*, 756–759.

Leuthold, B, & Leuthold, W. (1972). Food habits of giraffe in Tsavo National Park, Kenya, *E. African. Wildlife Journal. 10*, 129–141.

Lindeman, B. (1996). Taste reception. *Physiological Reviews, 76*, 719–766.

Loewi, O. (1953). *From the Workshop of Discoveries*. Lawrence, KS: University of Kansas Press.

Logan, C. G. & Grafton, S. T. (1995). Functional anatomy of human eyeblink conditioning determined with regional cerebral glucose metabolism and positron-emission tomography. *Proceedings of the National Academy of Sciences, USA, 92*, 7500–7504.

Lohse, P., Lohse, P., Chahrikh-Zadeh, S., & Seidel, D. (1997). The acid lipase family: Three enzymes, one highly conserved gene structure. *Journal of Lipid Research, 38*, 880–891.

Lorenz, K. Z. (1965). *Evolution and the Modification of Behaviour*. Chicago: University of Chicago Press.

MacLean, P. D. (1949). Psychosomatic disease and the "visceral brain": Recent developments bearing on the Papez theory of emotion. *Psychosomatic Medicine, 11*, 338–353.

MacLean, P. D. (1958). Contrasting function of the limbic and neocortical systems of the brain and their relevance to psychophysiological aspects of medicine. *American Journal of Medicine, 25*, 611–626.

MacLean, P. D. (1970). The limbic brain in relation to the psychoses. In P. Black (ed.), *Physiological Correlates of Emotion*. New York: Academic Press.

Macmillan, M. (1986). A wonderful journey through skull and brains: the travels of Mr. Gage's tamping iron. *Brain and Cognition, 5*, 67–107.

Macmillan, M. (2000). Restoring Phineas Gage: A 150th retrospective. *Journal of the History of the Neurosciences, 9(1)*, 46–66.

Maguire, E. A., Frackowiak, R. S. J., & Frith, C. D. (1997). Recalling routes around London: Activation of the right hippocampus in taxi drivers. *Journal of Neuroscience, 17*, 7103–7110.

Marsden, C. D. (1987). What do the basal ganglia tell premotor cortical areas? *CIBA Foundation Symposium, 132*, 282–300.

Matsunami, H., Montmayeur, J.-P., & Buck, L. B. (2000). A family of candidate taste receptors in human and mouse. *Nature, 404*, 601–604.

Matuszewich, L., Lorrain, D. S., & Hull, E. M. (2000). Dopamine release in the medial preoptic area of female rats in response to hormonal manipulation and sexual activity. *Behavioural Neuroscience, 114*, 772–782.

Maurice, D. M. (1998). The Von Sallman lecture of 1996: An ophthalmological explanation of REM sleep. *Experimental Eye Research, 66*, 139–145.

Mayer, E. (1942). *Systematics and the Origin of Species.* New York: Columbia University Press.

McBurney, D. H. (1984). Taste and olfaction: sensory discrimination. In I. Darian-Smith, (ed.) *Handbook of Physiology. Section 1: The Nervous System, Vol. III, Part 2.* Bethesda: American Physiological Society.

McCarley, R. W. & Hobson, J. A. (1981). The neurobiological origins of psychoanalytic dream theory. *American Journal of Psychiatry, 134*, 1211–1221.

McCloud, S. (2006). *Making Comics.* New York: Harper.

McConnell, J. V. (1962). Memory transfer through cannibalism in planarians. *Journal of Neuropsychiatry, 3* (suppl. 1), 42–48.

McDougall, W. (1908). *An introduction to Social Psychology.* London: Methuen.

McKeever, .W. F., Seitz, K. S., Krutsch, A. J., & Van Eys, P. L. (1995). On language laterality in normal dextrals and sinistrals: Results from the bilateral object naming latency task. *Neuropsychologia, 33*, 1627–1635.

Meddis, R., Pearson, A. J. D., & Langford, G. (1973). An extreme case of healthy insomnia. *EEG and Clinical Neurophysiology, 35*, 213–214.

Michael, R., Gagnon, J., Laumann, E., & Kolata, G. (1994). *Sex in America.* Boston: Little, Brown.

Miller, G. A. (1958). The magical number seven plus or minus two. Some limits on our capacity for processing information. *Psychological Review, 63*, 81–97.

Millhorn, D. E., Bayliss, D. A., Erickson, J. T., Gallman, E. A., Szymeczek, C. L., Czyzyk-Kreska, M., & Dean, J. B. (1989). Cellular and molecular mechanisms of chemical synaptic transmission. *American Journal of Physiology, 6* (part 1), L289–L310.

Milner, B. (1970). Memory and the temporal regions of the brain. In K. H. Pribram and D. E. Broadbent (eds.), *Biology and Memory.* New York: Academic Press.

Mink, J. W. (1999). Basal ganglia. In M. J. Zigmond, F. E. Bloom, S C. Landis, J. L. Roberts, and L. R. Squire (eds.) *Fundamental Neuroscience.* San Diego: Academic Press.

Monti-Bloch, L., Jennings-White, C., Dolberg, D. S., & Berliner, D. L. (1994). The human vomeronasal system, *Psychoneuroendocrinology, 19*, 673–689.

Mrosovsky, N. (1990). *Rheostasis: The Physiology of Change.* New York: Oxford University Press.

Murphy, M. G. & O'Leary, J. L. (1973). Hanging and climbing functions in raccoon and sloth after total cerebellectomy. *Archives of Neurology, 28*, 111–117.

Murphy, M. R., Checkley, S. A., Seckl, J. R., & Lightman, S. L. (1990). Neloxone inhibits oxytocin release at orgasm in man. *Journal of Clinical Endocrinology & Metabolism, 71*, 1056–1058.

Naylan, T. (1999). Frontal lobe function: Mr. Phineas Gage's famous injury. *Journal of Neuropsychiatry and Clinical Neuroscience, 11(2),* 280–283.

Nebes, R. D. (1974). Hemisphere specialisation in commissurotomized man. *Psychological Bulletin, 81*, 1–14.

Nelson, D. O. & Prosser, C. L. (1981). Intracellular recordings from thermosensitive preoptic neurons. *Science, 213*, 787–789.

Nesse, R. M. (1990). Evolutionary explanations of emotions. *Human Nature, 1*, 261–289.

Nesse, R. M. & Williams, G. C. (1994). *Why We Get Sick.* New York: Times Books, Random House.

Papez, J. W. (1937). A proposed mechanism of emotion. *Archives of Neurology and Psychiatry, 38*, 725–743.

Parent, M. B., Habib, M. K., & Baker, G. B. (1999). Task-dependent effects of the antidepressant/anti-panic drug phenelzine on memory. *Psychopharmacology, 142*, 280–288.

Patrick, C. J. & Iacono, W. G. (1989). Psychopathy, threat, and polygraph test accuracy. *Journal of Applied Psychology, 74*, 347–355.

Pavlov, I. (1927). *Conditoned Reflexes*. Oxford: Oxford University Press.

Pedersen, F. A. (1991). Secular trends in human sex ratios: Their influence on individual and family behaviour. *Human Nature, 2*, 271–291.

Pellew, R. (1984). The feeding ecology of a selective browser, the giraffe (*Giraffa camelopardalis tippelskirchi*). *J. Zool.*, London, *202*, 57–81.

Penfield, W. & Rasmussen, T. (1950). *The Cerebral Cortex of Man*. New York: Macmillan.

Penton-Voak, I. S., Perrett, D. I., Castles, D. l., Kobayashi, T., Burt, D. M., Murray, L. K., & Minamisawa, R. (1999). Menstrual cycle alters face preference. *Nature, 339*, 741–742.

Peters, R. H., Sensenig, L. D., & Reich, M. J. (1973). Fixed-ratio performance following ventromedial hypothalamic lesions in rats. *Physiological Psychology, 1*, 136–138.

Pincher, C. (1949). Evolution of the Giraffe. *Nature, 164*, 29–30.

Pinker, S. (1997). *How the Mind Works*. London: Penguin.

Plotkin, H. (1997). *Evolution in Mind*. St. Ives: Penguin.

Pouget, A., Dayan, P., & Zemel, R. (2000). Information processing with population codes. *Nature Reviews Neuroscience, 1*, 125–132.

Prescott, T. J., Redgrave, P., & Gurney, K. (1999). Layered control of architectures in robots and vertebrates. *Adaptive Behaviour, 7*, 99–127.

Quadagno, D. M., Briscoe, R., & Quadagno, J. S. (1977). Effect of perinatal gonadal hormones on selected nonsexual behaviour patterns: A critical assessment of the non-human and human literature. *Psychological Bulletin, 84*, 62–80.

Ramachandran, V. S. (1992). Perception: a biological perspective. In G. A. Carpenter and S. Grossberg (eds.) *Neural Networks for Vision and Image Processing*. Cambridge MA: The MIT Press.

Refinetti, R. & Menaker, M. (1992). The circadian rhythm of body temperature. *Physiology and Behavior, 51*, 613–637.

Refinetti, R. & Carlisle, H. J. (1986). Complementary nature of heat production and heat intake during behavioural thermoregulation in the rat. *Behavioral and Neural Biology, 46*, 64–70.

Reiner, A., Medina, L., & Veenman, C. L. (1998). Stuctural and functional evolution of the basal ganglia in vertebrates. *Brain Research Reviews, 28*, 235–285.

Rickard, T. C. & Grafman, J. (1998). Losing their configural mind; Amnesic patients fail on transverse patterning. *Journal of Cognitive Neuroscience, 10*, 509–524.

Richter, C. P. (1922). A behavioristic study of the activity of the rat. *Comparative Psychology Monographs, 1*, 1–55.

Richter, C. P. (1936). Increased salt appetite in adrenalectomized rats. *American Journal of Physiology, 115*, 155–161.

Richter, C. P. (1967). Psychopathology of periodic behaviour in animals and man. In J. Zubin and H. F. Hunt, (eds.) *Comparative Psychopathology*. New York: Grune & Stratton.

Rommel, S. A., Pabst, D. A., & McLelland, W. A. (1998). Reproductive thermoregulation in marine mammals. *American Scientist, 86*, 440–448.

Roozendal, B., Phillips, R. G., Power, A. E., Brooke, S. M., Sapolsky, R. M., & McGaugh, J. L. (2001). Memory retrieval impairment induced by hippocampal CA3 lesions is blocked adrenocortical suppression. *Nature Neuroscience, 4*, 1169–1171.

Rösler, A., & Witztum, E. (1998). Treatment of men with paraphilia with a long-acting analogue of gonadotropin-releasing hormone. *New England Journal of Medicine, 338*, 416–422.

Rozin, P. (1990). Getting to like the burn of chilli pepper. In B.G. Green, J. R. Mason, & M. R. Kare (eds.), *Chemical Senses* (Vol. 2). New York: Dekker.

Rozin, P. & Kalat, J. W. (1971). Specific hungers and poison avoidance as adaptive specializations of learning. *Psychological Review, 78*, 459–486.

Rozin, P. & Zellner, D. (1985). The role of Pavlovian conditioning in the acquisition of food likes and dislikes. *Annals of the New York Academy of Science, 443*, 189–202.

Sacks, O. (1984). *A Leg to Stand On.* New York: Touchstone.

Sacks, O. (1985). *The Man Who Mistook His Wife For a Hat and Other Clinical Tales.* New York: Simon & Shuster.

Satinoff, E. (1964). Behavioral thermoregulation in response to local cooling of the rat brain. *American Journal of Physiology, 206*, 1389–1394.

Satinoff, E., McEwen, G. N. Jr., & Williams, B. A. (1976). Behavioral fever in newborn rabbits. *Science, 193*, 1139–1140.

Schachter, S. & Singer, J. E. (1962). Cognitive, social, and physiological determinants of emotional state. *Psychological Review, 69*, 379–399.

Schulkin, J. (1991). *Sodium Hunger: The Search for a Salty Taste.* Cambridge: Cambridge University Press.

Sclater, A. (2003). The extent of Charles Darwin's knowledge of Mendel. *Georgia Journal of Science, 61*, 134.

Scott, T. R. (1990). Gustatory control of food selection. In E. M. Sticker (ed.), *Handbook of Behavioural Neurobiology,* Vol. 10, *Neurobiology of Food and Fluid Intake.* Basle: Karger.

Scott, T. R. & Plata-Salaman, C. R. (1991). Coding of taste quality. In T. N. Getchell (ed.) *Smell and Taste in Health and Disease.* New York: Raven Press.

Scoville, W. B. & Milner, B. (1957). Loss of recent memory after bilateral hippocampal lesions. *Journal of Neurology, Neurosurgery and Psychiatry, 20*, 11–21.

Seeley, R. J., Kaplan, J. M., & Grill, H. J. (1995). Effect of occluding the pylorus on intraoral intake: A test of the gastric hypothesis of meal termination. *Physiology and Behaviour, 58*, 245–249.

Shik, M. L. & Orlovosky, G. N. (1976). Neurophysiology of locomotor automatism. *Physiological reviews, 56*, 465–501.

Siegel, J. M. (1995). Phylogeny and the function of REM sleep. *Behavioural Brain Research, 69*, 29–34.

Simmons, R. & Scheepers, L. (1996). Winning by a neck: sexual selection in the evolution of the giraffe. *The American Naturalist, 148*, 771–786.

Simon, E. (2000). Interface properties of circumventricular organs in salt and fluid balance. *News in Physiological Sciences, 15*, 61–67.

Simpson, G. G. (1944). *Tempo and Mode in Evolution.* New York; Columbia University Press.

Shapiro, C. M., Bortz, R., Mitchell, D., Bartel, P., & Jooste, P. (1981). Slow wave sleep: A recovery period after exercise. *Science, 214, 1253–1254.*

Sjöström, M., Friden, J., & Ekblom, B. (1987). Endurance, what is it? Muscle morphology after an extremely long distance run. *Acta Physiologica Scandinavica, 130*, 513–520.

Slob, A. K., Bax, C. M., Hop, W. C. J., Rowland, D. L., & van der Werff ten Bosch, J. J. (1996). Sexual arousability and the menstrual cycle. *Psychoneuroendocrinology, 21*, 545–558.

Smith, G. P. (1998). Pregastric and gastric satiety. In G. P. Smith (ed.), *Satiation: From Gut to Brain.* New York: Oxford University Press.

Solms, M. (1997). *The Neuropsychology of Dreams.* Mahwah NJ: Erlbaum.

Spiegel, T. A. (1973). Caloric regulation of food intake in man. *Journal of Comparative and Physiological Psychology, 84*, 24–37.

Stelar, J. R. & Stellar, E. (1985). *The Neurobiology of Motivation and Reward.* New York: Springer-Verlag.

Stern, K. & McClintock, M. K. (1998). Regulation of ovulation by human pheromones. *Nature, 392*, 177–179.

Stickgold, R., James, L., & Hobson, J. (2000). Visual discrimination learning requires sleep after training. *Nature Neuroscience, 3*, 1237–1238.

Stickgolg, R., Whidbee, D., Schirmer, B., Patel, V., & Hobson, J. (2000). Visual discrimination task improvement: A multi-step process occurring during sleep. *Journal of Cognitive Neuroscience, 12*, 246–254.

Strack, F., Martin, L. L., & Stepper, S. (1988). Inhibiting and facilitating conditions of the human smile: a nonobtrusive test of the facial feedback hypothesis. *Journal of Personality and Social Psychology, 54*, 768–777.

Stricker, E. M. (1969). Osmoregulation and volume regulation in rats: Inhibition of hypovolemic thirst by water. *American Journal of Physiology, 217,* 98–105.

Sutton, L. C., Lea, E., Will, M. J., Schwartz, B. A., Hartley, C. E., Poole, J. C., Watkins, L. R., & Maier, S. F. (1997). Inescapable shock-induced potentiation of morphine analgesia. *Behavioral Neuroscience, 111,* 1105–1113.

Ratiu, P., Talos, I., Haker, S., Lieberman, D., & Everett, P. (2004). The tale of Phineas Gage, digitally remastered. *Journal of Neurotrauma, 21,* 637–643.

Stein, B. E. & Meradith, M. A. (1990). Multisensory integration: Neural and behavioural solutions for dealing with stimuli from different sensory modalities. *Annals of the New York Academy of Sciences, 608,* 51–70.

Thompson, R. F. (1986). The neurobiology of learning and memory. *Science, 233,* 941–947.

Tinbergen, N. (1951). *The Study of Instinct.* New York: Oxford University Press.

Toates, F. (2001). *Biological Psychology: An integrative Approach.* Harlow: Pearson.

Tomkins, S. S. (1962). *Affect, Imagery, Consciousness, Vol. I: The Positive Effects.* New York: Springer-Verlag.

Tomkins, S. S. (1980). Affect as amplification: Some modifications in theory. In R. Plutchik and H. Kellerman (eds.). *Emotion; Theory, Research, and Experience, Vol. I: Theories of Emotion.* New York: Academic Press.

Uchida, N., Takahashi, Y. K., & Mori, K. (2000). Odor maps in the mammalian olfactory bulb: Domain organization and odorant structural features. *Nature, 3,* 1035–1043.

Udry, J. R. & Morris, N. M. (1968). Distribution of coitus in the menstrual cycle. *Nature, 220,* 593–596.

Wallesch, C.-W., Hensikson, L., Kornhuber, H.-H., & Paulson, O. B. (1985). Observations on regional cerebral blood flow in cortical and subcortical structures during language production in normal man. *Brain and Language, 25,* 224–233.

Webb, W. B. (1974). Sleep as an adaptive response. *Perceptual and Motor Skills, 38,* 1023–1027.

Weinberger, N. M., Javid, R. and Lepan, B. (1995). Heterosynaptic long-term facilitation of sensory-evoked responses in the auditory cortex by stimulation of the magnocellular medial geniculate body in guinea pigs. *Behavioral Neuroscience, 109*(1), 10–17.

Wilkinson, G. W. (1984). Reciprocal food sharing in the vampire bat. *Nature, 308,* 181–184.

Williams, R. W. & Herrup, K. (1988). The control of neuron number. *Annual Review of Neuroscience, 11,* 423–453.

Wilson, E. O. (1975). *Sociobiology: The New Synthesis.* Cambridge, MA: Harvard University Press.

Wong, G. T., Gannon, K. S., & Margolskee, R. F. (1996). Transduction of bitter and sweet taste by gustaducin. *Nature, 381,* 796–800.

Woodruff-Pak, D. S., Papka, M., & Ivry, R. B. (1996). Cerebellar involvement in eyeblink classical conditioning in humans. *Neuropsychology, 10,* 443–458.

Woolnough, A. P. & du Toit J.T. (2001). Vertical zonation of browse quality in tree canopies exposed to a size-structured guild of African browsing ungulates, *Oecologia, 129,* 585–590.

Van Wyk, P. H. & Geist, C. S. (1984). Psychosocial development of heterosexual, bisexual and homosexual behaviour. *Archives of Sexual Behaviour, 13,* 505–544.

Young, T. & Isbell, L. (1991). Sex differences in giraffe feeding ecology: energetic and social constraints. *Ethology, 87,* 79–89.

Young, W. C., Goy, R. W., & Phoenix, C. H. (1964). Hormones and sexual behaviour. *Science, 143,* 212–218.

Zeki, S. (1993). *A Vision of the Brain.* Oxford: Blackwell.

Zola, S. M., Squire, L. R., Teng, E., Stefanacci, L., Buffalo, E. A., & Clark, R. E. (2000). Impaired recognition memory in monkeys after damage limited to the hippocampus. *Journal of Neuroscience, 29,* 451–463.

Subject Index

Note: page numbers in **bold** refer to comic panels.

CPSIA information can be obtained
at www.ICGtesting.com
Printed in the USA
LVHW061114160422
716063LV00003B/73